Clinical Nutrition for Sugical Patients

Mary Marian, MS, RD
Clinical Nutrition and Lecture
University of Arizona College of Medicine &
The AZ Cancer Center
Tucson, AZ

Mary Russell, MS, RD, LDN, CNSD
Interim Director, Nutrition Services
University of Chicago Hospitals
Chicago, IL

Scott A. Shikora, MD, FACS
Chief, Bariatric Surgery
Tufts-New England Medical Center
Professor of Surgery at Tufts University School of Medicine
Boston, MA

JONES AND BARTLETT PUBLISHERS
Sudbury, Massachusetts
BOSTON   TORONTO   LONDON   SINGAPORE

World Headquarters

Jones and Bartlett Publishers
40 Tall Pine Drive
Sudbury, MA 01776
978-443-5000
info@jbpub.com
www.jbpub.com

Jones and Bartlett Publishers
Canada
6339 Ormindale Way
Mississauga, Ontario L5V 1J2
Canada

Jones and Bartlett Publishers
International
Barb House, Barb Mews
London W6 7PA
UK

Jones and Bartlett's books and products are available through most bookstores and online book-sellers. To contact Jones and Bartlett Publishers directly, call 800-832-0034, fax 978-443-8000, or visit our website www.jbpub.com.

Substantial discounts on bulk quantities of Jones and Bartlett's publications are available to corporations, professional associations, and other qualified organizations. For details and specific discount information, contact the special sales department at Jones and Bartlett via the above contact information or send an email to specialsales@jbpub.com.

This publication is designed to provide accurate and authoritative information in regard to the Subject Matter covered. It is sold with the understanding that the publisher is not engaged in rendering legal, accounting, or other professional service. If legal advice or other expert assistance is required, the service of a competent professional person should be sought.

Production Credits
Publisher: Michael Brown
Associate Editor: Katey Birtcher
Production Director: Amy Rose
Production Editor: Tracey Chapman
Associate Production Editor: Rachel Rossi
Marketing Manager: Wendy Thayer
Manufacturing Buyer: Therese Connell
Composition: Publishers' Design and Production Services, Inc
Cover Design: Kristin E. Ohlin
Cover Image: © Clive Tooth/ShutterStock, Inc.
Printing and Binding: Malloy, Inc.
Cover Printing: Malloy, Inc.

Library of Congress Cataloging-in-Publication Data
Marian, Mary, 1956–
  Clinical nutrition for surgical patients / Mary Marian, Scott A. Shikora, and Mary Russell.
    p. ; cm.
  Includes index.
  ISBN-13: 978-0-7637-3881-5
  ISBN-10: 0-7637-3881-6
  1. Surgery—Nutritional aspects.   I. Shikora, Scott A., 1959–   II. Russell, Mary, 1951–   III. Title.
  [DNLM: 1. Nutrition Therapy. 2. Surgical Procedures, Operative. 3. Perioperative Care—methods.
WB 400 M333c 2007]
  RD52.N88M37 2007
  617'.919—dc22

2007001643

6048
Printed in the United States of America
11 10 09 08 07   10 9 8 7 6 5 4 3 2 1

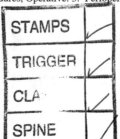

STAMPS

TRIGGER

CLA

SPINE

Dedication

This book is dedicated to:

~Our families for their continued love and support~

~To Our Colleagues and Friends in the field of preventive
and therapeutic nutrition~

Contents

*Scott A. Shikora, MD, FACS; Leonardo Claros, MD; and
Margaret Furtado, MS, RD, LD/N*

Preface

The role of nutrition in the care of surgical patients continues to expand. This has been increasingly evident in the past few decades with continued advances in the provision of specialized nutrition support, including the development and refinement of commercially-prepared nutrition products. Despite these advances, many surgical patients present with malnutrition preoperatively, or become malnourished postoperatively. Malnutrition is associated with an increase in infectious complications, length of hospital stay and cost of medical care, and reduced quality of life.

This book begins with a thorough review of the basics of medical nutrition therapy for surgical patients, including nutritional assessment, the role of surgical diets, and the indications and contraindications for specialized nutrition support. Subsequent chapters address specific medical and surgical conditions and disease states that present specific challenges with provision of nutrition support. Evidence-based recommendations and application to clinical practice provide the foundation for the text.

As the healthcare delivery system expands into the community and other care settings, the number of healthcare professionals providing nutritional care for surgical patients continues to expand as well. It is important for all practitioners to have the most up-to-date knowledge in order to provide optimal care. This text will benefit not only acute care professionals but also practitioners outside acute care centers who provide care to surgical patients.

This text was developed through the collaboration of a number of distinguished professionals who are among the most knowledgeable practitioners in the field of specialized nutrition support, and in particular in provision of this care to surgical patients. Their enthusiasm and expertise is evident throughout this book. There are few resources currently available that provide medical nutrition therapy information solely for surgical patients. It is our hope that this book fills that gap and becomes the preeminent resource for practitioners providing interdisciplinary nutrition care to patients in the perioperative period.

Mary Marian, MS, RD
Mary K. Russell, MS, RD, CNSD
Scott A. Shikora, MD, FACS

Foreword

The challenge to surgeons of providing supportive nutrition care to their surgical patients was the impetus for the development of parenteral and tube enteral nutrition over the last 40 years (1,2). Prior to that time many disease states such as cancer and inflammatory bowel disease made oral nutrition impossible and led to severe malnutrition that significantly increased the morbidity and mortality of needed surgery. In addition, complications of surgery were often associated with prolonged gastrointestinal tract dysfunction leading to increasing malnutrition, impaired wound healing, reduction in immune function and, if left untreated, death.

The critical need for maintaining and improving the surgical patients' nutrition status has been recognized for decades (3). Improvements in delivery techniques, nutrient solutions and identifying the nutrient and metabolic needs of surgical patients has led to rapid advances in the field of clinical nutrition for surgical patients. The ability to adequately address the nutrition needs of the complicated surgical patient has been felt by many to allow for safer convalescence from surgical procedures or associated complications (4).

The editors and contributing authors of this text are recognized expert clinicians in the management of the nutrition needs of surgical patients. They have provided guidance for assessing a patient's nutrition status and its severity and determining the metabolic requirements for maintaining or improving the surgical patient's nutrition status. A variety of nutrition support techniques are described and their roles in managing many types of surgical patients are outlined. Any clinician caring for surgical patients will benefit from the wealth of current information provided in this text.

Ezra Steiger MD, FACS, CNSP
Director, Intestinal Rehabilitation Program
The Cleveland Clinic – Digestive Disease Center
Cleveland, OH

REFERENCES

1. Dudrick SJ, Wilmore DW, Vars HM, Rhoads JE. Long-term total parenteral nutrition with growth, development, and positive nitrogen balance. *Surgery*. 1968; 64:134–142.

2. Stephens RV, Randall T. Use of a concentrated, balanced liquid elemental diet for nutritional management of catabolic states. *Ann Surg*. 1969;170:642–667.

3. Studley HO. Percentage of weight loss: A basis indicator of surgical risk in patients with chronic peptic ulcer. *JAMA*. 1936;106:458–460.

4. Fazio VW, Coutsoftides T, Steiger E. Factors influencing the outcome of treatment of small bowel cutaneous fistula. *World Journal of Surgery*. 1983; 7:481–488.

Contributors

David August, MD
Professor, Dept. of Surgery &
Robert Wood Johnson Medical School-
    UMDNJ
Chief, Surgical Oncology
The Cancer Institute of New Jersey

Peter Beyer, MS, RD, CNSD
Associate Professor, Dietetics &
    Nutrition
The University of Kansas Medical
    Center

**Joseph I. Boullata, PharmD, RPh,
    BCNSP**
Associate Professor – Pharmacology &
    Therapeutics
University of Pennsylvania, School of
    Nursing
Pharmacy Specialist, Clinical Nutrition
    Support Services
Hospital of University of Pennsylvania

Leonardo Claros, MD
Co-Director, Center for Weight Control
Caritas Saint-Elizabeth's Medical

**Charlene Compher, PhD, RD, FADA,
    CNSD**
Assistant Professor in Nutrition Science
University of Pennsylvania, School of
    Nursing

Sara DiCecco, MS, RD, LD
Clinical Dietitian
Department of Dietetics &
The William J. von Liebig Transplant
    Center
Mayo Clinic Rochester

Margaret Furtado, MS, RD, LD/N
Clinical Dietitian
Massachusetts General Hospital Weight
    Center

Dema Halasa-Esper, MS, RD, CNSD
Dietitian Specialist
University of Pittsburgh Medical Center
    Presbyterian

**Jeanette Hasse, PhD, LD, RD, FADA,
    CNSD**
Transplant Nutrition Specialist
Baylor University School of Medicine

Maureen Huhmann, MS, RD
Instructor, Department of Primary Care
Clinical Nutritionist
The Cancer Institute of New Jersey

Gordon L. Jensen, MD, PhD
Director, Vanderbilt Center for Human
    Nutrition
Professor of Medicine, Vanderbilt
    University

Jennifer Lefton, MS, RD, LD/N, CNSD
Clinical Dietitian
Nutrition Services, Jackson Memorial
  Hospital

Ainsley Malone, MS, RD, LD, CNSD
Nutrition Support Dietitian
Mt. Carmel West Hospital, Department of
  Pharmacy

Mary Marian, MS, RD
Clinical Nutritionist
University of Arizona – College of Medi-
  cine & AZ Cancer Center

Steve McClave, MD
Professor of Medicine, Director of Clinical
  Nutrition
University of Louisville School of Medicine
Division of Gastroenterology/Hepatology
Digestive Health Center, University
  Hospital

Kelly O'Donnell MS, RD, CNSD
Surgery Nutrition Support Specialist
University of Virginia Health System

Mary Russell, MS, RD, LDN, CNSD
Interim Director
Nutrition Services
University of Chicago Hospitals

Scott A. Shikora, MD, FACS
Professor of Surgery
Tufts University School of Medicine
Chief, Bariatric Surgery
Tufts-New England Medical Center

Marsha Stieber, MSA, RD, CNSD
Dietetic Internship Director
Arizona Department of Health Services

Jennifer Tomesko, MS, RD, CNSD
Clinical Nutrition Manager, Sodexho

Roopa Vemulapalli, MD
Department of Gastroenterology,
  Hepatology & Nutrition
St. Michael's Medical Center

Kate Willcutts, MS, RD, CNSD
Assistant Clinical Nutrition Manager/
  Nutrition Support Specialist
University of Virginia Hospital
Assistant Professor, School of Nursing

Marion Winkler, MS, RD, CNSD
Nutrition Support Service
Division of Surgical Research

About the Authors

Mary Marian is currently a clinical nutrition research specialist and clinical lecturer with the College of Medicine and Arizona Cancer Center at the University of Arizona in Tucson, Arizona. Additionally, she is a faculty member for the Program in Integrative Medicine at the University of Arizona and at the University of Phoenix. Her areas of focus include nutrition for disease prevention, nutrition support, and integrative medicine. Mary has been a clinical dietitian for over 20 years. After completing her dietetic internship, Mary was a Clinical Dietitian and Clinical Nutrition Manager at University Medical Center in Tucson. Her clinical responsibilities included providing nutritional care to medical, surgical, trauma, and pediatric intensive care patients in addition to general surgery patients, liver and kidney transplants, and patients with cystic fibrosis. After leaving UMC, Mary has been involved with teaching medical students, residents, and fellows about the role of medical nutrition therapy in disease prevention and treatment at the College of Medicine. She also provides medical nutrition therapy for cancer survivors through the AZ Cancer Center at the Univeristy of Arizona. Mary is involved with many local and national nutrition organizations. She has also published many chapters and articles in peer-reviewed publications, and has served as an editor or co-editor for several textbooks and publications. Mary has also been a speaker on various nutrition topics at many local, state, national, and international conferences including visits to Cuba and Brazil.

Mary Krystofiak Russell, MS, RD, LDN, CNSD, is currently serving as the Interim Director, Nutrition Services, University of Chicago Hospitals, Chicago Illinois. Previously, she was the director and interim director of the Nutrition Services Department of Duke University Hospital, Durham, North Carolina. Previous to that experience, Mary gained 13 years of progressive experience at Duke as a dietitian clinician, including 10 years on the adult Nutrition Support Service, and extensive experience with surgery, trauma, transplant, and medical intensive care unit patients. She is the author or co-author of multiple articles and chapters on nutrition support topics. She has spoken at numerous local, regional, national, and international meetings. Additional past experiences also include her extensive professional involvement as chair of A.S.P.E.N. Dietetics Practice section, and as Professional Issues delegate, Clinical Nutrition, for the American Dietetic Association (ADA) House of Delegates. She has also served as a past president of North Carolina Dietetic Association and past chair, Dietitians in Nutrition Support Dietetic Practice Group of the ADA.

Dr. Scott Shikora is a Professor of Surgery at Tufts University School of Medicine and the Chief of Bariatric Surgery at Tufts-New England Medical Center in Boston. He attended medical school at Columbia University College of Physicians & Surgeons. He did his surgical residency and Nutrition Support fellowship at New England Deaconess Hospital in Boston. He is a past president of the American Society for Parenteral and Enteral Nutrition and is on the Executive Council for the American Society for Bariatric Surgery. Dr Shikora is an Associate Editor of two surgical journals and has co-edited two nutritional textbooks.

CHAPTER 1

Nutrition Assessment and Requirements

Gordon Jensen, MD, PhD

INTRODUCTION

Although often overlooked, undernutrition has been characterized and reported for more than 50 years (1–5). Diminished intake, malabsorption or maldigestion, increased nutrient utilization, excessive losses, and altered metabolism are potential etiologies for undernutrition. Gastrointestinal surgery may predispose patients to undernutrition risk during the perioperative period. Undernourished patients are at particular risk for developing complications during their medical or surgical treatments (3). The inflammatory stress state associated with surgery and illness may alter a patient's nutritional needs. Patients who are undernourished before surgery tend to have higher rates of complications, which may include poor wound healing, compromised immune status, impairment of organ functions, and increased mortality (6–9). These complications can lead to prolonged hospital stays and increased expenditure of health care dollars (6–12).

Depending on the criteria used, undernutrition occurs in one third or more of patients in acute or chronic care settings (13–17). Determining which patients are undernourished or at risk for undernutrition and should receive perioperative nutrition intervention is a priority. A basic understanding of undernutrition syndromes is a prerequisite (18). This chapter will highlight practical nutrition assessment techniques suitable for routine clinical practice.

COMPONENTS OF COMPREHENSIVE NUTRITION ASSESSMENT

The first step in nutrition assessment of surgical patients is to identify patients who are undernourished or are at risk for developing undernutrition during their perioperative period. Undernutrition may be evidenced by weight loss as a result of their disease states, increased metabolic needs, and/or compromised nutrient intake. Special attention should be given to patients who may have a prolonged recovery with difficulty eating or tolerating oral nutrition, such as patients with advanced age or those who require extensive abdominal surgery procedures. Many surgical procedures can affect a patient's ability to chew, swallow, digest, and absorb nutrients and can also be associated with prolonged physical immobility (19). Therefore, careful consideration should be given to the postoperative management of these patients in order to minimize the risk of developing undernutrition and to support the recovery process.

The spectrum of undernutrition syndromes can include states of starvation (marasmus) or conditions that involve reduced visceral protein status. Cachexia is the loss of body cell mass with an underlying inflammatory condition. Decreased albumin or prealbumin may be indicators of protein undernutrition but in health care settings are more often manifestations of inflammatory stress response (20–24). Patients may exhibit manifestations of both of these types of syndromes, depending on the duration of starvation and the degree of underlying stress response. Marasmus is associated with a decline in skeletal muscle and subcutaneous fat as evidenced by weight loss. Typical disease states may include anorexia nervosa, malabsorption, or esophageal cancer. Classic Kwashiorkor, observed in children in underdeveloped populations, was originally characterized as hypoalbuminemia, edema, fatty liver, and anorexia resulting from a diet deficient in protein but with appreciable grain food intake. The mechanism by which Kwashiorkor occurs has not been fully elucidated; however, stress response to a parasitic or infectious condition may often be a contributor. Hypoalbuminemia in western health care has been described as "Kwashiorkor-like" but in reality the only common feature is usually inflammatory stress response. The cytokines that mediate response to stress or injury also reduce albumin and prealbumin levels by altering synthetic and catabolic rates for these acute phase reactants. The high prevalence of reduced visceral proteins observed in modern acute and chronic care settings is often associated with inflammatory phenomenon (22–24).

A cytokine-mediated acute phase metabolic response may be precipitated by inflammatory disease, illness, or injury (23,25–32). The inflammatory cytokines interleukin-1 (IL-1), interleukin-6 (IL-6), and tumor necrosis factor (TNF) may mediate changes in metabolism indirectly by altering the secretion of hormones and directly by affecting target organs. The resulting hormonal milieu favors a catabolic state. It is noteworthy that TNF was originally named cachectin for its suspected role in cachexia (27). These three cytokines are believed to have key roles in triggering the acute phase metabolic response. Manifestations of this response may include elevation in resting energy expenditure, a net export of amino acids from muscle to liver, an increase in gluconeogenesis, an expansion of the extracellular fluid compartment, and a shift toward the production of positive acute-phase reactants. These acute-phase reactants include antibodies, complement, C-reactive protein, and fibrinogen. A decline in the synthesis of negative acute-phase reactants like albumin, transferrin, prealbumin, and retinol-binding protein is observed. In simplistic terms, the body down regulates albumin synthesis so that urgently needed proteins for immune, clotting, and wound-healing functions can be made. Although over the short run this is likely an adaptive response, when the underlying stressor is severe, protracted, or repeated, adverse outcomes will ultimately result.

Five broad categories may be used to describe undernutrition: wasting (marasmus), sarcopenia, cachexia, protein-energy undernutrition (PEU), and failure to thrive (18,23,33–36). Table 1–1 lists the key characteristics for each syndrome. In order to select helpful interventions and management, the practitioner should identify the relevant undernutrition syndrome. Syndromes may overlap and underlying disease conditions may result in more than one type of syndrome.

Nutrition screening detects the risk for undernutrition. Nutrition assessment tools and techniques are used to evaluate the nutritional status of patients and to diagnose undernutrition syndromes. Conditions of undernutrition involve complex differential diagnosis and require evaluation to determine underlying etiologies. Because no single clinical or laboratory indicator provides a measure of comprehensive nutritional status, it is necessary to gather information from multiple different sources including historical, physical, anthropometric, and laboratory data.

Table 1–1 Key Characteristics of Undernutrition Syndromes

Undernutrition Syndrome	Characteristics
Wasting (marasmus)	Loss of body cell mass without underlying inflammatory condition. Visceral proteins preserved. Extracellular fluid not increased.
Sarcopenia	Aging-related muscle loss without other precipitating causes.
Cachexia	Loss of body cell mass with underlying inflammatory condition. Decline in visceral proteins. Increased extracellular fluid.
Protein-energy undernutrition	Clinical and laboratory evidence for reduced dietary intake of protein and energy. Reduced visceral proteins. In practice this term is often mistakenly applied to patients who manifest reduced visceral proteins in the setting of inflammatory response but without compromised nutrition intake.
Failure to thrive	Weight loss and decline in physical and/or cognitive functioning with signs of hopelessness and helplessness.

Source: Adapted with permission from Jensen GL. *Physicians' Information and Education Resource.* Philadelphia, Pa.: American College of Physicians-American Society of Internal Medicine.

HISTORICAL DATA

Many types of helpful data can be obtained from the patient, caregivers, and the medical record (See Table 1–2). The patient's weight history, medical and surgical history, medication history, and dietary practice history will aid the practitioner in determining the presence or risk of undernutrition.

Weight History

One of the most important historical elements is prior weight loss, including volitional weight reduction. The amount and duration of the weight loss should be noted. A weight loss of 10% or greater over the previous 6 months is of clinical significance.

Table 1–2 History and Physical Examination Elements for Undernutrition Syndromes

History
- Body weight changes
- Medical and surgical conditions; chronic disease
- Constitutional signs and symptoms
- Eating difficulties and gastrointestinal complaints
- Eating disorders
- Medication use
- Dietary practices and use of supplements
- Influences on nutritional status

Physical examination
- Body mass index (BMI)
- Weight loss, loss of subcutaneous fat, loss of muscle mass
- Weakness or loss of strength
- Peripheral edema
- Hair examination
- Skin examination
- Eye examination
- Perioral examination
- Extremity examination
- Mental status and nervous system examination
- Functional assessment

Source: Adapted with permission from Roy MA, Jensen GL. "Nutrition Screening and Assessment." In: Lang R, Hensrud DD, eds. *Clinical Preventive Medicine.* Chicago, Ill.: AMA Press; 2004:173–181. Further details on these elements can be found in Jensen GL: *Physicians' Information and Education Resource.* Philadelphia, Pa.: American College of Physicians-American Society of Internal Medicine.

Medical/Surgical History

Chronic diseases, medical conditions or treatment, and surgical interventions may adversely impact nutritional status. Often the treatments for these diseases necessitate dietary restrictions or limitations that further compromise nutritional status. Treatments may also be associated with an inability to ingest or absorb nutrients. For some patients, increased energy demands without a compensatory increase in food energy intake may result in undernutrition. Conversely, the course and treatment of specific acute and chronic diseases may be undesirably affected by compromised nutritional status

Medication History

A careful medication history is important because many drugs can compromise nutritional status by interfering with food intake or with the absorption, metabolism, and excretion of nutrients (37). Interactions between nutrients and medications may also impact the absorption, metabolism, and excretion of the medications (38). Some examples of nutrient interactions with drugs are highlighted in Table 1–3; however, many other potential interactions have been identified.

Diet History

Food choices and dietary habits are impacted by a variety of environmental, cultural, and socioeconomic factors, and may profoundly affect nutritional status. Dietary assessment can be used to detect inadequate or imbalanced food or nutrient intakes;

Table 1–3 Common Drug-Nutrient Interactions

Drug	Nutrient Lost
Aluminum (magnesium hydroxide antacids)	Phosphate
Cholestyramine (bile resin)	Fat-soluble vitamins
	Folate
Omeprazole (acid-pump inhibitor)	Vitamin B$_{12}$
Methotrexate (chemotherapy; folate antagonist)	Folate
Isoniazid (antituberculosis; B$_6$ antagonist)	Pyridoxine
Coumadin	Vitamin K
Lasix (diuretic)	Calcium
	Potassium
	Magnesium
	Zinc

Source: Adapted with permission from Jensen GL. *Physicians' Information and Education Resource.* Philadelphia, Pa.: American College of Physicians-American Society of Internal Medicine.

however, dietary intake information should be interpreted carefully and in combination with other indicators of nutritional status. Dietary intake instruments are subject to random and systematic errors. The selection of dietary assessment methodology depends on the skills of the assessor, the feasibility in the context of clinical assessment, and the patient-specific characteristics (39). Table 1–4 summarizes different methods of dietary assessment.

Table 1–4 Dietary Assessment Methods

Method and Classification	Procedure	Characteristics	Limitations	Precision
Food record or diary *Prospective Quantitative*	The subject records all food and beverages as eaten for a specified period of time (usually 3–14 days). Portion size, cooking methods and brand names (if possible) are recorded.	Does not rely on memory	Requires numerate and literate subjects. Subject may modify eating patterns to simplify process or to impress investigator. Subject's compliance decreases with longer time frames. Underreporting common.	2 to 5 days of records are recommended for favorable precision and compliance
24-hour recall *Retrospective Quantitative*	The subject reports to an interviewer all foods and beverages consumed in the previous 24 h. Portion size, cooking methods and brand names (if possible) are recorded.	Rapid Inexpensive Low respondent burden	Requires trained interviewer. Relies on memory. Single recall unlikely to represent usual intake. Underreporting common.	Higher precision with multiple replicate recalls, three non-consecutive random days to include a weekend day are recommended

Table 1–4 Continued

Method and Classification	Procedure	Characteristics	Limitations	Precision
Food frequency questionnaire (FFQ) Retrospective *Qualitative or quantitative*	The subject self-reports (or reports to an inter-viewer) the frequency of consumption (day, week, month, year) for a compre-hensive or specific list of food items. In semiquanti-tative FFQs, usual portion size can be quantified with or without the use of food models.	Rapid Low respon-dent burden Can capture the intake of infrequently consumed nutrients.	Can be expensive Broad time frame, usually averaged over months.	Probably adequate for general assessment but accuracy lower than other methods.

Source: Adapted from Gibson RD. *Principles of Nutritional Assessment.* New York: Oxford University Press; 1990, and Roy MA, Jensen GL. Nutrition Screening and Assessment. In: Lang RS, Hensrud DD, eds. *Clinical Preventive Medicine.* 2nd ed. Chicago, Ill.: AMA Press; 2004:173–179.

PHYSICAL EXAMINATION

A complete physical examination can help to identify undernutrition or the pres-ence of specific nutrient deficiencies. Key findings on physical exam include mus-cle wasting, subcutaneous fat loss, and skin changes. The presence of peripheral edema, which may accompany hypoalbuminemia, should be noted. Areas of the body where cell replacement occurs at a high rate such as hair, skin, mouth, and tongue, are most likely to show signs of undernutrition and warrant close exami-nation. Table 1–2 highlights important physical examination elements.

ANTHROPOMETRIC DATA

Anthropometrics are physical measurements that provide an indirect assessment of body size and composition. The investigator compares measurements with standards (for the same gender and age). Trends may be evaluated by comparison with previous measurements taken on the same individual. Detection of undernutrition and obesity may be possible by identifying variations in the amount and proportion of measurements. Common anthropometric measurements include height, weight, skin folds, and circumferences. Appropriate training and skill are required for reliable measurements.

Height

Height measurements are essential in the determination and interpretation of other anthropometric measurements and indices. A wall-mounted stadiometer may be used to measure height for individuals who are able to stand unassisted. Height can be estimated by doubling the arm-span measurement from the patient's sternal notch to the end of the longest finger for adults who are bedridden or wheelchair bound. Stature of older persons can also be estimated using knee height (measured with a caliper device) (40).

Men: Stature (cm) = [2.02 × knee height (cm)] – (0.04 × age) + 64.19
Women: Stature (cm) = [1.83 × knee height (cm)] – (0.24 × age) + 84.88

Weight

Ideal reference tables such as the Metropolitan Height and Weight Tables (41) were developed using healthy populations, limiting their application to hospitalized patients or other population groups. Usefulness may also be confounded by a subjective interpretation of the patient's frame size, which may vary by observer. The body mass index (BMI), defined as weight (kg) over height (m²), measures body size and is an indirect measure of body fatness. BMI is extensively used as a reference for healthy populations; the relation between BMI and outcome in acute illness/surgery has been subject to limited investigation. The National Institutes of Health have released guidelines for body size classification (42).

BMI <18.5 = underweight, at risk of undernutrition
BMI 18.5 to 24.9 = desirable
BMI 25 to 29 = overweight
BMI ≥30 = obese

Skin Folds and Circumferences

Skin folds and circumference measurements have limited practical utility in patient care settings because highly trained personnel are required to achieve acceptable reliability. The NHANES III Anthropometric Procedures video can aid the practitioner who wishes to use these procedures (43).

Other Body Composition Assessment Tools

High-technology body-composition assessments tools are available but are primarily used in research settings because they are impractical for routine clinical use (see Table 1–5). These tools include water displacement, bioelectrical impedance analysis, dual-energy X-ray absorptiometry, computer tomography (CT), magnetic resonance imaging (MRI), total body counting of the naturally occurring potassium isotope, and air plethysmography.

LABORATORY DATA

Laboratory studies can be useful in the determination of a patient's nutritional status. However, patients with low visceral proteins may or may not be undernourished. Additional evidence suggesting loss of body cell mass or compromised dietary intake is required to diagnose an undernutrition syndrome.

Hypoalbuminemia is commonly considered an indicator of undernutrition; however, it should be interpreted with great caution. Albumin lacks specificity and sensitivity for this application (20–23,44–46). Underlying injuries, disease, or inflammatory conditions are often accompanied by low levels of serum albumin, and levels are slow to recover due to the protracted 2 to 3 week half-life of albumin. The usual threshold for reduced albumin is ≤35 gm/L, but ≤38 gm/L may be an appropriate risk screen for older persons (47). Albumin synthetic functions tend to be fairly well preserved in aging patients (48–50). In acute and chronic care settings, the prevalence of low albumin (≤35 gm/L) is approximately 25%–53% of patients (51–55). Prevalence of low albumin (≤35 gm/L) in the community setting is dependent on the population being studied but is generally less than 10% unless

Table 1–5 Body Composition Studies for Nutritional Syndromes

- Anthropometrics
- Bioelectrical impedance
- Water displacement
- Whole-body counting and isotope dilution techniques
- Air plethysmography
- Dual-energy X-ray absorptiometry (DXA)
- Computed tomography (CT) or magnetic resonance imaging (MRI)

Source: Adapted with permission from Roy MA, Jensen GL. Nutrition Screening and Assessment. In: Lang R, Hensrud DD, eds. *Clinical Preventive Medicine.* Chicago, Ill.: AMA Press; 2004:173–181. Further details on these studies can be found in Jensen GL. *Physicians' Information and Education Resource.* Philadelphia, Pa.: American College of Physicians-American Society of Internal Medicine.

the population sample is frail or homebound (10,47,50,55). Prealbumin possesses similar limitations as albumin as an indicator of nutritional status, because it may also be confounded by response to injury, disease, or inflammation; however, its shorter half-life of 2 days may make it a more useful marker to follow for short-term trends (56).

Individuals with profound marasmus due to semistarvation may exhibit normal visceral proteins as long as they are not stressed by disease, inflammation, or injury. Examples include anorexia nervosa (57) or depression. Obese persons in diet programs with low protein and energy intakes and resulting weight loss will generally have normal visceral proteins (58). Albumin has been found to lack sensitivity in comparison to reference measures of body composition. Despite erosion in body cell mass, changes in albumin may not be observed (59). Changes in dietary intake have related inconsistently to visceral protein status. A major confounder is that patients who are sick or injured tend to eat less. Other disease states that impact upon albumin synthesis or losses may confound interpretation including liver disease, nephrotic syndrome, or protein-wasting enteropathy. Fluid status may limit interpretation including those derangements associated with acute fluid resuscitation, volume overload, dehydration, diuretic use, congestive heart failure, ascites, renal failure, or dialysis.

Low albumin has been consistently associated with adverse outcomes that include greater in-hospital complications, longer hospital stays, more frequent readmissions, and increased in-hospital mortality as well as mortality at 90 days and 1 year (60–73). Low albumin also is predictive of mortality among residents of chronic care facilities (74–76). Low albumin in the community setting is predictive of not only mortality but also functional limitation (77–79). The combination of low albumin and low cholesterol may be particularly useful in the identification of older persons at risk for subsequent mortality and functional decline (80). Utility of albumin as a prognostic indicator reflects its use as a powerful proxy measure for underlying disease burden, inflammatory condition, or injury. In general, the lower the visceral proteins, the bigger the insult that the patient has suffered and the worse the prognosis.

Other Biological Markers

Adverse outcomes including mortality are associated with hypocholesterolemia (81). Inflammatory cytokines likely mediate a decline in cholesterol levels (82). Low cholesterol concentration correlates poorly with dietary intake (83). C-reactive protein (CRP) is a positive acute-phase reactant that is elevated in inflammatory states (84–86). It can be useful to help ascertain whether active inflammation is contributing to reduced visceral protein status (23). Although measuring CRP levels is not warranted in all patients, the measurement of CRP may aid in the appropriate interpretation of reduced visceral proteins. Table 1–6 addresses a variety of laboratory and other tests used to evaluate nutritional disorders.

Table 1–6 Laboratories and Other Studies for Nutritional Syndromes

Test	Notes
Albumin	Lacks sensitivity and specificity for undernutrition. Potent risk indicator for morbidity and mortality. Proxy measure for underlying injury, disease or inflammation. Half-life is 14–20 days. Also consider liver disease, nephrotic syndrome, and protein-wasting enteropathy.
Prealbumin	Sensitive to short-term changes in inflammation and protein nutriture with half-life of 2–3 days. Otherwise suffers the same limitations of albumin with limited sensitivity and specificity for undernutrition. Levels may be decreased in liver failure and increased in renal failure.
Transferrin	Acute phase reactant also altered by perturbation in iron status. Half-life is 8–10 days. Lacks sensitivity and specificity for undernutrition.
Retinol-binding protein	Responds to very short-term changes in nutritional status but utility is also limited by response to stress and inflammation. Half-life is 12 hours. Also affected by vitamin A deficiency and renal disease.
C-reactive protein	C-reactive protein is a positive acute phase reactant. It should be elevated if an active inflammatory process is manifest. Useful in discerning inflammatory contribution to reduced visceral proteins.
Cholesterol	Low cholesterol (<160 mg/dl) is often observed in undernourished persons with serious underlying disease. It is unrelated to dietary intake in many clinical settings. Increased complications and mortality are observed. It appears that low cholesterol is again a nonspecific feature of poor health status that reflects cytokine-mediated inflammatory condition. Vegans may also exhibit low cholesterol.
Carotene	Nonspecific indicator of malabsorption and poor nutritional intake.
Cytokines	Research is exploring prognostic use of cytokine measurements as indicators of inflammatory status.

(continues)

Table 1–6 Continued

Test	Notes
Electrolytes, BUN, and Cr	Monitor for abnormalities consistent with under- or overhydration status and purging (contraction alkalosis). BUN may also be low in the setting of markedly reduced body cell mass.
CBC with differential	Screen for nutritional anemias (iron, B_{12}, and folate), lymphopenia (undernutrition) and thrombocytopenia (vitamin C and folate).
Total lymphocyte count	Relative lymphopenia (total lymphocyte count <1200/mm^3) is a nonspecific marker for undernutrition.
Helper/suppressor T cell ratio	Ratio may be reduced in severely undernourished patients. Not specific for nutritional status.
Nitrogen balance	24-hour urine can be analyzed for urine urea nitrogen (UUN) to determine nitrogen balance and give indication of degree of catabolism and adequacy of protein replacement. Requires accurate urine collection and normal renal function. Nitrogen balance = (protein / 6.25) – (UUN+4).
Urine 3-methylhistidine	Indicator of muscle catabolism and protein sufficiency. Released upon breakdown of myofibrillar protein and excreted without reutilization. Urine measurement requires a meat-free diet for 3 days prior to collection.
Creatinine height index (CHI)	CHI = (24-hour urinary creatinine excretion / ideal urinary creatinine for gender and height) × 100. Indicator of muscle depletion. Requires accurate urine collection and normal renal function.
Prothrombin time / INR	Nonspecific indicator of vitamin K status.
Specific nutrients	When suspected, a variety of specific nutrient levels may be measured: thiamine, riboflavin, niacin, folate, pryridoxine, vitamins A, C, D, E, B_{12}, zinc, iron, selenium, carnitine, and homocysteine-indicator of B_{12}, folate, and pyridoxine status
Skin testing—recall antigens	Delayed hypersensitivity testing. While undernourished patients are often anergic, this is not specific for nutritional status.

Table 1–6 Continued

Test	Notes
Electrocardiogram	Severely undernourished patients with reduced body cell mass may exhibit low voltage and prolonged QT interval. These findings are not specific for undernutrition.
Video fluoroscopy	Helpful to evaluate suspected swallowing disorders.
Endoscopic and X-ray studies of gastrointestinal tract	Useful to evaluate impaired function, motility, and obstruction.
Fat absorption	72-hour fecal fat can be used to quantitate degree of malabsorption.
Schilling test	Identify the cause for impaired vitamin B_{12} absorption.
Indirect calorimetry	Metabolic cart can be used to determine resting energy expenditure (REE) for accurate estimation of energy needs.

Source: Adapted with permission from Jensen GL. *Physicians' Information and Education Resource.* Philadelphia, Pa.: American College of Physicians-American Society of Internal Medicine.

NUTRITION SCREENING AND ASSESSMENT TOOLS

Young and middle-aged adults generally do not require frequent nutrition screening unless disease or eating disorders are present. Older patients, particularly those who are homebound, frail, chronically ill, or hospitalized, should be screened more often because the prevalence of undernutrition is higher in these populations.

The lack of any single screening or assessment measure that is a valid indicator of comprehensive nutritional status has prompted the development of multi-item screening and assessment tools (Table 1–7). Patients in acute or chronic care settings have been most extensively investigated while those in community settings have received less scrutiny. It is not established whether these multi-item tools actually have appropriate specificity and sensitivity to identify undernourished persons for many clinical applications (87,88).

The Subjective Global Assessment (SGA) includes assessments of weight change, dietary intake, gastrointestinal symptoms, functional capacity, presence of disease, and physical exam (89). SGA divides patients into three classes: Class A, well nourished; Class B, moderately (or suspected of being) undernourished; and class C, severely undernourished. It requires trained practitioners for administration and has demonstrated good interrater reliability. It has proven a useful predictor of

Table 1–7 Common Nutrition Screening and Assessment Tools and Properties

Name of Tool	Purpose	Administration Method
Ambulatory Patients		
Mini-Nutritional Assessment Short-Form (MNA-SF)	Screen nutritional status	Trained clinician
Mini-Nutritional Assessment (MNA)	Assess nutritional status	Trained clinician
Nutrition Screening Initiative (NSI) checklist	Encourage those at risk to seek help	Self-administered
Nutrition Screening Initiative—Level I screen	Assess for further evaluation and intervention	Trained clinician
Nutrition Screening Initiative—Level II screen	Collect diagnostic information for evaluation and intervention	Trained clinician
Hospitalized Patients		
Subjective Global Assessment (SGA)	Assess nutritional status	Trained clinician
Nutrition Risk Index (NRI)	Predict operative complications	Predictive equation using laboratories and anthropometrics
Hospital Prognostic Index (HPI)	Predict sepsis and mortality	Predictive equation using laboratory and clinical data
Prognostic Nutritional Index (PNI)	Predict operative complications	Predictive equation using laboratory and clinical data
Prognostic Inflammatory and Nutritional Index (PINI)	Predict mortality and risk of complications	Predictive equation using laboratories

Source: Adapted from Roy MA, Jensen GL. Nutrition Screening and Assessment. In: Lang RS, Hensrud DD, eds. *Clinical Preventive Medicine.* Chicago, Ill.: AMA Press; 2004:173–179.

postoperative complications and provides one of the better validated measures of nutritional status (3,89).

The Mini-Nutritional Assessment (MNA) is a clinical assessment tool consisting of 18 items designed to assess the nutritional status of older persons (90–92). The MNA classifies older persons into three levels of nutritional status on a scale ranging from 0 to 30. A score of 24 or more indicates satisfactory nutritional status, a score of 17 to 23.5 indicates risk of undernutrition, and a score below 17 suggests protein-energy undernutrition. Extensive cross-validation studies have been completed with the MNA. Scores were significantly correlated with dietary intake and anthropometric and laboratory nutritional parameters (93). Although the MNA is probably the most studied tool, its utility has also been questioned (94). A shorter version of the MNA has only six items and can be used as a screening tool (95).

The Prognostic Nutritional Index (PNI) incorporates laboratory measurements to predict outcomes (96,97).

$$PNI\ (\%) = 158 - 16.6\ (Alb) - 0.78\ (TSF) - 0.20\ (Tfn) - 5.8\ (DH)$$

NOTE: Abbreviations: Alb = albumin, TSF = triceps skin fold, Tfn = transferrin, DH = delayed hypersensitivity

Elevated PNI correlates with increased morbidity and mortality in elective gastrointestinal and oncologic surgeries (97).

Certain surgical patients will have diagnoses that should alert the clinician as nutrition risk indicators. These diagnoses may include severe acute or chronic pancreatitis, enterocutaneous fistula, mesenteric ischemia, complications of inflammatory bowel disease, motility disorders, and short-bowel syndrome. Other patients may develop perioperative complications including critical illness, severe gastrointestinal hemorrhage, or gastrointestinal ileus or obstruction that require protracted *nil per os* (NPO) status or repeated surgical interventions that place them at elevated nutritional risk.

DETERMINATION OF REQUIREMENTS

Energy Needs

Calorie needs are dependent on the patient's size, body composition, clinical condition, concurrent organ failure, and activity level. Accurate determination of the appropriate energy needs is crucial for meeting metabolic demands and helping to prevent erosion of lean body mass. Overzealous feeding is associated with significant risks including difficulties with glucose control and excessive carbon dioxide production (98). Hyperglycemia should be avoided because of recent investigation that found strong associations with adverse outcomes in critically ill surgical patients (99). Calorie goals for stressed patients are frequently estimated at 25–35 kcal/kg body weight/day. An adjusted body weight must be used for obese individuals. The Harris-Benedict equations are also often used to estimate basal energy expenditure (BEE) (100).

Males*: BEE (kcal) = 66.5 + [13.8 × weight (kg)] + [5 × height (cm)] − 6.8 × age (y)]
Females*: BEE (kcal) = 655.1 [9.6 × weight (kg)] + [1.8 × height (cm)] − [4.7 × age (y)]

The BEE is then adjusted for the perceived degree of stress (101). Recent trends of providing fewer calories to seriously ill patients in order to prevent complications such as hyperglycemia, hypercapnia, and hepatic steatosis have been described as "permissive underfeeding" (102,103). Trials have been conducted in obese hospitalized patients using hypocaloric regimens. These studies suggested that most patients achieved positive nitrogen balance and improved clinically with high-protein, hypocaloric parenteral nutrition formulations without experiencing significant adverse effects (104–107). It is not clear whether permissive underfeeding offers similar benefits to nonobese critically ill surgical patients, but this question is subject to active investigation.

Indirect calorimetry may be considered when an accurate assessment of energy needs is desired (108). Such patients might include those who are otherwise difficult to assess or those who will require protracted nutrition support (109–111). A metabolic cart is used to measure oxygen consumption (VO_2) and carbon dioxide production (VCO_2). Estimated resting energy expenditure (REE) is determined using the modified Weir equation. Respiratory quotient (RQ) is determined as RQ $= VCO_2/VO_2$. The RQ gives an indication of net substrate oxidation, with RQ >1.0 consistent with carbohydrate oxidation associated with overfeeding. An RQ <0.68 is consistent with lipid oxidation or starvation ketosis. Elevated FiO_2 requirements ($>0.60\%$) or gas leaks are common limitations to reliable measurements by this approach.

Protein Requirements

Determining appropriate protein goals is important in order to help maintain lean body mass and to promote positive nitrogen balance (112). Note that for the patient with robust inflammatory response, achievement of positive nitrogen balance may not be a realistic goal. Baseline requirements are adjusted by a subjective assessment of the patient's degree of catabolism and an evaluation of renal and hepatic functions. Typical stress needs are on the order of 1.5–1.8 gm protein/kg body weight/day. Subsequently, the protein prescription should be adjusted based on clinical response and continued reevaluation. Reductions in protein doses may be warranted in patients with significant hepatic failure with encephalopathy (113). Reductions may also be indicated for renal insufficiency, depending on the severity of renal failure and whether dialysis is initiated (114). For the morbidly obese patient, ideal body weight should be used to estimate protein needs (107).

CONCLUSION

An understanding of clinical nutrition is crucial to the principles of optimal care of the surgical patient. This chapter has introduced assessment considerations and tools to identify patients who are undernourished or are at risk for developing undernutrition during the perioperative period. The use of key historical elements and a systems approach to physical examination are promoted. The lack of any single clinical or laboratory measure that provides a comprehensive assessment of nutritional status means that it is necessary to capture information from a variety of historical, physical examination, anthropometric, dietary intake, and biochemical sources. Albumin and prealbumin lack sensitivity and specificity as indicators of nutritional status. The appropriate interpretation of albumin and prealbumin levels requires careful consideration of all confounding variables. A low albumin or prealbumin level should not be simply equated with undernutrition without also documenting qualifying alternatives. In critically ill patients, these proteins may best be used as proxy indicators for disease, inflammatory condition, or injury, such that those patients with reduced visceral proteins are likely to be stressed and to therefore be at risk to develop nutritional concerns. Practical nutrition assessment should include a comprehensive approach. Clinical judgment from an experienced practitioner is perhaps the most important element of assessment.

REFERENCES

1. Bistrian BR, Blackburn GL, Hallowell E, Heddle R. Protein status of general surgical patients. *JAMA*. 1974;230:858–860.

2. Bistrian BR, Blackburn GL, Sherman M, Scrimshaw NS. Therapeutic index of nutritional depletion in hospitalized patients. *Surg Gynecol Obstet*. 1975;141:512–516.

3. Detsky AS, Smalley PS, Chang J. Is this patient malnourished? *JAMA*. 1994;271:54–58.

4. Burger GC, Drummond JC, Stanstead HR. *Malnutrition and Starvation in Western Netherlands, September 1944–July 1945*. The Hague, Netherlands: General Printing Office; 1948.

5. Keys A, Brozel J, Henschel A, Mickelsen O, Taylor HL. *The Biology of Human Starvation*. Vol. 1 and 2. Minneapolis: University of Minnesota Press; 1950.

6. Klein S, Kinney J, Jeejeebhoy K, et al. Nutrition support in clinical practice: Review of published data and recommendations for future research directions. *JPEN*. 1997;21:133–156.

7. Souba WW. Nutritional support. *N Engl J Med*. 1997;336:41–48.

8. Sullivan DH, Sun S, Walls RC. Protein-energy undernutrition among elderly hospitalized patients: A prospective study. *JAMA*. 1999;281:2013–2019.

9. Institute of Medicine. *The Role of Nutrition in Maintaining Health in the Nation's Elderly: Evaluating Coverage of Nutrition Services for the Medicare Population*. Washington, D.C.: National Academy Press; 2000.

10. Jensen GL, Kita K, Fish J, Heydt D, Frey C. Nutrition risk screening characteristics of rural older persons: Relation to functional limitations and health care charges. *Am J Clin Nutr*. 1997;66: 819–828.

11. Jensen GL, Friedmann JM, Coleman CD, Smiciklas-Wright H. Screening for hospitalization and nutritional risks among community-dwelling older persons. *Am J Clin Nutr*. 2001;74:201–205.

12. Bales CW. What does it mean to be at "nutritional risk"? Seeking clarity on behalf of the elderly. *Am J Clin Nutr*. 2001;74:155–156.

13. Sullivan DH, Moriarty MS, Chernoff R, Lipschitz DA. Patterns of care: An analysis of the quality of nutritional care routinely provided to elderly hospitalized veterans. *JPEN*. 1989;13:249–254.

14. Mowe M, Bohmer T. The prevalence of undiagnosed protein-calorie undernutrition in a population of hospitalized elderly patients. *J Am Geriatr Soc*. 1991;39:1089–1092.

15. Constans T, Bacq Y, Brechot JF, et al. Protein-energy malnutrition in elderly medical patients. *J Am Geriatr Soc*. 1992;40:263–268.

16. Burns JT, Jensen GL. Malnutrition among geriatric patients admitted to medical and surgical services in a tertiary care hospital: Frequency, recognition, and associated disposition and reimbursement outcomes. *Nutrition*. 1995;11(suppl 2):245–249.

17. Messner RL, Stephens N, Wheeler WE, Hawes MC. Effect of admission nutritional status on length of hospital stay. *Gastroenterol Nurs*. 1991;13:202–205.

18. Roubenoff R, Heymsfield SB, Kehayias JJ, Cannon JG, Rosenberg IH. Standardization of nomenclature of body composition in weight loss. *Am J Clin Nutr*. 1997;66:192–196.

19. Bengmark S. Theory and therapeutics. In: Shikora S, Martindale RG, Schwaitzberg SD, eds. *Nutritional Considerations in the Intensive Care Unit: Science, Rationale, and Practice*. Dubuque, Iowa: Kendall/Hunt Publishing Co.; 2002;365–380.

20. Fuhrman MP, Charney P, Mueller CM. Hepatic proteins and nutrition assessment. *J Am Diet Assoc*. 2004;104:1258–1264.

21. Johnson AM. Low levels of plasma proteins: Malnutrition or inflammation? *Clin Chem Lab Med*. 1999;37:91–96.

22. Gabay C, Kushner I. Acute-phase proteins and other systemic responses to inflammation. *N Engl J Med*. 1999;340:448–454.

23. Jensen GL. Inflammation as the key interface of the medical and nutrition universes: A provocative examination of the future of clinical nutrition and medicine. *JPEN*. 2006;30:453–463

24. Don BR, Kaysen G. Serum albumin: Relationship to inflammation and nutrition. *Seminars in Dialysis* 2004;17:432–437.

25. Kushner I. Regulation of the acute phase response by cytokines. *Perspect Biol Med*. 1993;36:611–622.

26. Roubenoff R. Inflammatory and hormonal mediators of cachexia. *J Nutr*. 1997;127(suppl):1014S–1016S.

27. Beutler B, Mahoney J, LeTrang N, et al. Purification of cachectin, a lipoprotein lipase suppressing hormone secreted by endotoxin-induced RAW 264.7 cells. *J Exp Med*. 1985;161:984–995.

28. Roubenoff R, Roubenoff RA, Cannon JG, et al. Rheumatoid cachexia: Cytokine driven hypermetabolism and loss of lean mass in chronic inflammation. *J Clin Invest*. 1994;93:2379–2386.

29. Roubenoff R, Roubenoff RA, Ward LM, Holland SM, Hellman DB. Rheumatoid cachexia: Depletion of lean body mass in rheumatoid arthritis. Possible associations with tumor necrosis factor. *J Rheumatol*. 1992;19:1505–1510.

30. Anker SD, Clark AL, Kemp M, et al. Tumor necrosis factor and steroid metabolism in chronic heart failure: Possible relation to muscle wasting. *J Am Coll Cardiol*. 1997;30:997–1001.

31. Cannon JG, Friedberg JS, Gelfand JA, et al. Circulating interleukin-1β and tumor necrosis factor-α concentrations after burn injury in humans. *Crit Care Med*. 1992;20:1414–1419.

32. Wolfe RR. Herman Award Lecture, 1966: Relation of metabolic studies to clinical nutrition— The example of burn injury. *Am J Clin Nutr*. 1996;64:800–808.

33. Rosenberg IH. Sarcopenia: Origins and clinical relevance. *J Nutr*. 1997;127(suppl 5):990S–991S.

34. Roubenoff R. Inflammatory and hormonal mediators of cachexia. *J Nutr*. 1997;127(suppl 5):1014S–1016S.

35. Lexell J. Human aging, muscle mass, and fiber type composition. *J Gerontol A Biol Sci Med Sci*. 1995;50(spec no):11–16.

36. Sarkisian CA, Lachs MS. "Failure to thrive" in older adults. *Ann Intern Med*. 1996;124:1072–1078.

37. ASPEN Board of Directors and the Clinical Guidelines Task Force. Guidelines for the use of parenteral and enteral nutrition in adult and pediatric patients. *JPEN*. 2002;26:1SA–138SA.

38. Chan L. Redefining drug-nutrient interactions. *NCP*. 2000;15:245–252.

39. Roy MA, Jensen GL. Nutrition screening and assessment. In: Lang R, Hensrud DD, eds. *Clinical Preventive Medicine*. Chicago, Ill.: AMA Press; 2004;173–181.

40. Chumlea WC, Roche AF, Steinbaugh ML. Estimating stature from knee height for persons 60 to 90 years of age. *J Am Geriatr Soc.* 1985;33:116–120.

41. Society of Actuaries and Association of Life Insurance Medical Directors. *1979 Build Study.* Chicago, Ill.: Metropolitan Life Insurance Company; 1980.

42. National Institute of Health. *Clinical Guidelines on the Identification, Evaluation, and Treatment of Overweight and Obesity in Adults.* Bethesda, Md.: NIH; 1998.

43. U.S. Department of Health and Human Services, National Health and Nutrition Examination Survey. *NHANES III Anthropometric Procedures* (videotape). Washington, D.C.: Government Printing Office; 1988.

44. Doweiko JP, Nompleggi DJ. The role of albumin in human physiology and pathophysiology, Part III: Albumin and disease states. *JPEN.* 1991;15:476–483.

45. Rall C, Roubenoff R, Harris T. Albumin as a marker of nutritional and health status. In: Rosenberg IH, ed. *Nutritional Assessment of Elderly Populations: Measure and Function.* 1st ed. New York, N.Y.: Raven; 1991.

46. Rothschild MA, Oratz M, Schreiber SS. Serum albumin. *Hepatology.* 1988;8:385–401.

47. Reuben DB, Moore AA, Damesyn M, et al. Correlates of hypoalbuminemia in community-dwelling older persons. *Am J Clin Nutr.* 1997;66:38–45.

48. Campion EW, deLabry LO, Glynn RJ. The effect of age on serum albumin in healthy males: Report from the Normative Aging Study. *J Gerontol.* 1988;43:M18–M20.

49. Cooper JK, Gardner C. Effect of aging on serum albumin. *J Am Geriatr Soc.* 1989;37:1039–1042.

50. Salive ME, Coroni-Huntley J, Phillips CL, et al. Serum albumin in older persons: Relationship with age and health status. *J Clin Epidemiol.* 1992;45:213–221.

51. Bienia R, Ratcliff S, Barbour GL, Kummer M. Malnutrition in the hospitalized geriatric patient. *J Am Geriatr Soc.* 1982;30:433–436.

52. Constans T, Bacq Y, Brechot JF, Guilmot JL, Choutet P, Lamisse F. Protein-energy malnutrition in elderly medical patients. *J Am Geriatr Soc.* 1992;40:263–268.

53. Sullivan DH, Walls RC, Bopp MM. Protein-energy undernutrition and the risk of mortality within one year of hospital discharge: A follow-up study. *J Am Geriatr Soc.* 1995;507–512.

54. Abbasi AA, Rudman D. Observations on the prevalence of protein-calories undernutrition in VA nursing homes. *J Am Geriatr Soc.* 1993;41:117–121.

55. Ritchie CS, Burgio KL, Locher JL, et al. Nutritional status of urban homebound older adults. *Am J Clin Nutr.* 1997;66:815–818.

56. Ingenbleek Y, Young V. Transthyretin (prealbumin) in health and disease: Nutritional implications. *Annu Rev Nutr.* 1994;14:495–533.

57. Halmi KA, Struss AL, Owen WP, Stegink LD. Plasma and erythrocyte amino acid concentrations in anorexia nervosa. *JPEN.* 1987;11:458–464.

58. Shetty PS, Jung RT, Watrasiewicz KE, James WPT. Rapid turnover transport proteins: An index of subclinical protein energy malnutrition. *Lancet.* 1979;230–232.

59. Forse RA, Shizgal HM. Serum albumin and nutritional status. *JPEN.* 1980;4:450–454.

60. Harvey KB, Moldwer LL, Bistrian BR, Blackburn GL. Biological measures for the formulation of a hospital prognostic index. *Am J Clin Nutr.* 1981;34:2013–2022.

61. Anderson CF, Moxness K, Meister J, Burritt MF. The sensitivity and specificity of nutrition-related variables in relationship to the duration of hospital stay and rate of complications. *May Clin Proc.* 1984;59:477–483.

62. Agarwal N, Acevedo F, Leighton LS, Cayten CG, Pitchumoni CS. Predictive ability of various nutritional variables for mortality in elderly people. *Am J Clin Nutr.* 1988;48:1173–1178.

63. Herrmann FR, Safran C, Levkoff SE, Minaker KL. Serum albumin level on admission as a predictor of death, length of stay, and readmission. *Arch Intern Med.* 1992;152:125–130.

64. Patterson BM, Cornell CN, Carbone B, Levine B, Chapman D. Protein depletion and metabolic stress in elderly patients who have a fracture of the hip. *J Bone Joint Surg*. 1992;74-A(2): 251–260.

65. Volkert D, Kruse W, Oster P, Schlierf G. Malnutrition in geriatric patients: Diagnostic and prognostic significance of nutritional parameters. *Ann Nutr Metab*. 1992;36:97–112.

66. McClave SA, Mitoraj TE, Thielmeier KA, Greenberg RA. Differentiating subtypes (hypoalbuminemic vs marasmic) of protein-calorie malnutrition: Incidence and clinical significance in a university hospital setting. *JPEN*. 1992;16(4):337–342.

67. Cederholm T, Jagren C, Hellstrom K. Outcome of protein-energy malnutrition in elderly medical patients. *Am J Med*. 1995;98:67–74.

68. Sullivan DH, Walls RC. The risk of life-threatening complications in a select population of geriatric patients: The impact of nutritional status. *J Am Coll Nutr*. 1995;14:29–36.

69. Burness R, Horne G, Purdie G. Albumin levels and mortality in patients with hip fractures. *NZ Med J*. 1996;109:56–57.

70. D'Erasmo E, Pisani D, Ragno A, et al. Serum albumin level at admission: Mortality and clinical outcome in geriatric patients. *Am J Med Sci*. 1997;314(1):17–20.

71. Friedmann JM, Jensen GL, Smiciklas-Wright H, McCamish MA. Predicting early nonelective hospital readmission in nutritionally compromised older adults. *Am J Clin Nutr*. 1997;65:1714–1720.

72. Marinella MA, Markert RJ. Admission serum albumin level and length of hospitalization in elderly patients. *Southern Med J*. 1998;91(9):851–854.

73. Incalzi RA, Capparella O, Gemma A, et al. Inadequate caloric intake: A risk factor for mortality of geriatric patients in the acute-care hospital. *Age Ageing*. 1998;27:303–310.

74. Henderson CT, Trumbore LS, Mobarhan S, et al. Prolonged tube feeding in long-term care: Nutritional status and clinical outcomes. *J Am Col Nutr*. 1992;11:309–325.

75. Rudman D, Feller AG, Nagrag HS, Jackson DL, Rudman IW, Mattson DE. Relation of serum albumin concentration to death rate in nursing home men. *J Parent Ent Nutr*. 1987;11:360–363.

76. Ferguson RP, O'Connor P, Crabtree B, et al. Serum albumin and prealbumin as predictors of clinical outcomes of hospitalized elderly nursing home residents. *J Am Geriatr Soc*. 1993;41: 545–549.

77. Klonoff-Cohen H, Barett-Connor EL, Edelstein SL. Albumin levels as a predictor of mortality in the healthy elderly. *J Clin Epidemiol*. 1992;45:207–212.

78. Corti M, Guralnik JM, Salive ME, Sorkin JD. Serum albumin level and physical disability as predictors of mortality in older persons. *JAMA*. 1994;227:1036–1042.

79. Sahyoun NR, Jacques PF, Dallal G, Russell RM. Use of albumin as a predictor of mortality in the community-dwelling and institutionalized elderly populations. *J Clin Epidemiol*. 1996;49:981–988.

80. Reuben DB, Ix JH, Greendale GA, Seeman TE. The predictive value of combined hypoalbuminemia and hypocholesterolemia in high functioning community-dwelling older persons. *J Am Geriatr Soc*. 1999;47:402–406.

81. Noel MA, Smith TK, Ettinger WH. Characteristics and outcomes of hospitalized older patients who develop hypocholesterolemia. *J Am Geriatr Soc*. 1991;39:455–461.

82. Ettinger WH, Harris T, Verdery RB, Tracy R, Kouba E. Evidence for inflammation as a cause of hypocholesterolemia in older people. *J Am Geriatr Soc*. 1995;43:264–266.

83. Goichot B, Schlienger JL, Grunenberger F, et al. Low cholesterol concentrations in free-living elderly subjects: Relations with dietary intake and nutritional status. *Am J Clin Nutr*. 1995;62: 547–553.

84. Pepys MB. C-reactive protein fifty years on. *Lancet*. 1981;653–656.

85. Rosenthal AJ, Sanders KM, McMurty CT, et al. Is malnutrition overdiagnosed in older hospitalized patients? Association between the soluble interleukin-2 receptor and serum markers of malnutrition. *J Gerontol A Biol Sci Med*. 1998;53:M81–M86.

86. Haupt W, Holzheimer RG, Riese J, et al. Association of low preoperative serum albumin concentrations and the acute phase response. *Eur J Surg.* 1999;165:307–313.

87. Sahyoun NR, Jacques PF, Dallal GE, Russell RM. Nutrition Screening Initiative Checklist may be a better awareness/educational tool than a screening one. *J Am Diet Assoc.* 1997;97:760–764.

88. Rush D. Nutrition screening in old people: Its place in a coherent practice of preventive health care. *Annu Rev Nutr.* 1997;17:101–125.

89. Detsky AS, McLaughlin JR, Baker JP, et al. What is subjective global assessment of nutritional status? *JPEN.* 1987;11:8–13.

90. Guigoz Y, Vellas B, Garry PJ. Assessing the nutritional status of the elderly: The Mini Nutritional Assessment as part of the geriatric evaluation. *Nutr Rev.* 1996;54 (1 pt 2):S59–S65.

91. Vellas B, Guigoz Y, Garry PJ, et al. The Mini Nutritional Assessment (MNA) and its use in grading the nutritional state of elderly patients. *Nutrition.* 1999;15:116–122.

92. Nestle Nutrition. MNA Mini-Nutritional Assessment. Available at: www.mna-elderly.com. Accessed October 15, 2005.

93. Vellas B, Guigoz Y, Baumgartner M, et al. Relationships between nutritional markers and the mini-nutritional assessment in 155 older persons. *J Am Geriatr Soc.* 2000;48:1300–1309.

94. de Groot LC, Beck AM, Schroll M, van Staveren WA. Evaluating the DETERMINE Your Nutritional Health Checklist and the Mini Nutritional Assessment as tools to identify nutritional problems in elderly Europeans. *Eur J Clin Nutr.* 1998;52:877–883.

95. Rubenstein LZ, Harker JO, Salva A, Guigoz Y, Vellas B. Screening for undernutrition in geriatric practice: Developing the short-form mini-nutritional assessment (MNA-SF). *J Gerontol A Biol Sci Med Sci.* 2001;56:M366–M372.

96. Mullen J, Buzby G, Waldman T, et al. Prediction of operative morbidity and mortality by preoperative nutritional assessment. *Surg Forum.* 1979;30:80–82.

97. Buzby GP, Mullen JL, Matthews DC, et al. Prognostic nutritional index in gastrointestinal surgery. *Am J Surg.* 1980;139:160–167.

98. Klein CJ, Stanek GS, Wiles CE. Overfeeding macronutrients to critically ill adults: Metabolic complications. *J Am Diet Assoc.* 1998;795–805.

99. Van den Berghe G, Wouters P, Weekers F, et al. Intensive insulin therapy in critically ill patients. *N Engl J Med.* 2001;345:1359–1367.

100. Harris JA, Benedict FG. *Biometric Studies of Basal Metabolism in Man.* Publication 279. Washington, D.C.: Carnegie Institute; 1979.

101. Long CL, Schaffel N, Geiger JW, et al. Metabolic response to injury and illness: Estimation of energy and protein needs from indirect calorimetry and nitrogen balance. *JPEN.* 1979;3:452–456.

102. McCowen K, Friel C, Sternberg J, et al. Hypocaloric total parenteral nutrition: Effectiveness in prevention of hyperglycemia and infectious complications—A randomized clinical trial. *Crit Care Med.* 2000;28:3606–3611.

103. Patino JF, de Pimiento SE, Vergara A, et al. Hypocaloric support in the critically ill. *World J Surg.* 1999;23:553–559.

104. Shikora SA, Jensen GL. Hypoenergetic nutrition support in hospitalized obese patients. *Am J Clin Nutr.* 1997;66:679–680.

105. Dickerson RN, Rosato EF, Mullen JL. Net protein anabolism with hypocaloric parenteral nutrition in obese stressed patients. *Am J Clin Nutr.* 1986;44:747–755.

106. Burge JC, Goon A, Choban PS, Flancbaum L. Efficacy of hypocaloric total parenteral nutrition in hospitalized obese patients: A prospective, double-blind randomized trial. *JPEN.* 1994;18:203–207.

107. Choban PS, Burge J, Scales D, Flancbaum L. Hypoenergetic nutrition support in hospitalized obese patients: A simplified method for clinical application. *Am J Clin Nutr.* 1997;66:546–550.

108. McClave SA, McClain CJ, Snider HL. Should indirect calorimetry be used as a part of nutritional assessment? *J Clin Gastroenterol.* 2001;33(1):14–19.

109. McClave SA, Snider HL. Use of indirect calorimetry in clinical nutrition. *Nutr Clin Pract.* 1992;7(5):207–221.

110. Brandi LS, Bertoline R, Calafa M. Indirect calorimetry in critically ill patients: Clinical applications and practical advice. *Nutrition.* 1997;13(4):349–358.

111. Flancbaum L, Choban PS, Sambucco S, et al. Comparison of indirect calorimetry, the Fick method, and prediction equations in estimating the energy requirements of critically ill patients. *Am J Clin Nutr.* 1999;69:461–466.

112. Frankenfield, D. Energy and macrosubstrate requirements. In: *The Science and Practice of Nutrition Support: A Case-Based Core Curriculum.* Dubuque, Iowa: Kendall/Hunt; 2001:31–52.

113. Teran JC, McCullough AJ. Nutrition in liver disease. In: *The Science and Practice of Nutrition Support: A Case-Based Core Curriculum.* Dubuque, Iowa: Kendall/Hunt; 2001:537–552.

114. Wolk R. Nutrition in renal failure. In: *The Science and Practice of Nutrition Support: A Case-Based Core Curriculum.* Dubuque, Iowa: Kendall/Hunt; 2001:575–600.

CHAPTER 2

Surgical Diets

Kate Willcutts, MS, RD, CNSD;
and Kelly O'Donnell, MS, RD, CNSD

INTRODUCTION

The traditional approach to diet advancement after surgery has been to keep patients *nil per os* (NPO), sometimes with nasogastric (NG) decompression, until the return of bowel function. Typically, the first postoperative meal after the return of bowel function has been a clear liquid diet. These practices are predicated on several unsubstantiated beliefs. One of these beliefs is that early removal of an NG tube and/or early initiation of anything, particularly solid food, via the GI tract will cause nausea, vomiting, and thus increase the risk of aspiration. Furthermore, after surgery to the GI tract, some surgeons are concerned that early removal of an NG tube and/or early nutrition via the GI tract will increase peristalsis and the volume of bowel contents, thus increasing risk of anastomotic and/or wound dehiscence (1). In the past, postoperative nausea, vomiting, and ileus were more prevalent. However, these problems are less common with improved use of the appropriate intraoperative and postoperative analgesia and antiemetic medications (2).

The choice of a clear liquid diet for the first postoperative diet is based on the theory that clear liquids are more easily tolerated than full liquids or solid food in the immediate postoperative period (3). Other reasons clear liquids may be used are that they provide oral hydration and minimize pancreatic and gastrointestinal secretions compared to regular foods (4). The traditional, slow postoperative diet advancement from clear liquids to full liquids to soft foods and then finally to a regular diet was designed with the intention of allowing the GI tract time to adapt to the more complex foods and hopefully reducing the incidence of nausea, vomiting, and diarrhea.

Little scientific evidence supports these practices. In fact, over the past decade, traditional diet advancement has been challenged mainly as a result of the increased use of laparoscopic surgery. Due to the minimally invasive nature of laparoscopic surgery, diets are typically advanced within 24–48 hours regardless of bowel function. This practice has been shown to be safe and effective (1,5,6). Based on the success of this practice, investigators have conducted many clinical trials to assess the feasibility of early postoperative feeding following open procedures. The vast majority of these trials have shown that early removal of NG tubes, earlier initiation of an oral diet, and quicker progression to a regular diet results in shorter lengths of stay and reduced hospital costs without an increase in complications including nausea, vomiting, anastomotic leaks, aspiration, wound dehiscence, mortality, or hospital readmission. The purpose of this chapter is to discuss the basis for traditional postoperative diet advancement and to present evidence that a more progressive approach is safe and effective.

ILEUS

The rate of diet advancement after surgery is dictated by the belief that an ileus is a natural consequence of the surgery. However, there is no standard definition for postoperative ileus and the exact etiology is unknown. It has been described as "an impairment of gastrointestinal motility after abdominal or other surgery and is characterized by abdominal distention, lack of bowel sounds, accumulation of gas and fluid in the bowel, and delayed passage of flatus" (p. 7). Possible factors contributing to a postoperative ileus include bowel manipulation, anesthesia, inflammatory response to surgery, and perioperative narcotics (7,8). An ileus may result in gas, abdominal distention, emesis, and pain. After surgery, motility usually returns within 6–12 hours in the small bowel, 12–24 hours in the stomach, and 48–72 hours in the colon (3,8).

USE OF POSTOPERATIVE NASOGASTRIC DECOMPRESSION

Pearl et al. demonstrated that the routine use of postoperative NG decompression for the treatment of postoperative ileus may not be necessary and may delay oral feeding (3). NG decompression was introduced in 1921 and thought to protect the anastomosis as well as decrease the duration of the ileus and incidence of wound complications (9). This, however, has never been proven. NG decompression may actually prolong an ileus by leading to fever and atelectasis (7). A prospective analysis of 4000 patients after laparotomy and colorectal resections found that there were significantly fewer days to oral intake and significantly fewer pulmonary complications in those without NG tubes (9).

IS THE GI TRACT WORKING YET?

Assessment of the resolution of ileus is often based on physical signs of bowel function including bowel sounds, passage of flatus, and bowel movements. Bowel sounds are a poor marker of bowel function for several reasons. They may or may not be present with bowel activity, and even in the presence of a prolonged ileus, the bowel moves (1). The presence of bowel sounds, in the presence of other signs of an ileus, may not indicate anterograde movement of endogenous bowel contents (10). In an unfed patient, 500–1000 mL of gastric fluid is secreted each day, and, in turn, it stimulates the secretion of pancreatic fluid, presenting the small intestine with 1–2 L of endogenous fluid (3). Therefore, withholding nutrition via the GI tract does not eliminate the passage of bowel contents past an anastomosis.

Schilder et al. demonstrated that bowel activity occurs before the passage of flatus (11). In another early postoperative feeding study, investigators found that bowel sounds were typically heard on postoperative day (POD) 1; however, 50% of patients in both the early fed group and the late fed group did not pass flatus (or did not report passing flatus) before being discharged from the hospital. The authors concluded that traditional physical signs of ileus resolution should not be the major factor in determining diet advancement (3). Reissman and colleagues (12) also found that the majority of patients receiving early postoperative feeds tolerated solid foods before their first bowel movement.

Currently, there is no good marker for measuring the return of bowel function (1). Patients after surgery have been successfully fed prior to the return of bowel sounds, flatus, and bowel movements. In fact, initiating feeding could stimulate the return of bowel function. It has been demonstrated that food intake can potentially increase colonic motility (13). Interestingly, Asao et al. simulated sham (or pretend) feeding with gum chewing and reported reduction in time to flatus by 1 day, time to first bowel movement by 2.7 days, and length of stay by about 1 day in adult patients after laparoscopic colectomies (14).

LOWER GI SURGERY

The traditional approach to feeding after elective colon surgery has been to wait until flatus or bowel movements have occurred before initiating an oral diet. As early oral feeding has proven to be safe in laparascopic-assisted colectomies (5), recent studies have focused on whether early feeding protocols in elective, open resections could be tolerated. DiFronzo and colleagues (15) instituted an early postoperative feeding protocol in 200 patients after elective open colon resection. Clear liquids were provided on the eve of POD 2 and a regular diet on POD 3. Nasogastric tubes were not used postoperatively. Overall, 86.5% of the patients tolerated early feeding with no increased incidence of complications. Male patients and those who underwent a total abdominal colectomy or proctocolectomy, were more likely to be intolerant to early feeding.

Several years later, in a nonrandomized study, DiFronzo and colleagues (5) analyzed whether using an early feeding protocol in elderly patients undergoing elective open colon resections would result in early hospital discharge and low morbidity compared to results reported after laparoscopy-assisted colectomies. Patients greater than 70 years old (n = 80) undergoing open colon resections received an early feeding regimen: no routine use of NG tube, clear liquids *ad libitum* on the eve of POD 2 and a regular diet the morning of POD 3. Results revealed that 89.6% of patients tolerated an early feeding regimen and the mean hospital stay was 3.6 days. Postoperative complications such as urinary retention, atrial fibrillation, and mental status changes were seen in 14.9% of patients. These results are comparable to previous studies done in patients undergoing laparoscopy-assisted colectomies.

Both Ortiz et al. (16) and Petrelli et al. (6) concluded that when patients undergoing elective open colon surgery were advanced from a liquid diet to a regular diet on POD 0 or 1, early oral feeding was safe with no significant complications. Petrelli observed that those patients who failed early feeding had significantly more blood loss during surgery. Similarly, Bufo and colleagues (17) concluded that, although the majority of patients tolerate an early regular diet, longer operative time, and increased blood loss during surgery were associated with diet intolerance after elective colorectal surgery. In a prospective, randomized study (12), 161 patients were assigned to either the early feeding group, which consisted of clear liquids POD 1 with advancement to a regular diet within 24 to 48 hours as tolerated, or the traditional diet group, who remained NPO until ileus resolved and whose diet was then advanced from liquids to regular. Resolution of ileus was defined as no abdominal distention, no emesis, and having a bowel movement. In both groups, the NG tube was pulled immediately after surgery. There was no difference in need for NG tube reinsertion, length of ileus, length of stay, or complications. A regular diet was tolerated earlier in the early feeding group.

Kasparek et al. (13) studied whether colonic motility was increased by the gastrocolonic response during the early postoperative period in patients undergoing colorectal surgery. Fifteen patients were given a liquid meal on POD 1 and high-fat, solid foods (53% fat) on POD 2 while four patients served as unfed controls. Manometry was used to measure colonic motility 60 minutes postprandially. The same experimental protocol was used on seven healthy volunteers. Results showed that colonic motility was increased significantly after the standard meal on day 1. However, on day 2, colonic motility did not increase significantly after the meal compared to baseline. In the unfed group, colonic motility remained unchanged during POD 1 and 2. In addition, 66% of the fed patients reported nausea after the meal on day 1 and 73% after the meal on day 2. The first bowel movement occurred between days 2 and 5 in the fed group and days 3 and 4 in the unfed group. This study demonstrated that a clear liquid diet after colorectal surgery increases colonic motility and perhaps that a lower fat diet may have a positive effect on motility without adverse side effects.

LOWER AND UPPER GI SURGERIES

The majority of postoperative feeding studies in patients after small bowel surgery also include patients who have had large bowel surgery. Lewis et al. conducted a systematic review and meta-analysis of controlled trials in elective gastrointestinal (small and large bowel) surgical patients to compare early (<24 hours after surgery) enteral (tube feeding or oral diet) feedings to NPO until gut function returned (18). The analysis included 11 randomized, controlled trials and more than 800 patients. Five of the trials included early oral diet and six included early tube feeding. The early fed patients had statistically fewer infections and shorter average lengths of stay. There was also a trend toward significance in risk reductions for anastomotic leaks and mortality. Despite the fact there was more emesis in the early fed patients, the authors concluded there was no clear benefit to NPO after elective GI surgery and that early feeding is safe and beneficial. Other researchers have come to similar conclusions. Bickel and colleagues (19) compared a liquid diet 4 hours after NGT removal and then slow diet advancement to starting a solid diet immediately after NGT removal based on the patient's desire for food and ability to take food. One hundred and seventy-one patients were studied after elective upper or lower GI surgeries. There was no difference in GI complications (vomiting, abdominal distention, intestinal obstruction, anastomotic leakage, upper GI bleeding, or anastomotic stenosis) between the groups. Of note, a few patients in the solid diet group initially chose to take only liquids due to nausea.

Behrus and colleagues (20) took a unique approach to evaluate postoperative feeding practices. In their study of elective upper or lower GI surgery patients, the control group (17 patients) received the standard clear liquid diet after flatus or stool, continued with clear liquids until 750 mL was consumed and tolerated, before advancing to a regular diet. These patients were discharged from the hospital after three solid meals were tolerated. The study group (27 patients) received clear liquids beginning on POD 2 at 30 mL per hour. On POD 3, they received unlimited clear liquids and were discharged from the hospital on POD 4 drinking only clear liquids. Their diet instructions were to begin solid food immediately on arrival at home. The subjects received close follow-up via telephone. Emesis and ileus were infrequent in both groups, however, the two (7%) patients in the study group who had emesis required NG tube placement. Surgical complications and hospital readmissions were higher in the standard group than in the early clear liquid group. However, neither of these differences was statistically significant. There was no significant difference in length of stay or costs, yet there was a trend toward shorter length of stay in the clear liquid group.

As with studies in colorectal surgery patients alone, these studies indicate that early initiation of enteral nutrition—whether tube feeding, clear liquids, or solid diet—is well tolerated in patients after both upper and lower GI surgery. To these authors' knowledge, no similar studies have been conducted in patients after only small bowel surgery.

GYNECOLOGICAL SURGERY

Many investigators have studied early oral intake after gynecologic (GYN) surgery. Schilder and colleagues (11) conducted a prospective, controlled trial with 96 patients. One group remained NPO until bowel sounds, stool, or flatus occurred and were then advanced to a regular diet. (Most of these patients were given clear liquids first and advanced to a regular diet when tolerated). The other group started clear liquids on POD 1, and after tolerating 500 mL advanced to a regular diet. There was a statistically significant reduction in length of stay in the earlier fed group and no difference in pain regimens, antiemetics, bowel regimens, or postoperative complications. There was more emesis in the earlier fed group but no increase in aspiration or wound dehiscence. The authors concluded that early diet advancement after gynecologic surgery reduces length of stay without adverse effects.

Steed and colleagues conducted a similarly designed study several years later (21). They also found that clear liquids on POD 1 with a regular diet thereafter resulted in a decreased length of stay after gynecologic surgery.

A randomized, controlled trial of 245 patients demonstrated that a regular diet on POD 1 versus clear liquids on POD 1 was tolerated with no difference in postop complications, time to flatus, bowel sounds, length of stay, aspiration, or anastomotic complications. There were more major postop complications in the early fed group but the difference was not significant (3). Macmillan and colleagues conducted a more aggressive randomized controlled trial of patients after open gynecologic surgery (8) in which the early feeding group received a low residue diet within 6 hours of arrival to the floor. The late feeding group received ice chips postoperatively and clear liquids when bowel sounds were detected. A regular diet was ordered after flatus or bowel movement. No difference was noted in perioperative complications, postoperative ileus, or gastrointestinal symptoms. Patients in the late feeding group complained of nausea more often. Another group found that solid foods eaten within 8 hours after cesarean section, versus the traditional diet advancement contingent on flatus or bowel movements, were well tolerated (22). Malhotra and colleagues (23) randomized postoperative cesarean section patients into the study group (who received fluids 6 hours postoperatively, irrespective of return of bowel sounds and solid food 24 hours after detection of bowel sounds) or the control group (who received intravenous fluid until bowel sounds returned followed by a gradual diet advancement). No significant difference was found in time to return of bowel sounds, flatus, first bowel movement, and mean time to ambulation or advancement to a soft diet. Nausea was slightly higher in the control group. The investigators concluded that early oral hydration is safe and helps patients return to a normal diet and early ambulation.

SURGICAL DIETS

Clear liquids consist of foods and beverages that are both clear and liquid at room temperature including juice, soda, broth, gelatin, and Popsicles, and excluding pulp-containing beverages and milk products (4). There are several protein-fortified clear liquid supplements available commercially. Disadvantages of clear liquids include nutritional inadequacy, increased risk of aspiration in patients with compromised gag reflex, hyperosmolarity, and poor palatability (4,24). Due to the lack of residue in a clear liquid diet, there is rationale for its use prior to elective GI surgery to help minimize bowel contents. However, there is little evidence to support the routine use of a clear liquid diet as the first postoperative diet. Several of the studies described earlier in this chapter showed no benefit to this practice (8,19,22). Jeffrey and colleagues (24) had similar results. In their study, 241 patients were randomized to receive a clear liquid diet or a regular diet as the first meal after elective or emergent abdominal surgery. The group receiving the regular diet consumed significantly more calories and protein and there was no significant difference between groups regarding diet tolerance. The authors recommended eliminating clear liquids as part of the routine management in patients undergoing abdominal surgery.

Some postoperative diet progressions advance from clear liquid to full liquids. Full liquids include all the items on the clear liquid diet as well as other liquids such as milk-based liquids, ice cream, pudding, custard, refined/strained hot cereals, and juices with pulp (25). With appropriate choices, the full liquid diet can be nutritionally complete. The specific liquids and semisolid foods allowed vary from institution to institution. Part of the reason for this variation is that, as with the clear liquid diet, there is no scientific evidence for the need for the full liquid diet in the postoperative period. In fact, many clinicians do not recommend the full liquid diet. Many nutrition care manuals no longer include it, due to its high lactose and sugar content that could contribute to GI intolerance (26).

The next step in the traditional postoperative diet advancement is to the "surgical soft" diet, also known as the soft diet, the soft/bland diet, or the low fiber diet. This diet eliminates "hard to digest" foods such as high fiber, gas-forming or spicy foods (25). There is no scientific evidence to support its use.

Some of the aforementioned studies have examined various postoperative diet progressions: transitioning from clear liquids to regular diet prior to discharge, clear liquids at discharge and advance to regular when the patient arrives at home, and starting a regular diet immediately postoperatively, allowing the patients to select their foods (3,19,24). In each of these studies, the most progressive study group fared as well as, if not better than, the traditional diet group. No scientific proof states that postoperative patients benefit from starting with clear liquids, and then advancing by steps to full liquids, a soft diet, and finally to a regular diet.

CONCLUSION

Published studies indicate that early removal of the NG tube, early feeding, and a quick transition to a regular diet is safe and tolerated in most patients after GI and GYN surgeries. For surgeries not involving the GI tract, the same approach would presumably be safer and even better tolerated. The patients who may not benefit from or tolerate this more progressive postoperative care are those who have had emergent GI surgery, required longer and more complicated surgeries, and/or lost large amounts of blood during surgery. In terms of the first postoperative meals, the ideal approach may be to allow patients to select their foods and beverages. Those patients who are nauseated or not hungry are more likely to choose clear liquids and those who are hungry and feeling well will choose from a regular diet.

REFERENCES

1. Schulman AS, Sawyer RG. Have you passed gas yet? Time for a new approach to feeding patients postoperatively. *Practical Gastroenterol* 2005;XXIX(10):82–88.
2. Bisgaard T, Kehlet H. Early oral feeding after elective abdominal surgery—What are the issues? *Nutrition.* 2002;18:944–948.
3. Pearl ML, Frandina M, Mahler L, et al. A randomized controlled trial of a regular diet as the first meal in gynecologic oncology patients undergoing intraabdominal surgery. *Obstet Gynecol.* 2002;100:230–234.
4. Hancock S, Cresci G, Martindale R. The clear liquid diet: When is it appropriate? *Current Gastro Reports.* 2002;4:324–331.
5. DiFronzo LA, Yamin N, Patel K, O'Connell TX. Benefits of early feeding and early hospital discharge in elderly patients undergoing open colon resection. *J Am Coll Surg.* 2003;197:747–752.
6. Petrelli NJ, Cheng C, Driscoll D, Rodgriguez-Bigas MA. Early postoperative oral feeding after colectomy: An analysis of factors that may predict failure. *Ann Surg Oncology.* 2001;8:796–800.
7. Kehlet H, Holte K. Review of postoperative ileus. *Am J Surgery.* 2001;182:3S–10S.
8. Macmillan SLM, Kammerer-Doak D, Rogers RG, Parker KM. Early feeding and the incidence of gastrointestinal symptoms after major gynecologic surgery. *Obstet Gynecol.* 2000;96:604–608.
9. Sands DR, Wexner SD. Nasogastric tubes and dietary advancement after laparoscopic and open colorectal surgery. *Nutrition.* 1999;15:347–350.
10. Tournadre JP, Barclay M, Fraser R, et al. Small intestinal motor patterns in critically ill patients after major abdominal surgery. *Am J Gastroenterol.* 2001;96:2418–2426.
11. Schilder JM, Hurteau JA, Look KY, et al. A prospective controlled trial of early postoperative oral intake following major abdominal gynecologic surgery. *Gyn Onc.* 1997;67:235–240.
12. Reissman P, Tiong-Ann T, Cohen SM, et al. Is early oral feeding safe after elective colorectal surgery? *Ann Surg.* 1995;222:73–77.
13. Kasparek MS, Mueller MH, Glatzle J, et al. Postoperative colonic motility increases after early food intake in patients undergoing colorectal surgery. *Surgery.* 2004;136:1019–1027.
14. Asao T, Kuwano H, Nakamura J, et al. Gum chewing enhances early recovery from postoperative ileus after laparoscopic colectomy. *J Am Coll Surg.* 2002;195:30–32.
15. DiFronzo LA, Cymerman J, O'Connell TX. Factors affecting early postoperative feeding following elective open colon resection. *Arch Surg.* 1999;134:941–946.
16. Ortiz H, Armendariz P, Yarnoz C. Early postoperative feeding after elective colorectal surgery is not a benefit unique to laparosopy-assisted procedures. *Int J Colorect Dis.* 1996;11:246–249.
17. Bufo AJ, Feldman S, Daniels GA, Lieberman RC. Early postoperative feeding. *Dis Colon Rectum.* 1994;37:1260–1265.
18. Lewis SJ, Egger M, Sylvester PA, Thomas S. Early enteral feeding versus "nil by mouth" after gastrointestinal surgery: Systematic review and meta-analysis of controlled trials. *BMJ.* 2001; 323:1–5.
19. Bickel A, Shtamler B, Mizrahi S. Early oral feeding following removal of nasogastric tube in gastrointestinal operations. *Arch Surg.* 1992;127:287–289.
20. Behrus KF, Kircher AP, Galanko JA, et al. Prospective randomized trial of early initiation and hospital discharge on a liquid diet following elective intestinal surgery. *J Gastrointest Surg.* 2000;4:217–222.
21. Steed HL, Capstick V, Flood C, et al. A randomized controlled trial of early versus "traditional" postoperative oral intake after major abdominal gynecologic surgery. *Am J Obstet Gynecol.* 2002;186:861–865.

22. Patollia DS, Hilliard RLM, Toy EC, Baker B. Early feeding after cesarean: Randomized trial. *Obstet Gynecol.* 2001;98:113–116.

23. Malhotra N, Khanna S, Pasrija S, et al. Early oral hydration and its impact on bowel activity after elective caesarean section—Our experience. *Eur J Obstet Gynecol Repr Biol.* 2005;120:53–56.

24. Jeffery KM, Harkins B, Cresci GA, Martindale RG. The clear liquid diet is no longer a necessity in the routine postoperative management of surgical patients. *Am Surg.* 1996;62:167–170.

25. Dudek SG. Feeding patients: Hospital food and enteral and parenteral nutrition. In: Dudek SG, ed. *Nutrition Essentials for Nursing Practice.* 5th ed. Philadelphia, Pa.: Lippincott, Williams, and Wilkins; 2006:417–419.

26. Grodner M, Long S, DeYoung S. Nutrition in patient care. In: Grodner M, Long S, DeYoung S, eds. *Foundations and Clinical Application of Nutrition: A Nursing Approach.* 3rd ed. St. Louis, Mo.: Mosby; 2004:417–418.

CHAPTER 3

Specialized Nutrition Support

Ainsley Malone, MS, RD, LD, CNSD

INTRODUCTION

Specialized nutrition support (*SNS*) is defined as the therapeutic provision of nutrients either enterally or parenterally. The use of SNS is uncommon in the majority of patients undergoing surgical procedures. Oral diet advancement following resolution of postoperative ileus will be the main source of nutrient intake for most patients. A select group of surgical patients will require the use of SNS because they are unable to consume sufficient quantities of nutrients orally.

The primary methods of specialized nutrition support are parenteral and enteral nutrition. *Parenteral nutrition* (*PN*) is defined as the provision of nutrients intravenously while *enteral nutrition* (*EN*) is described as the provision of nutrients via the gastrointestinal tract. Parenteral and enteral nutrition support have been utilized effectively in the surgical population both pre- and postoperatively. Parenteral nutrition support is reserved for patients with significant gastrointestinal dysfunction. The purpose of this chapter is to

1. Review the indications for SNS (both PN and EN) in the surgical population.
2. Outline components of PN and EN formulations.
3. Review the acute complications of PN and EN therapy.

GENERAL INDICATIONS FOR SNS

It is well accepted that adequate nutrient intake is essential to promote surgical recovery and minimize the risk of postoperative complications. The period of time in which an individual can tolerate minimal or no nutrient intake postoperatively without experiencing complications including infection, prolonged hospital stay, and wound healing issues is unknown. In the early 1990s, adult surgical patients, evaluated retrospectively, were found to have a longer hospital length of stay if they experienced a longer period of *nil per os* status (1). Guidelines from the American Society for Parenteral and Enteral Nutrition (ASPEN) recommend that SNS should be utilized in patients who cannot achieve their nutrient requirements orally for a period of approximately 7 to 14 days or in those patients in whom inadequate intake is expected over this same time period (2).

Several factors including the surgical patient's overall clinical and nutritional status are important considerations when evaluating the need for SNS. Patients with preoperative malnutrition are at an increased risk of postoperative morbidity and mortality when compared to well-nourished patients (3) and therefore may benefit from earlier initiation of SNS. Minimizing the risk of further decline in a patient's nutritional status during the hospital course by initiating SNS is important in improving overall patient outcome. Altered diet schedules in the preoperative period are frequent, resulting in an overall poor nutrient intake and possibly contributing to nutritional decline. Patients experiencing moderate to severe metabolic stress such as critically ill surgical patients are also at increased nutrition risk. The initiation of SNS in this patient population should be considered if it is anticipated that nutrient requirements will not be met orally for 5 to 10 days (2).

GENERAL CONTRAINDICATIONS FOR SNS

The decision to initiate SNS must be made in consideration of any identified contraindications. Most importantly, the benefits of SNS must outweigh its potential burdens. Hemodynamically unstable patients undergoing fluid resuscitation as well as terminally ill cancer patients exemplify situations where burden will exceed benefit. SNS may extend life but it cannot prevent death from a terminal illness or a rapid clinical decline. Generally, initiating SNS in these settings is not indicated (4).

PARENTERAL NUTRITION

In the late 1960s, Dudrick and colleagues reported the successful infusion of hypertonic parenteral nutrients in surgical patients with nonfunctional GI tracts (5). These pioneers recognized the important role of nutrition in minimizing both infectious and noninfectious complications in their patient population. Early use of PN demonstrated benefits in patients with enterocutaneous fistulas as well as in children with short bowel syndrome (6). These advances marked the beginning of what is now lifesaving practice when used appropriately in surgical patients.

DEFINITIONS

PN is defined as the intravenous administration of nutrients. PN can be administered centrally via a large diameter vein, such as the superior vena cava or via a peripheral vein. Central PN (CPN) has often been referred to as *total parenteral nutrition* or *hyperalimentation*. It is comprised of a high dextrose concentration, amino acids, and vitamins and minerals resulting in a hypertonic (1300–1800 mOsm/L) formulation requiring infusion through a central vein. PN can also be infused peripherally (PPN) but must be a lower concentration to promote tolerance by the peripheral vein. The maximum osmolarity for a PPN formula is suggested to be approximately 900 mOsm/L. Figure 3–1 outlines a method for calculating the osmolarity of a PN formula. Disdavantages in using PPN include (1) the inability to provide a concentrated formula and thus the need to provide a large fluid volume, (2) difficulty in achieving increased nutrient requirements in hypercatabolic patients, and (3) a limited tolerance by the peripheral vein and the need for frequent changes in peripheral access (7). Advantages in using PPN include avoiding the risks associated with central intravenous access and the ability to provide fluid volumes to meet an individual's overall fluid requirements. Other considerations for peripheral versus central access are outlined in Table 3–1.

Figure 3–1 Osmolarity Calculations for Parenteral Solutions

The osmolarity of 1 L of parenteral nutrient solution can be estimated according to the following calculations:

- Amino acids—multiply the concentration by 100
- Dextrose—multiply the concentration by 50
- Electrolytes—multiply the number of milliquivalents/liter as follows:
  - Sodium × 2
  - Potassium × 2
  - Magnesium × 1
  - Calcium × 1.4

Example
- Amino acids 3.5%   3.5 × 100 = 350 mOsm
- Dextrose 7.5%   7.5 × 50 = 375 mOsm
- Sodium 35 mEq   35 × 2 = 70 mOsm
- Potassium 20 mEq   20 × 2 = 40 mOsm
- Magnesium 8 mEq   8 × 1 = 8 mOsm
- Calcium 5 mEq   5 × 1.4 = 7 mOsm
- **Total**   **850 mOsm**

Source: Reprinted with permission from Skipper A. Parenteral nutrition. In: Matarese LE, Gottschlich MM, eds. *Contemporary Nutrition Support Practice: A Clinical Guide.* 2nd ed. Philadelphia, Pa.: WB Saunders; 2003:227–241.

Table 3–1 Criteria for Peripheral versus Central Parenteral Nutrition (8)

Peripheral	*Central*
Length of therapy <5–7 days	Length of therapy >5–7 days
Not hypermetabolic	Hypermetabolic
No fluid restriction	Fluid restriction
	Intolerance/allergy to IV lipids
	Poor peripheral access
	Central access already in place

Source: Reprinted with permission. DeChicco RS, Matarese LE. Determining the Nutrition Support Regimen. In: Matarese LE, Gottschlich MM, eds. *Contemporary Nutrition Support Practice: A Clinical Guide.* 2nd ed. Philadelphia, Pa.: WB Saunders; 2003:227–241.

INDICATIONS FOR PN

The excitement generated by Dudrick and colleagues with the advent of PN led to its use in many patients without regard to whether a true indication existed. Subsequently, a great deal of study has focused on identification of the patient in whom PN is most appropriate, with respect to improved clinical outcome. PN is costly and may result in serious metabolic and infectious complications (7). Its use must be limited to those patients who can achieve a benefit.

The primary determinant of the need for PN will center on the patient's GI function. If the GI tract is functioning well, PN is not indicated (2). Multiple conditions can exist in the surgical patient where the GI tract is either nonfunctional or poorly functional. The ASPEN guidelines outline clinical scenarios in which PN is indicated (Table 3–2). The challenge facing the clinician making decisions about which route to use for SNS occurs when patients demonstrate partial GI function or in whom full function is not anticipated to return in a reasonable period of time. Normal postoperative ileus will typically resolve within a 3–5 day period and therefore does not warrant PN initiation (9). Prolonged ileus, however, can delay the return of bowel function and may be a consideration for initiation of PN. The ASPEN guidelines identify that PN is indicated in patients in whom the GI tract is not functional and from whom adequate oral intake is not expected for 7 to 14 days. When consideration is given to altered diet schedules preoperatively and lack of bowel function return in the presence of malnutrition, PN is warranted in the surgical patient who fails to demonstrate good bowel function within 5 to 7 days postoperatively (2).

The malnourished patient is at increased risk for nutrition-related complications and should be considered a primary candidate for PN in the presence of GI dysfunction. The Veterans Affairs Total Parenteral Nutrition Cooperative Study demonstrated that severely malnourished patients who received PN experienced

Table 3–2 General Indications for PN

- Nonfunctional GI tract
- Inaccessible GI tract
- Pancreatitis with intolerance to enteral nutrition
- Short bowel syndrome if nutritional requirements cannot be met by oral or enteral nutrition
- Inflammatory bowel disease with intolerance to enteral nutrition
- Gastrointestinal fistulas in which enteral intake must be restricted
- Burn patients in whom enteral nutrition is contraindicated or unlikely to meet nutritional requirements
- Postoperative patients in whom enteral or oral intake is not expected for 7–10 days

Source: Adapted from: A.S.P.E.N. Board of Directors and Clinical Guidelines Task Force. Guidelines for the use of parenteral and enteral nutrition in adult and pediatric patients. American Society for Parenteral and Enteral Nutrition. *JPEN.* 2002;26:1SA–138SA.

---

fewer noninfectious complications compared to those who received standard therapy (10). These results were not seen with mildly or moderately malnourished patients; however, this along with other similar studies did not control for hyperglycemia, a potentially confounding variable now known to be of significance. Initiation of PN in these patients should be considered earlier (5 to 7 days earlier than in the normally nourished patient to minimize further nutritional decline and its risk of increased morbidity [7]).

SPECIFIC INDICATIONS FOR PARENTERAL NUTRITION

For a more detailed review of PN use in selected surgical conditions or disease states, refer to the appropriate chapter in this text.

PANCREATITIS

SNS is not indicated in patients with mild to moderate pancreatitis. These patients generally have a self-limiting disease course and are able to resume oral nutrition within 5 to 7 days (11). Until recently, PN was considered the SNS method of choice in severe acute pancreatitis (12). Current evidence, however, suggests that EN, specifically in the jejunum, is well tolerated and promotes improved clinical outcome (13–15). Patients with ileus or who demonstrate intolerance to EN will require PN use (16). Complications of acute pancreatitis such as enterocutaneous fistula may require initiation of PN. See Chapter 12 for additional recommendations regarding nutrition support and pancreatitis.

INFLAMMATORY BOWEL DISEASE

The routine use of PN as a treatment modality for inflammatory bowel disease (IBD) is not effective and should not be utilized (17). Prospective studies have not confirmed that bowel rest combined with PN will promote IBD remission (18,19). If a patient with IBD requires SNS, EN should be utilized. There is a role for PN in IBD patients who are malnourished and require surgical intervention. Reduced postoperative complications and hospital length of stay have been demonstrated in malnourished IBD patients receiving preoperative PN (20). In addition, PN and bowel rest is suggested for IBD patients who develop enterocutaneous fistulae (17). IBD patients who demonstrate significant GI dysfunction such as bowel obstruction or intractable diarrhea will also require the use of PN. Chapter 11 provides a more in-depth discussion of this topic.

ENTEROCUTANEOUS FISTULAE

Whether PN and bowel rest promote spontaneous closure of enterocutaneous fistulae (ECF) is unknown. There are no known prospective randomized trials comparing PN with no SNS on ECF closure (21). Enterocutaneous fistulae drainage coupled with food restriction, however, can lead to profound nutrient depletion and increased morbidity and mortality. Patients with ECF involving the esophagus, stomach, or duodenum can be fed with EN by obtaining access distal to the site of the fistula. PN should be reserved for malnourished patients and/or those with high output ECF (>500 mL/day) requiring bowel rest (21).

SHORT BOWEL SYNDROME

Short bowel syndrome (SBS) results from a loss of bowel function from either resection or dysfunction of remaining bowel such that nutrient and fluid requirements cannot be achieved through the use of standard oral nutrition and/or EN (22). Specific definitions exist for SBS, which involve the remaining length of the small bowel and the presence or absence of the colon. Patients with less than 100 cm of small bowel distal to the Ligament of Treitz and without a colon will most likely require PN for an indefinite time period. The need for long-term PN is not uncommon in this setting. Those with as little as 50 cm of small bowel combined with a functional colon may successfully tolerate oral nutrition and/or EN. For those with varying degrees of remaining anatomy, initial postoperative PN is often utilized with close monitoring of the response to advancing oral intake (23). See Chapter 13 for a more in-depth discussion of short bowel syndrome.

CANCER

Cancer patients are at an increased nutrition risk due to an underlying altered metabolism coupled with a reduced nutrient intake (24). Routine use of PN in the cancer patient requiring surgical intervention is not indicated (25). Malnourished patients undergoing surgical intervention may benefit from preoperative PN if EN is contraindicated or if enteral access cannot be achieved. As in other surgical settings, postoperative PN is indicated in patients who experience GI dysfunction and in whom adequate oral nutrition or EN cannot be achieved within 7 to 10 days (2).

PREOPERATIVE SNS

Malnourished surgical patients experience an increased incidence of postoperative complications and are therefore appropriate candidates for preoperative SNS (3,26). Several studies have demonstrated favorable outcomes in malnourished surgical patients with the use of preoperative PN (10,27,28). Reduced infectious complications were demonstrated in severely malnourished patients undergoing major abdominal or thoracic surgery who received preoperative PN for 1 to 2 weeks (10). It appears that preoperative PN must be provided for a period of 7 to 14 days to achieve benefit. Whether the underlying surgical procedure can be safely delayed for this time period must be considered (26).

Preoperative EN using immune-enhancing enteral formulas may be an effective modality in the malnourished GI cancer patients. Recent research evaluating preoperative administration of immune-enhancing enteral nutrition has demonstrated reduced infectious complications and hospital length of stay in malnourished cancer patients undergoing major GI surgical procedures (29,30).

CONTRAINDICATIONS FOR PN

The absolute contraindication for PN is the presence of a functional GI tract. Patients who exhibit normal GI function should not receive PN and should be supported with EN if they are unable to achieve nutrient requirements orally (2). EN is preferred over PN for several reasons including reduced infectious complications, preservation of intestinal function, and reduced cost (31,32). A classic study by Moore and colleagues in 1989 demonstrated reduced infectious complications in trauma patients who received EN compared to PN (33). This has been validated by others supporting use of EN as the first approach in patients who require SNS (9,34). However, an exception to this contraindication is the patient in whom successful enteral access cannot be achieved.

As just outlined, hemodynamic instability is a contraindication for SNS initiation. In the case of PN, the patient must be able to tolerate the fluid and macronutrient levels necessary to provide adequate nutrients. Patients should be metabolically stable prior to PN initiation because the provision of PN can exacerbate existing metabolic abnormalities. Table 3–3 outlines clinical conditions in which tentative use of PN is warranted. It may require postponing the initiation of PN until the patient is fluid resuscitated and hemodynamic and metabolic stability have been achieved (7).

Table 3–3 Clinical Conditions Warranting Prudent Use of Parenteral Nutrition

Condition	Suggested Criteria
Hyperglycemia	Glucose >300 mg/dL
Azotemia	BUN >100 mg/dL
Hyperosmolality mOsm/kg	Osmolality >350
Hypernatremia	Na >150 mEq/L
Hypokalemia	K <3 mEq/L
Hyperchloremia	Cl >115 mEq/L
Hypophosphatemia	P04 <2 mg/dL
Hypochloremia	Cl <85 mg/dL

Source: Reprinted with permission: Mirtallo JM. Introduction to Parenteral Nutrition. In: Gottschlich MM, ed. *The Science and Practice of Nutrition Support: A Case-Based Core Curriculum.* Dubuque, Iowa: Kendall/Hunt Publishing; 2001:211–223.

COMPONENTS OF PARENTERAL NUTRITION

PN components are intravenous forms of macronutrients and micronutrients including dextrose, amino acids, vitamins, minerals, and lipid emulsions. PN formulations are created to provide varying components of nutrients that will achieve the needs of each individual patient.

Dextrose

Commercial carbohydrate is available in the form of anhydrous dextrose monohydrate. This form of dextrose provides 3.4 kcals/gm. A variety of concentrations ranging from 5% to 70% is available for compounding PN formulas. Higher dextrose concentrations (>10%) are reserved for CPN due to their propensity for causing thrombophlebitis in the peripheral vein (7). There are no specific recommendations for a minimum dextrose intake; however, a 100-gm/day intake is often suggested to suppress both gluconeogenesis and protein catabolism. The maximum glucose oxidation rate of 5 mg/kg/minute suggests that providing greater dextrose amounts can lead to hyperglycemia and lipogenesis (35,36).

Amino Acids

Crystalline amino acids (CAA) provide the protein source in PN formulations and yield 4 kcals/gm. Manufacturers of CAA offer varying mixtures of essential and nonessential amino acids in concentrations ranging from 3% to 20%. The nitrogen content will vary depending on the amino acid profile. See Table 3–4 for amino acid profiles of several commercial solutions. In addition to the amino acids, these solu-

Table 3–4 Examples of Crystalline Amino Acid Formulations (37)

	Travasol	*FreAmine III*	*Aminosyn II*
Manufacturer	Clintec	B.Braun	Abbott
Concentration	10%	10%	10%
Nitrogen (g/100 mL)	1.65	1.53	1.53
Essential amino acids (mg/100 mL)			
Isoelucine	600	690	660
Leucine	730	910	1000
Lysine	580	730	1050
Methionine	400	530	172
Phenylalanine	560	560	298
Threonine	420	400	400
Tryptophan	180	150	200
Valine	580	660	500
Nonessential amino acids (mg/100 mL)			
Alanine	2070	710	993
Arginine	1150	950	1018
Histidine	480	280	300
Proline	680	1120	722
Serine	500	590	530
Taurine	0	0	0
Tyrosine	40	0	270
Glycine	1030	1400	500
Glutamic acid	0	0	738
Aspartic acid	0	0	700
Cysteine	0	<24	0
Electrolytes (mEq/L)			
Sodium	0	10	45.3
Potassium	0	0	0
Chloride	40	<3	0
Acetate	87	~89	71.8
Phosphate (mmol/L)	0	10	0

Source: Drug facts and comparisons, Facts and Comparisons 4.0. http://onlinefactsandcomparisons.com/index.aspx. Accessed October 10, 2005.

tions also include varying amounts of electrolytes, either those inherent to the CAA or as added components.

Several specialized CAA solutions are available for use in patients with renal and hepatic disease. The hepatic formulations contain high amounts of the branched chain amino acids (BCAA), leucine, isoleucine, and valine, and reduced amounts of the aromatic amino acids (AAA), tyrosine, phenylalanine, and tryptophan. It has been suggested that, due to the preferential movement of the BCAAs across the blood-brain barrier, the use of high BCAA formulations may improve the neurologic sequelae observed in hepatic encephalopathy (38). Renal formulas provide only essential amino acids, suggesting this will support urea recycling, improve nitrogen balance, and reduce or eliminate the need for dialysis (38). Little evidence supports using these specialized formulas. With their significantly greater cost and little evidence for efficacy, use of specialized CAA formulas is not recommended (38,39).

Glutamine, an amino acid important for immune function, has recently received attention as an additive to PN formulas (40,41). Glutamine is not a stable product, and thus a commercially available glutamine product that can be added to PN formulas is not available. Research studies demonstrating benefit of added glutamine in selected populations have used preparations of powdered glutamine that must be reconstituted.

Fat

Intravenous fat emulsions (IVFE) are utilized as both an energy source and as a source of essential fatty acids. Commercial IVFE available in the United States are aqueous emulsions of safflower or soybean oil and are comprised primarily of long-chain triglycerides. Additional components include egg yolk phospholipids and glycerol; the latter contributes additional energy resulting in an energy content of 10 kcals per gram. Refer to Table 3–5 for the fatty acid profiles of selected IVFE. IVFE are available in 10%, 20%, and 30% concentrations. All are available for infusion but the 30% formulation may only be used for compounding of total nutrient admixtures (TNA).

Table 3–5 Fatty Acid Content of Intravenous Lipid Emulsions (37)

	Intralipid		Liposyn II		Liposyn III	
Manufacturer	Clintec		Hospira		Hospira	
Concentration %	10	20	10	20	10	20
Oil %						
Safflower			5	10		
Soybean	10	20	5	10	10	20
Fatty acid content %						
Linolenic	50	50	65.8	65.8	54.5	54.5
Oleic	26	26	17.7	17.7	22.4	22.4
Palmitic	10	10	8.8	8.8	10.5	10.5
Linoleic	9	9	4.2	4.2	8.3	8.3
Stearic	3.5	3.5	3.4	3.4	4.2	4.2

Source: Drug facts and comparisons, Facts and Comparisons 4.0. http://onlinefactsandcomparisons.com/index.aspx. Accessed October 10, 2005.

Recommendations for optimal intakes of lipids vary. Providing IVFE as a minimum of 10% of the total daily energy intake is necessary to meet the requirement of the essential fatty acids and linoleic and linolenic acids (42). The increased use of lipids as an energy source gained popularity when adverse effects of high-dextrose PN formulas were reported in the 1980s (43). Providing lipids of approximately 30% to 50% of total calories at that time was not uncommon. Recent evidence demonstrates a potential negative impact with the high use of omega-6 fatty acids, the primary fatty acids of currently available parenteral fat emulsions. High amounts of omega-6 fatty acids are associated with aggravation of inflammatory states such as acute respiratory distress syndrome and sepsis (44,45). Current recommendations for IVFE are to not exceed 1 gm/kg/day or 25% to 30% of total calories (46). In patients with triglyceride-induced pancreatitis or those in whom serum triglycerides are over 400 mg/dl, IVFE should be avoided (16).

Electrolytes

Electrolytes are added to the PN formula to meet requirements of each specific patient. Electrolyte requirements can vary greatly depending on, among other factors, body weight, organ function, degree of catabolism, presence of malnutrition, electrolyte losses, and administered medications. Table 3–6 outlines electrolyte daily requirement ranges for adults. Electrolyte management strategies vary with some practitioners using PN as a vehicle for providing additional electrolytes while others use separate intravenous doses to meet increased electrolyte requirements (47). Some PN commercial formulations provide added electrolytes intended to meet the requirements of most patients receiving PN. These are often utilized by hospital pharmacy departments that do not offer automated PN compounding systems

Table 3–6 Standard Daily Electrolyte Additions to Adult PN Formulations*

Electrolyte	Standard Requirements
Calcium	10–15 mEq
Magnesium	8–20 mEq
Phosphorous	20–40 mmol
Sodium	1–2 mEqkg
Potassium	1–2 mEq/kg
Acetate	As needed to maintain acid-base balance
Chloride	As needed to maintain acid-base balance

*Standard intake ranges based on generally healthy people with normal losses.

Source: Reprinted with permission from: Task Force for the Revisions of Safe Practices for Parenteral Nutrition. Safe practices for parenteral nutrition. *JPEN.* 2004;28:S39–S69.

and thus compound PN solutions manually. Regardless of how electrolytes are provided, frequent monitoring of serum electrolytes, especially upon PN initiation, is essential to identify real and/or potential alterations and to correct them as they occur (48).

Vitamins and Trace Elements

Parenteral vitamin preparations are available to meet the requirements as outlined by the American Medical Association (AMA) and recently updated by the Food and Drug Association (FDA) (49). Table 3–7 specifies the daily requirements for adult parenteral vitamins. This update added a requirement for vitamin K, not previously included in multivitamin preparations. Multivitamin preparations are available with and without vitamin K. The need for daily vitamin administration was highlighted in the late 1980s when, during a national IV vitamin shortage, several cases of thiamin deficiency were reported (50).

Trace element requirements are outlined in Table 3–8. Commercially available products include single-entity or combination preparations. The multiple preparation products provide trace element amounts that meet requirements as outlined by the AMA. For those with excessive GI losses, additional amounts of zinc are added. Reduction in manganese and copper intakes should be considered in patients with hepatobiliary disease due to impaired excretion (51). Recent attention has been generated regarding the aluminum load of PN formulas especially for those who

Table 3–7 Daily Requirements for Adult Parenteral Vitamins

Vitamin	Requirement
Thiamin (B_1)	6 mg
Riboflavin (B_2)	3.6 mg
Niacin (B)	40 mg
Folic acid	600 mcg
Pantothenic acid	15 mg
Pyridoxine (B_6)	6 mg
Cyanocobalamin (B_{12})	5 mcg
Biotin	60 mcg
Ascorbic acid (C)	200 mg
Vitamin A	3300 IU
Vitamin D	200 IU
Vitamin E	10 IU
Vitamin K	150 mcg

Source: Reprinted with permission from: Task Force for the Revisions of Safe Practices for Parenteral Nutrition. Safe practices for parenteral nutrition. *JPEN.* 2004;28:S39–S69.

Table 3–8 Daily Trace Element Supplementation to Adult PN Formulations*

Trace Element	Standard Intake
Chromium	10–15 mcg
Copper	0.3–0.5 mg
Iron	Not routinely added
Manganese	60–100 mcg#
Selenium	20–60 mcg
Zinc	2.5–5 mg

*Standard intake ranges based on generally healthy people with normal losses.

#The contamination level in various components of the PN formulation can significantly contribute to total intake. Serum concentrations should be monitored with long-term use.

Source: Reprinted with permission from: Task Force for the Revisions of Safe Practices for Parenteral Nutrition. Safe practices for parenteral nutrition. *JPEN.* 2004;28:S39–S69.

are at an increased risk for aluminum toxicity such as neonates requiring long-term PN. Because there is risk of aluminum toxicity in some populations, it is recommended that aluminum intake be minimized when at all possible (52).

Medications

In addition to the nutrients provided in PN, the PN formula can be utilized as a medium for the delivery of certain medications. Specifically, insulin, the histamine receptor agonist, famotidine, and octreotide are medications that can be added directly to the PN formula. The primary advantage of adding these to PN is that it minimizes the need for these agents to be provided via separate administration.

PARENTERAL NUTRITION PREPARATION

Methods utilized by pharmacy departments to compound PN formulas vary from institution to institution. Compounding by an automatic compounding device is common when high volumes of individual PN formulas are required. Manual compounding is more prevalent in facilities where PN is less utilized. Many institutions have elected to outsource their PN preparation by utilizing an outside compounding facility to prepare and deliver PN formulas. Additionally, pharmacy departments may purchase premixed formulas with macro- and micronutrients amounts designed to meet general nutrient requirements. Irrespective of which method is utilized, strict adherence to compounding and inspection protocols by the pharmacist is necessary for a visual assessment of incompatibility (51).

PN formulas may be prepared in either a two-in-one or three-in-one format. The two-in-one preparation combines dextrose and CAA base solutions and other additives in single or multiple containers for infusion. IVFE is infused separately, either daily or intermittently, as a piggyback infusion. In a three-in-one preparation (total nutrient admixture, or TNA), all three macronutrients are compounded together in the same container. Advantages and disadvantages exist for both preparation methods. Table 3–9 describes advantages and disadvantages of the TNA preparation system.

COMPLICATIONS OF PARENTERAL NUTRITION

PN is an important therapy for those with a nonfunctioning GI tract; however, it is not without risk of adverse effects. A meta-analysis by Heyland and colleagues in 1998 involving both surgical and critically ill patients found that PN was asso-

Table 3–9 Advantages and Disadvantages of the Total Nutrient Admixture System

Advantages	Disadvantages
All components aseptically compounded by the pharmacy	All components aseptically compounded by the pharmacy
Preparation is more efficient for pharmacy personnel, especially if automated	Larger particle size of admixed lipid emulsion precludes use of 0.22 micron (bacteria eliminating) filter and requires a larger pore filter
Less manipulation of the system during administration	Admixed lipid emulsion is less stable and more prone to separation of lipid components
Less risk of contamination during administration	
Less nursing time needed for 1 bag/ day and no piggyback to administer	Admixtures are more sensitive to destabilization with certain electrolyte concentrations
Less supply and equipment expense for only one pump and IV tubing	Difficult to visualize precipitate or particulate material in the opaque admixture
More convenient storage, fewer supplies, easier administration in home care settings	
Glucose and venous access tolerance may be better in some situations	Catheter occlusion is more common with daily lipid administration
More cost-effective	Less desirable in pediatric settings due to pH and compatibility considerations

Source: Reprinted with permission: Barber JR, Miller SJ, Sacks GS. Parenteral feeding formulations. In: Gottschlich MM, ed. *The Science and Practice of Nutrition Support: A Case-Based Core Curriculum.* Dubuque, Iowa: Kendall/Hunt Publishing; 2001:251–268.

ciated with poorer outcomes compared with patients not receiving PN (53). In the Veterans Administration Cooperative study, mildly or moderately malnourished patients who received PN experienced a greater number of infectious complications than did the control group who did not receive PN (10). More recently, Braunschweig and colleagues demonstrated in 2001 that PN patients experienced significantly more hyperglycemia than those patients who did not receive PN (34).

Complications can be categorized as nutrient related or related to long-term administration such as in those who require PN for greater than 3 months. Nutrient-related complications include, among others, hyperglycemia, refeeding syndrome, and lipid metabolism abnormalities. Complications associated with long-term PN infusion include steatosis, cholestasis, and metabolic bone disease (54).

Nutrient-Related Complications

Hyperglycemia is the most common metabolic complication associated with PN administration (54,55). Previous recommendations for glycemic management in PN suggested maintaining blood glucose levels <200 mg/dL (56). The landmark study by Van den Berg et al. demonstrating improved mortality in critically ill patients with tight glycemic control of 80–110 mg/dL (57) led to recent recommendations that glucose levels in those receiving PN be maintained at <150 mg/dL (58).

Multiple strategies exist for managing hyperglycemia in PN patients. Limiting dextrose intake to ≤4 mg/kg/min is associated with reduced hyperglycemia incidence (36). Initiating PN with a reduced amount of dextrose in the first 24 hours (150–200 g) has also been suggested (54,55). Most PN protocols utilize sliding scale insulin as a method to control glucose in PN patients who experience hyperglycemia. Insulin, either added to the PN formula or infused separately, often is required in addition to the previous measures, to improve glycemic control. One suggested strategy is to add 0.1 units of regular insulin per gram of dextrose per day to the PN formula with incremental increases of 0.05 units per gram of dextrose as needed (58). An additional strategy is to add two thirds of the previous day's sliding scale insulin requirements (59). Regardless of the strategy utilized, when insulin is added to PN formulas, close monitoring of glucose levels is necessary to minimize hypoglycemia. As the patient's clinical status improves, glucose levels often decrease, which can predispose the patient to the risk of hypoglycemia if insulin adjustments in the PN formula are not made.

Hypoglycemia following PN weaning and discontinuation is not a common occurrence (60). Current recommendations are to taper the PN formula for 1 to 2 hours prior to discontinuation (21). However, if PN is abruptly discontinued, it is suggested that a 10% dextrose solution be infused at the same hourly rate as the PN solution to minimize the risk of a hypoglycemic event.

Hyperlipidemia can occur in patients receiving PN, especially in those with decreased lipid clearance such as the critically ill. To minimize the incidence in this setting, IVFE should be infused continuously over a 24-hour period (54,55). Triglyceride levels of <400 mg/dl are acceptable with continuous IVFE infusion. Changing the IVFE to intermittent (i.e., 3 days/week) is an alternative infusion method if triglyceride levels exceed 400 mg/dL. With intermittent IVFE infusion, triglyceride levels of <250 mg/dL 4 hours following infusion are acceptable. Higher levels will necessitate decreasing the lipid dose (61). Hypertriglyceridemia is not a contraindication to IVFE use in pancreatitis. IVFE may be utilized in this setting provided triglycerides remain <400mg/dL (16).

Refeeding Syndrome

Refeeding syndrome is defined as severe electrolyte and fluid shifts that may result from refeeding after severe weight loss (protein-calorie malnutrition) (62). It is more common in the elderly, although mortality figures are difficult to accurately establish due to patients' underlying disease states (63). Anorexia nervosa and alcoholism are the two most common clinical scenarios that can present with refeeding syndrome, as are oncology patients undergoing chemotherapy, the refeeding of malnourished individuals, and selected postoperative patients. Other patients at risk include stressed and depleted patients; those who have been not been fed for 7–10 days, and elderly individuals with chronic medical conditions and poor nutrient intake (64).

Complications may result if refeeding is initiated using an excessively rapid repletion of carbohydrate. A sudden shift to glucose as the predominant fuel will be associated with a high demand for production of phosphorylated glycolytic intermediates as well as a shift away from fat metabolism, a process to which these patients would have adapted (65). The rapid reintroduction of large amounts of carbohydrate feedings can result in fluid and electrolyte abnormalities, including hypophosphatemia, hypokalemia, and hypomagnesmia. Hypophosphatemia is the hallmark of the refeeding syndrome and has been reported in patients being repleted both parenterally and enterally. Severe hypophosphatemia is associated with hematologic, neuromuscular, cardiac, and respiratory dysfunction (66).

Table 3–10 further outlines the physiologic and metabolic sequelae of the refeeding syndrome. Close monitoring of serum phosphate, magnesium, potassium, and glucose are imperative when any form of SNS is initiated, particularly in malnourished patients (66).

The refeeding syndrome can be life threatening if not treated promptly. Several recommendations have been made to minimize the risk of refeeding syndrome. Table 3–11 outlines specific measures that should be utilized when initiating PN in patients at risk. In addition to close monitoring of electrolyte levels, use of conservative calorie estimation and gradual introduction of dextrose (over a 2- to 3-day period) should be considered the standard approach in patients at risk for refeeding syndrome (64,67). After electrolytes and fluid status have stabilized, consideration can be given to advancing the energy intake (67).

Hepatobiliary Complications

Liver function abnormalities have been associated with PN therapy. Elevated liver function tests (LFTs) (aspartate aminotransferase, alkaline phosphatase, and

Table 3–10 Physiologic and Metabolic Sequelae of Refeeding Syndrome

Organ System	Effects of Hypophosphatemia (<2.5 mg/dL)	Effects of Hypokalemia (<3.5 mEq/dL)
Cardiac	Changes in myocardial function Arrhythmia Heart failure Sudden death	Orthostatic hypotension Altered sensitivity to digoxin Arrhythmia Electrocardiogram changes Cardiac arrest
Hematologic	Changes in red blood cell morphology White blood cell dysfunction Hemolytic anemia Thrombocytopenia, platelet dysfunction	
Hepatic	Liver dysfunction	
Neuromuscular	Confusion, coma, weakness Lethargy, paresthesia Cranial nerve palsy, seizures Guillain-Barré-like syndrome Rhabdomyolysis	Areflexia, hyporeflexia Paresthesia, rhabdomyolysis Weakness, paralysis Paresthesias Respiratory depression
Respiratory	Acute respiratory failure	
Gastrointestinal	Constipation, ileus Increased hepatic encephalopathy	
Metabolic		Glucose intolerance Hypokalemic metabolic acidosis
Renal		Reduced urinary concentrating ability Polyuria, polydypsia Nephropathy with reduced urinary concentrating ability Myoglobinuria due to rhabdomyolysis

Organ System	Effects of Hypomagnesemia (<1.7 mg/dL)	Effects of Glucose/ Fluid Intolerance
Cardiac	Arrhythmia Tachycardia Torsade de pointes	Congestive heart failure Sudden death

(*continues*)

Table 3–10 Continued

Organ System	Effects of Hypomagnesemia (<1.7 mg/dL)	Effects of Glucose/ Fluid Intolerance
Hemodynamic		Dehydration
		Fluid overload
		Hypotension
Neuromuscular	Ataxia	Hyperosmolar nonketotic
	Confusion	coma
	Hyporeflexia	
	Irritability	
	Muscular tremors	
	Paresthesias	
	Personality changes	
	Seizures	
	Tetany	
	Weakness	
	Vertigo	
Pulmonary		Carbon dioxide retention
		Respiratory depression
Gastrointestinal	Abdominal pain	Fatty liver
	Anorexia	
	Diarrhea, constipation	
Metabolic		Hyperglycemia
		Hypernatremia
		Ketoacidosis
		Metabolic acidosis
Renal		Osmotic diuresis
		Prerenal azotemia

Source: Reprinted with permission: Russell M, Cromer M, Grant J. Complications of enteral nutrition therapy. In: Gottschlich MM, ed. *The Science and Practice of Nutrition Support: A Case-Based Core Curriculum*, Dubuque, Iowa: Kendall/Hunt Publishers; 2001:189.

bilirubin) with infusion of PN for less than 1 month are transient and do not reflect permanent liver damage (68). Prevention of overfeeding, cycling of PN infusion, and providing a 70%/30% dextrose-to-fat ratio are suggested strategies to minimize the occurrence of elevated LFTs (42,59). Patients who require long-term PN therapy are at greater risk of permanent hepatic dysfunction and should therefore be monitored closely for LFT elevation with subsequent referral for medical treatment if necessary (42).

Metabolic Bone Disease

Premature neonates and those requiring long-term PN are at risk for developing metabolic bone disease (MBD). Multiple factors contributing to its development

Table 3–11 Recommendations to Reduce the Risk of Refeeding Syndrome

- Understand the syndrome
- Recognize individuals at risk
  - ◦ anorexia nervosa
  - ◦ classic kwashiorkor or marasmus
  - ◦ chronic malnutrition
  - ◦ chronic alcoholism
  - ◦ morbid obesity with massive weight loss
  - ◦ prolonged fasting
  - ◦ prolonged IV hydration
  - ◦ significant stress and depletion
  - ◦ NPO for 7–10 days
- Correct phosphorus, magnesium, and potassium abnormalities before initiating nutrition support (via enteral, oral or parenteral route)
- Utilize initial calorie assessments for maintenance of current body weight and not repletion (25–30 kcal/kg usual body weight)
- Restrict fluid to 1.2–1.5 liters per day
- Begin with hypocaloric feedings, approximately 20 kcal/kg of body weight per day
- Monitor electrolytes daily for the first 3 days of feeding and continue until measurements are stable
- Monitor pulse rate, intake and output, weight, and electrolyte levels closely
- Provide appropriate vitamin supplementation
- Gradually advance infusion rate to goal
- After several days of feeding tolerance and stable laboratory values, prescribed calories can be increased for repletion (30–35 kcal/kg ideal body weight)

Source: Reprinted with permission: Russell M, Cromer M, Grant J. Complications of enteral nutrition therapy. In: Gottschlich MM, ed. *The Science and Practice of Nutrition Support: A Case-Based Core Curriculum.* Dubuque, Iowa: Kendall/Hunt Publishers; 2001:189.

---

include, among others, excessive amino acid intake, inadequate phosphorous intake, inactivity, and the use of specific medications such as corticosteroids and heparin (69,70). Interventions are aimed at minimizing the development and progression of MBD and include monitoring of bone mineral density, providing adequate amounts of calcium, phosphorous, and vitamin D, and limiting aluminum exposure (70).

ENTERAL NUTRITION

The use of EN has increased steadily in the last 2 decades, owing to the recognition of its benefits coupled with improved enteral access devices and placement methods. If the GI tract is functional, it should be the primary route for SNS. Deciding when to initiate EN, what access route to use, and what formula to initiate are key components in EN decision making.

BENEFITS OF ENTERAL NUTRITION

It is commonly recognized that EN provides multiple benefits to the patient, which have the potential to improve clinical outcome (2). Specific demonstrated benefits, among others, include attenuation of the catabolic response (71), maintenance of absorptive capabilities of the GI tract (72), decreased incidence of hyperglycemia when compared with PN (34), and reduced hospital length of stay and cost (2,73). Perhaps the most significant potential benefit in providing EN involves the preservation of intestinal barrier function. This benefit is thought to be the underlying mechanism for the reduced infectious complications seen with EN (Figure 3–3) (9,29). EN has been shown to maintain intestinal integrity, which may prevent the occurrence of bacterial translocation and the passage of bacteria across the intestinal wall, ultimately leading to fewer infections (73–75).

INDICATIONS FOR ENTERAL NUTRITION

EN is the preferred feeding modality when the gastrointestinal tract is functional and the patient is unable to adequately consume an oral diet. Increased nutrient requirements due to wound healing and/or the patient's underlying disease state, coupled with a lack of appetite, often make it difficult for patients to consume adequate nutrients orally. It is not necessary, however, that patients have a fully functioning GI tract to successfully tolerate EN. In patients with partial GI tract function such as in pancreatitis and inflammatory bowel disease, hydrolyzed formulas can be successfully utilized and tolerated (3). In patients with some degree of bowel dysfunction, selection of appropriate EN candidates requires a thorough and objective evaluation of bowel function. Performing a physical exam in conjunction with clinical status evaluation is necessary to assess whether ileus is present (77). When the GI

Figure 3–3 Patients Who Should Receive Early Enteral Nutrition with an Immune Enhancing Formula

---

- Patients undergoing elective gastrointestinal (GI) surgery
  - Moderately or severely malnourished patients undergoing major elective upper GI procedures on the esophagus, stomach, pancreas, and hepatobiliary tree
  - Severely malnourished patients undergoing lower GI surgery
- Patients with blunt and penetrating torso trauma
  - Trauma patients with an injury severity score ≥18
  - Patients with injuries to two or more body systems
  - Patients with an abdominal trauma index ≥ 20
  - Patients with severe injuries to the colon, pancreas and duodenum, and stomach

Adapted from: Kudsk KA, Schloerb PR, DeLegge MH, et al. Consensus recommendations from the U.S. summit on immune-enhancing enteral therapy. *JPEN*. 2001;25:S61–S62.

---

tract is dysfunctional, EN is contraindicated. Refer to Table 3–12 for specific contraindications to the use of EN.

EARLY ENTERAL FEEDING IN THE POSTOPERATIVE PATIENT

Early enteral feeding, specifically via the duodenum or jejunum, is desirable in the critically ill postoperative patient when it is evident that there will be a delay in the achievement of adequate oral intake. The exact definition of "early" has been debated but most clinicians would agree that initiating EN within the first 24 to 48 hours postoperatively meets the definition (78). This time period is consistent with the observation that the small bowel continues to function postoperatively in the face of gastric and colonic ileus (78).

Multiple benefits of early postoperative EN have been demonstrated. Studies evaluating early jejunal feedings in upper GI surgical patients have reported a lower incidence of postoperative infections (71,79) and improved wound healing (74). Pancreatic surgery patients receiving postoperative jejunal feedings demonstrated reduced complications and readmissions compared to those who received no feedings (80). A meta-analysis conducted by Moore and colleagues of prospective trials evaluating early EN versus PN demonstrated a reduced incidence of infections with the use of EN (31).

In the presence of hemodynamic instability, the concern related to risk of bowel necrosis has led to a debate regarding safety in the use of early EN. Bowel ischemia due to EN rarely occurs (81). However, it is prudent to identify patients who may be at increased risk and consider these factors when deciding to initiate EN. Does the patient have abdominal pain, distention, and increased nasogastric tube out-

Table 3–12 Contraindications for Enteral Nutrition (76)

- Nonoperative mechanical GI obstruction
- Intractable vomiting/diarrhea refractory to medical management
- Severe short bowel syndrome with failure of EN
- Persistent postoperative ileus
- Distal high-output fistulas
- Severe GI bleeding
- Severe GI malabsorption
- Inability to gain access to the GI tract
- Need is expected for less than 5–7 days for malnourished patients or 7–10 days if adequately nourished
- Aggressive nutrition intervention is not warranted or desired by the patient or proxy.

Source: Adapted from Marian M. Patient selection and indications for enteral feedings. In: Charney P, Malone A, eds. *A Pocket Guide to Enteral Nutrition.* American Dietetic Association; 2005:1–25.

put? Is the patient hypotensive (82,83)? Recommendations for EN use in patients at increased risk for bowel necrosis include initiation with close monitoring of GI function, limiting the use of EN to those patients receiving stable doses of inotropic agents, volume repletion, and sustaining a mean arterial pressure of ≥70 mm Hg. Additionally, small bowel feedings should be utilized with an isotonic, fiber-free formula (83), particularly in those with evidence of poor gastric emptying.

ENTERAL FORMULAS

Enteral formulas can be classified as intact, elemental, or specialized. Many formulas are available within each category, often containing significant differences in nutrient composition. Standard formulas often can meet a patient's nutrient requirements and frequently cost less than specialized formulas. Tables 3–13 through 3–19 outline enteral formulas currently in use.

Table 3–13 Intact Nutrient Standard Formulas

Product	Manufacturer	Kcals/ml	% CHO Kcals	% PRO Kcals	% FAT Kcals	Comments
Compleat®	Novartis	1.07	53	16	31	Unflavored 4.3 gm fiber/L (soluble and insoluble)
Fibersource®	Novartis	1.2	57	14	29	Unflavored 10 gm fiber/L (sol and insol)
Fibersource HN®	Novartis	1.2	53	18	29	Unflavored 10 gm fiber/L (sol and insol)
Isocal®	Novartis	1.06	51	12.8	37.2	Unflavored
Isocal HN®	Novartis	1.06	46	16	38	Unflavored
Isosource®	Novartis	1.2	57	14	29	Unflavored
Isosource HN®	Novartis	1.2	53	18	29	Unflavored
Isosource VHN®	Novartis	1	50	25	25	Unflavored 10 gm fiber/L (sol and insol) High protein

Table 3–13 Continued

Product	Manufacturer	Kcals/ml	% CHO Kcals	% PRO Kcals	% FAT Kcals	Comments
Isosource® 1.5	Novartis	1.5	44	18	38	8 gm fiber/L (sol and insol)
Jevity®	Ross Products	1.06	54.3	16.7	29	Mild flavor 14.4 gm fiber/L
Jevity® 1.2	Ross Products	1.2	53.6	17	29.4	Unflavored 12 gm fiber/L (sol and insol) Contains fructo-oligosacch-arides
Jevity® 1.5	Ross Products	1.5	53.6	17	29.4	Unflavored 12 gm fiber/L (sol and insol) Contains fructo-oligosacch-arides
Nutren® 1.0	Nestle	1	51	16	33	Unflavored
Nutren® 1.0 with fiber	Nestle	1	51	16	33	Unflavored 14.0 gm fiber/L
Osmolite®	Ross Products	1.06	57	14	29	Mild flavored
Osmolite® 1 cal	Ross Products	1.06	54.3	16.7	29	Mild flavored
Osmolite® 1.2 cal	Ross Products	1.06	54.3	16.7	29	Mild flavored
Osmolite® 1.5 cal	Ross Products	1.2	54.3	16.7	29	Unflavored
Probalance®	Nestle	1.2	52	18	30	Vanilla 10 gm fiber/L (sol and insol)
Promote®	Ross Products	1	52	25	23	Vanilla High protein
Promote® with fiber	Ross Products	1	50	25	25	Vanilla 14.4 gm fiber/L (sol and insol) High protein

(continues)

Table 3–13 Continued

Product	Manufacturer	Kcals/ml	% CHO Kcals	% PRO Kcals	% FAT Kcals	Comments
Replete®	Nestle	1	45	25	30	Vanilla High protein Fortified with vitamins A, C, zinc, and β-carotene
Replete® with fiber	Nestle	1	45	25	30	Vanilla High protein 14.0 gm fiber/L Fortified with vitamins A, C, zinc, and β-carotene
Novasource® 2.0	Novartis	2.0	43	18	39	Vanilla Contains arginine
Nutren® 1.0	Nestle	1	51	16	33	Vanilla
Nutren® 1.0 fiber	Nestle	1	51	16	33	Vanilla 14 gm fiber/L (insol and sol)
Nutren® 1.5	Nestle	1.5	45	16	39	Vanilla
Nutren® 1.5 fiber	Nestle	1.5	45	16	39	Vanilla 14 gm fiber/L (insol and sol)
Traumacal®	Novartis	1.5	38	22	40	Vanilla
Twocal HN®	Ross Products	2	43.2	16.7	40.1	Vanilla Contains fructo-oligosacch-arides
Ultracal®	Novartis	1.06	50	17	35	Unflavored 14.4 gm dietary fiber/L

Source: Reprinted from Consensus recommendations from the U.S. Summit on Immune-Enhancing Enteral Therapy. *JPEN.* 2001:25(suppl):S61–S62; with permission from the American Society for Parental and Enteral Nutrition (A.S.P.E.N.). A.S.P.E.N. does not endorse the use of this material in any form other than its entirety.

Table 3–14 Defined or Elemental Formulas

Product	Manufacturer	Kcals/ml	% CHO Kcals	% PRO Kcals	% FAT Kcals	Comments
F.A.A.®	Nestle	1	70	20	10	100% FAA
Optimental®	Ross Products	1	54.5	20.5	25	Vanilla Fortified with arginine Contains fructo-oligosacch-arides
Peptamen®	Nestle	1	51	16	33	MCT/LCT 70/30
Peptamen® with FOS	Nestle	1	51	16	33	MCT/LCT 70/30 Contains fructo-oligosacch-arides
Peptamen® 1.5	Nestle	1.5	49	18	33	MCT/LCT 70/30
Peptamen® VHP	Nestle	1	42	25	33	MCT/LCT 70/30
Peptinex®	Novartis	1	65	20	15	Vanilla Peptides FAA (16%)
Peptinex® DT	Novartis	1	65	20	15	Greater % of smaller peptides FAA (40%) 10 gm fiber (soluble)/L
Subdue®	Novartis	1	50	20	30	Orange-vanilla and chocolate Peptides
Subdue® plus	Novartis	1.5	50	20	30	Unflavored Peptides
Tolerex®	Novartis	1	91	8	1	Powder form Protein is 100% FAA
Vivonex® plus	Novartis	1	76	18	6	Powder form Protein is 100% FAA
Vivonex® RTF	Novartis	1	70	20	10	Liquid form Protein is 100% FAA
Vivonex® TEN	Novartis	1	82	15	3	Powder form Protein is 100% FAA
Vital® HN	Ross	1	73.8	16.7	9.5	Powder form Peptides and FAA

Table 3–15 Enteral Products Designed for Renal Disease (84)

Product	Manufacturer	Kcals/ ml	Protein* (gm)	Potassium (mEq)*	Phosphorus (mg)*	Magnesium (mg)*
Renal Formulas						
Nepro®	Ross Products	2	35.0	14	343	108
NovaSource® Renal	Novartis Nutrition	2	37.0	14	325	100
Suplena®	Ross Products	2	15.0	14	365	108
Nutren® Renal	Nestle Clinical Nutrition	2	17.0	Negligible	Negligible	Negligible
Renalcal®	Nestle Clinical Nutrition	2	17	16	350	100
Suplena®	Ross Products	2	15	14.3	365	107

*per 1000 kcals

Source: Reprinted from McClave SA, DeMeo MT, DeLegge MH, et al. North American Summit on Aspiration in the Critically Ill Patient: Consensus statement. *JPEN.* 2002;26(suppl):S80–S85, with permission from the American Society for Parenteral and Enteral Nutrition (A.S.P.E.N.). A.S.P.E.N. does not endorse the use of this material in any form other than its entirety.

Standard Formulas

Standard formulas are used in most patients requiring tube feedings. Nutrient sources provided are essentially equal to those consumed by healthy individuals. Additional product types include those with supplemental fiber and those with greater nutrient concentration. Use of formulas of varying nutrient density may be of clinical significance. Close evaluation of fluid requirements and free water provided by the formula should be undertaken (85).

Fiber Formulas

Dietary fiber is defined as structural and storage polysaccharides in plants not digested by human enzymes. Sources of fiber in enteral formulas include, among others, soy polysaccharide, hydrolyzed guar gum, and oat fiber, which may aid in the management of diarrhea and overall gastrointestinal tract health (86). Use of a fiber-containing formula can be considered in enterally fed patients who develop diarrhea. It should be remembered, however, that many other factors may be responsible for the etiology of an individual's diarrhea and not primarily the enteral

Table 3–16 Enteral Formulas Designed for Hepatic Disease (84)

Product	Manufacturer	Kcals/ ml	% CHO Kcals	% FAT Kcals	% PRO Kcals	Comments
Hepatic-Aid® II	Hormel Healthlabs	1.2	57.3	27.7	15.0	• Increased levels of leucine, isoleucine and valine • Minimal phenylalanine, tryptophan and tyrosine content • Contains negligible amounts of vitamins and minerals
Nutren® Hepatic	Nestle Clinical Nutrition	1.5	77.0	11.0	12.0	• Contains standard amounts of vitamins and minerals • 50% BCAA and 50% AAA • 66% of fat is MCT

Source: Reprinted from McClave SA, DeMeo MT, DeLegge MH, et al. North American Summit on Aspiration in the Critically Ill Patient: Consensus statement. *JPEN* 2002;26(suppl):S80–S85, with permission from the American Society for Parenteral and Enteral Nutrition (A.S.P.E.N.). A.S.P.E.N. does not endorse the use of this material in any form other than its entirety.

Table 3–17 Enteral Formulas Designed for Diabetes Mellitus

Product	Manufacturer	Kcals/ ml	% CHO Kcals	% PRO Kcals	% FAT Kcals	Fiber (gm/1000 ml)
Diabetisource® AC	Novartis Nutrition	1	36.0	20.0	44.0	4.3
Glucerna® Select	Ross Products	1	22.8	20.0	49.0	21.1
Glytrol®	Nestle Clinical Nutrition	1	40.0	18.0	42.0	15.0
Resource® Diabetic	Novartis Nutrition	1.06	36.0	24.0	40.0	12.8

Table 3–18 Formulas Designed for Pulmonary Disease

Product	Manufacturer	Kcals/ml	% CHO Kcals	% PRO Kcals	% FAT Kcals
COPD Formulas					
NovaSource® Pulmonary	Novartis Nutrition	1.5	40.0	20.0	40.0
Nutren® Pulmonary	Nestle Clinical Nutrition	1.5	27.0	18.0	55.0
Pulmocare®	Ross Products	1.5	28.2	16.7	55.1
ARDS Formula					
Oxepa®*	Ross Products	1.5	28.1	16.7	55.2

*Supplemented with eicosapentanoic and gamma-linolenic acids as well as vitamins C, E and beta-carotene

Table 3–19 Formulas Designed for Immune Enhancement

Product	Manufacturer	Kcals/ml	% CHO Kcals	% PRO Kcals	% FAT Kcals	Comments
Crucial®	Nestle Clinical Nutrition	1.5	33.7	23.5	39.0	Hydrolyzed protein, fortified with arginine (15.0 g/L), vitamins A, C, zinc and β-carotene MCT/LCT 50/50, marine oil as source of n-3 fatty acids
Impact®	Novartis Nutrition	1.5	53	22	25	Fortified with arginine and nucleotides Menhaden oil as source of n-3 fatty acids
Impact® 1.5	Novartis Nutrition	1.5	38	22	40	Fortified with arginine and nucleotides Menhaden oil as source of n-3 fatty acids

Table 3–19 Continued

Product	Manufacturer	Kcals/ml	% CHO Kcals	% PRO Kcals	% FAT Kcals	Comments
Impact® Glutamine	Novartis Nutrition	1.3	46	24	30	Fortified with arginine and nucleotides Menhaden oil as source of n-3 fatty acids Impact Glutamine fortified with 15.0 g/L of glutamine and 10.0 g/L fiber
Impact® with Fiber	Novartis Nutrition	1	53	22	25	Fortified with arginine and nucleotides Menhaden oil as source of n-3 fatty acids Impact with Fiber provides 10.0 g/L fiber
Perative®	Ross Products	1.3	54.5	20.5	25	Peptides Fortified with arginine
Pivot® 1.5	Ross Products	1.5				Protein in peptide form Fortified with arginine and glutamine

formula (85). Fiber formulas can also be beneficial in the patient who experiences constipation. Fiber increases fecal weight, thereby promoting increased stooling. These are commonly used in patients requiring long-term EN (87).

Elemental Formulas

Elemental formulas (see Table 3–14) are those with "predigested" or hydrolyzed macronutrients. Nutrients include peptides, hydrolyzed proteins containing a mixture of di- and tripeptides, along with a fat source of primarily medium-chain triglycerides. A small amount of long-chain triglycerides are provided to supply essential fatty acids. The primary indication for an elemental formula is the presence of gastrointestinal dysfunction. Elemental formulas are indicated in patients with malabsorption, pancreatic dysfunction, short bowel syndrome, or other evidence of gastrointestinal disease. In those with normal gastrointestinal function, however, standard enteral formulas should be routinely utilized (85).

Specialized Formulas

Specialized formulas encompass a wide range of products and are designed for a variety of clinical conditions or disease states. Currently, there are over 35 enteral formulas designed for a particular condition or disease state. Evidence supporting their routine use is limited (85,88). In addition, the cost of specialized formulas is considerably higher than that of standard formulas, an important consideration in enteral formula selection.

Renal formulas (see Table 3–15) are best used in patients in whom dialysis is delayed or not planned. In this setting, a calorically dense, reduced protein formula is appropriate. These formulas also offer alterations in electrolyte composition, primarily in potassium, magnesium, and phosphorus content. Patients undergoing renal replacement therapy, however, often have significantly increased protein requirements that are unable to be achieved with a renal formula. Standard calorically dense formulas are frequently appropriate for these patients.

Similarly to PN formula, hepatic enteral formulas (see Table 3–16) provide increased amounts of BCAA and reduced amounts of AAA with the rationale that this alteration will minimize hepatic encephalopathy (HE) (38). The routine use of BCAA-enriched enteral formulas does not appear to be clinically beneficial in patients with advanced liver disease and/or hepatic encephalopathy. Standard enteral formulas can successfully be used with most patients (39). However, in those patients who are refractory to routine drug therapy for HE and are unable to tolerate standard protein intakes without precipitation of HE, the use of BCAA-enriched enteral formulas may be of benefit (85).

Enteral formulas for diabetes mellitus (see Table 3–17) have been designed to assist in the control of blood glucose levels. Formula characteristics include the addition of soluble fiber and an altered carbohydrate-to-fat ratio. Few randomized, controlled trials evaluate diabetic formulas; the routine use of a diabetic formula does not appear warranted. However, in specific instances when blood glucose control becomes problematic, despite appropriate pharmacologic intervention and the avoidance of overfeeding, use of a diabetic formula may offer an advantage in facilitating improved glucose control (88).

Enteral formulas for chronic pulmonary disease (see Table 3–18) provide an increased amount of lipid and a decreased amount of carbohydrate compared to standard formulas. Substituting a portion of carbohydrate calories with fat calories is thought to limit carbon dioxide production resulting in improved ventilatory status in those with marginal pulmonary function. Research demonstrating whether chronic pulmonary enteral products offer a clinical advantage to the patient with chronic pulmonary disease is inconclusive (89–93). The routine use of a pulmonary formula in patients with chronic pulmonary disease does not appear warranted due to lack of supporting evidence (91).

An enteral formula specifically designed for acute respiratory distress syndrome (ARDS) offers a modified lipid component designed to potentially modulate the inflammatory cascade that occurs in this setting. Limited evidence demonstrates improved clinical outcome with this type of formula (94,95). Despite the lack of controlled trials, there is a possible benefit in using an ARDS formula. Further validation studies are needed (91).

Immune-enhancing formulas (IEF) (see Table 3–19) are those designed to enhance the immune system by offering specific nutrients such as arginine, nucleotides, and n-3 fatty acids known to promote beneficial immune effects. The evidence demonstrating an advantage with these formulas in selected patient populations is conflicting (96–99). Table 3–20 outlines those patients who should receive an immune-enhancing formula. More recently, the American Dietetic Association's Evidence Analysis Critically Ill Workgroup concluded that IEFs have limited impact on hospital length of stay and are not associated with decreased infectious complications in critically ill ICU patients, a group that often includes complicated surgical patients (100).

GASTROINTESTINAL COMPLICATIONS OF ENTERAL NUTRITION

Nausea and Vomiting

Nausea and/or vomiting occur in approximately 12% to 20% of patients who receive EN (102,103). Multiple etiologies exist with delayed gastric emptying representing the most commonly identified problem (104). Slowed gastric emptying may occur with hypotension, sepsis, stress, diabetes, electrolyte abnormalities, anesthesia, and surgery. In addition, many medications, such as morphine, can reduce gastric motility (105). Strategies for managing delayed gastric emptying include

Table 3–20 Patients Who Should Receive Early Enteral Nutrition with an Immune Enhancing Formula (101)

- Patients undergoing elective gastrointestinal (GI) surgery
  - ○ Moderately or severely malnourished patients undergoing major elective upper GI procedures on the esophagus, stomach, pancreas, and hepatobiliary tree
  - ○ Severely malnourished patients undergoing lower GI surgery
- Patients with blunt and penetrating torso trauma
  - ○ Trauma patients with an injury severity score ≥18
  - ○ Patients with injuries to two or more body systems
  - ○ Patients with an abdominal trauma index ≥ 20
  - ○ Patients with severe injuries to the colon, pancreas and duodenum, and stomach

Source: Adapted from: Kudsk KA, Schloerb PR, DeLegge MH, et al. Consensus recommendations from the U.S. summit on immune-enhancing enteral therapy. *JPEN.* 2001;25:S61–S62.

reducing or discontinuing all narcotic medications, switching to a low-fat and/or isotonic formula, reducing the rate of infusion by 20–25 mL/hr, or administering a prokinetic agent (e.g., metoclopromide or erythromycin) (104,106).

GASTRIC RESIDUAL VOLUME

The measurement of gastric residual volumes (GRVs) in the patient receiving enteral tube feeding is recommended as a determinant of enteral tolerance. The rationale for this practice is flawed because studies have shown that GRVs do not correlate with altered gastric emptying (107,108). Despite this, the use of GRVs will most likely continue to be utilized as a measure to assess enteral feeding tolerance (107). The practice of measuring and assessing GRVs should focus not on single measurements but rather on serial trends and in correlation with clinical assessment (108). In a recent summit on aspiration in the critically ill patient, recommendations were made regarding the interpretation and use of GRVs in monitoring enteral tube feeding. Table 3–21 outlines these recommendations. The importance of rational interpretation of GRVs in relation to patient clinical status cannot be overemphasized.

ASPIRATION

Aspiration and aspiration pneumonia are the most serious complications of enteral tube feedings (104). *Aspiration* is defined as the inhalation of material into the airway and can include, among others, saliva, nasopharyngeal secretions, and liquids, including enteral feeding formulas. Aspiration rates range from 0%–95%, depending on the population being studied (104). Multiple risk factors exist for aspiration

Table 3–21 Recommendations for Interpretation and Response to Gastric Residual Volumes (GRV) (109,110)

- Abrupt cessation should occur for overt regurgitation or aspiration
- GRVs should always be used with clinical assessment
- Feeds should not be stopped for GRVs <400–500 ml
- GRVs > 500 ml should result in withholding of feeds and reassessment of tolerance
- GRVs < 500 ml should be returned to the patient
- GRVs between 200 and 500 ml should prompt careful bedside evaluation
- GRVs < 200 ml should prompt ongoing evaluation of aspiration risk

Source: Adapted from McClave SA, Snider HL. Clinical use of gastric residual volumes as a monitor for patients on enteral tube feeding. *JPEN.* 2002;26:S43–S50 and McClave SA, Snider HL, Lowen CC, et al. Use of residual volume as a marker for enteral feeding intolerance: Prospective blinded comparison with physical examination and radiographic findings. *JPEN.* 1992;16:99–105.

in patients receiving enteral tube feeding (see Tables 3–22 and 3–23). Measures recommended to minimize aspiration risk include elevating the head of the bed between 30° to 45°, providing good oral care, and regularly assessing EN tolerance and tube placement/position. Additional recommendations include the use of prokinetics, placement of a small bowel feeding tube with the tip at or below the Ligament of Treitz, and the use of continuous enteral tube feeding infusion (66,77).

DIARRHEA

Diarrhea is the most commonly reported GI side effect in patients receiving EN (111). There is no universally accepted definition of diarrhea (112); however, a clinically useful definition is any abnormal volume or consistency of stool. Common causes of diarrhea in patients receiving EN include medications (liquid medications in a sorbitol base, antibiotics, etc.), infection (*C. difficile* and nonclostridial

Table 3–22 Major Risk Factors for Aspiration in Critically Ill Patients (84)

- Documented previous episode of aspiration
- Decreased level of consciousness (sedation, increased intracranial pressure)
- Neuromuscular disease and structural abnormalities of the aerodigestive tract
- Endotracheal intubation
- Vomiting
- Persistently high gastric residual volumes
- Need for prolonged supine position

Source: Reprinted with permission: McClave SA, DeMeo MT, DeLegge MH, et al., North American summit on aspiration in the critically ill patient consensus statement. *JPEN.* 2002;26:S80–S85.

Table 3–23 Additional Risk Factors for Aspiration in Critically Ill Patients (84)

- Presence of a nasoenteric tube
- Noncontinuous or intermittent feeding
- Abdominal or thoracic surgery or trauma
- Delayed gastric emptying
- Poor oral care
- Age
- Inadequate nursing staff
- Large size or diameter of feeding tube
- Malpositioned feeding tube
- Transport

Source: Reprinted with permission: McClave SA, DeMeo MT, DeLegge MH, et al., North American summit on aspiration in the critically ill patient consensus statement. *JPEN.* 2002;26:S80–S85.

bacteria), and intolerance due to the make-up of the formula (osmolarity, fat content) or specific components in the formula (lactose). Refer to Table 3–24 for additional causes. If clinically significant diarrhea develops during EN, consider the following options: Assess the patient for infectious or inflammatory causes, fecal impaction, use of diarrheogenic medications, and so forth; change to an enteral formula with added fiber; initiate an antidiarrheal agent (once *C. difficile* has been ruled out or is being treated); or discontinue EN and initiate PN (66).

CONSTIPATION

Constipation, the accumulation of excess colonic waste, is more prevalent in patients requiring long-term enteral feedings than in the acute surgical patient (111). Multiple potential causes of constipation exist (see Table 3–25) including lack of fiber, insufficient water, impaction, and decreased bowel motility (66). Preventative measures to minimize the development of constipation include ensuring adequate fluid intake either by providing additional boluses of water or by formula dilution and using a fiber formula (66). If, despite the use of fiber or administration of increased fluids, constipation is not resolved, the use of stool softeners such as docusate or other agents such as laxatives, prokinetics, or enemas may be necessary (113).

Table 3–24 Potential Causes of Diarrhea in the Enterally Fed Patient

Unrelated to Tube Feeding Formula
- Medications
- Antibiotics
- Enteric Pathogens
- Preexisting medical condition
- Hypoalbuminemia
- Inflammatory syndromes and/or sepsis

Related to Tube Feeding Formula/Administration
- Overly rapid infusion rate
- Overly rapid initiation and/or progression
- Microbial contamination
- Lack of fiber
- High fat content of formula
- Osmolality of formula

Source: Reprinted with permission: Lefton J. Management of common gastrointestinal complications in tube-fed patients. *Support Line.* 2002;24(1):19–25.

Table 3–25 Potential Causes of Constipation in Tube-Fed Patients

- Inadequate fluid
- Immobilization
- Neuromuscular disorders
- Inadequate fiber intake
- Hypothryoidism
- Hypokalemia
- History of laxative misuse
- Gastrointestinal motility disorders
- Anticholinergics
- Nonsteroidal anti-inflammatory agents
- Bile acid sequestrants
- Furosemide
- Nitroglycerin
- Antidepressants
- Opioids
- Calcium channel blockers
- Chemotherapeutic agents (vincristine)
- Impaction

Source: Reprinted with permission: Lefton J. Management of common gastrointestinal complications in tube-fed patients. *Support Line.* 2002;24(1):19–25.

CONCLUSION

Malnutrition is associated with poor outcomes. Initiating SNS in the surgical patient becomes a necessity when nutrient intake—for whatever reason—does not match requirements. Poor nutrient intake increases the patient's risk for nutrition-related complications, which, in turn, can result in a negative clinical outcome. Whether PN or EN is utilized as the SNS therapy of choice will depend on a number of factors including GI function and overall clinical status. EN is superior to PN with regards to reduced complications and the potential for improved outcome. No matter what SNS method is utilized, monitoring for metabolic complications in PN and gastrointestinal complications in EN is essential to optimize overall nutrition care and maximize the patient's potential for a positive clinical outcome.

REFERENCES

1. Shaw-Stiffel TA, Zarny LA, Pleban WE, et al. Effect of nutrition status and other factors on length of hospital stay after major gastrointestinal surgery. *Nutrition.* 1993;9:140–145.

2. American Society for Parenteral and Enteral Nutrition Board of Directors and Clinical Guidelines Task Force. Guidelines for the use of parenteral and enteral nutrition in adult and pediatric patients. *JPEN*. 2002;26:18SA–19SA.

3. Mullen JL, Gertner MH, Buzby GP, et al. Implications of malnutrition in the surgical patient. *Arch Surg*. 1979;114:121B–125B.

4. O'Sullivan-Maillet J. Ethical considerations. In: Matarese LE, Gottschlich MM, eds. *Contemporary Nutrition Support Practice: A Clinical Guide*. 2nd ed. Philadelphia, Pa.: WB Saunders; 2003:625–635.

5. Dudrick SJ, Wilmore DW, Vars HM, et al. Can intravenous feeding as the sole means of nutrition support growth in the child and restore weight loss in an adult? An affirmative answer. *Ann Surg*. 1969;169:974–984.

6. Kinney JM. History of parenteral nutrition with notes on clinical biology. In: Rombeau JL, Rolandelli RH, eds. *Clinical Nutrition-Parenteral Nutrition*. 3rd ed. Philadelphia, Pa.: WB Saunders; 2001;1–20.

7. Mirtallo JM. Introduction to parenteral nutrition. In: Gottschlich MM, ed. *The Science and Practice of Nutrition Support: A Case-Based Core Curriculum*. Dubuque, Iowa: Kendall/Hunt Publishing; 2001:211–223.

8. DeChicco RS, Matarese LE. In: Matarese LE, Gottschlich MM, eds. *Contemporary Nutrition Support Practice: A Clinical Guide*. 2nd ed. Philadelphia, Pa.: WB Saunders; 2003:227–241.

9. Kudsk KA, Croce MA, Fabian TC, et al. Enteral versus parenteral feeding: Effects on septic morbidity after blunt and penetrating abdominal trauma. *Ann Surg*. 1992;215:503–511.

10. Veterans Affairs Total Parenteral Nutrition Cooperative Study Group. Perioperative total parenteral nutrition in surgical patients. *N Engl J Med*. 1993;325:525–532.

11. Sax HC, Warner BW, Talamini MA, et al. Early total parenteral nutrition in acute pancreatitis: Lack of beneficial effects. *Am J Surg*. 1987;153:117–124.

12. ASPEN Board of Directors. Guidelines for use of parenteral and enteral nutrition in adult and pediatric patients. *JPEN*. 1993;17(4 suppl):25SA–26SA.

13. Marik PE, Zaloga GP. Meta-analysis of parenteral nutrition versus enteral nutrition in patients with acute pancreatitis. *BMJ*. 2004;328:1407.

14. Abou-Assi S, O'Keefe SJ. Nutrition support during acute pancreatitis. *Nutrition*. 2002;18:938–943.

15. McClave SA, Greene LM, Snider HL, et al. Comparison of the safety of early enteral vs. parenteral nutrition in mild acute pancreatitis. *JPEN*. 1997;21:14–20.

16. ASPEN Board of Directors and Clinical Guidelines Task Force. Guidelines for the use of parenteral and enteral nutrition in adult and pediatric patients. *JPEN*. 2002;26:68SA–69SA.

17. ASPEN Board of Directors and Clinical Guidelines Task Force. Guidelines for the use of parenteral and enteral nutrition in adult and pediatric patients. *JPEN*. 2002;26:73SA–74SA.

18. McIntyre PB, Powell-Tuck J, Wood SR, et al. Controlled trial of bowel rest in the treatment of severe acute colitis. *Gut*. 1986;27:481–485.

19. Dickenson RJ, Ahston MG, Axon ATR, et al. Controlled trial of intravenous hyperalimentation and total bowel rest as an adjunct to the routine therapy of acute colitis. *Gastroenterology*. 1980;79:1199–1204.

20. Rombeau JL, Barot LR, Williamson CE, et al. Preoperative total parenteral nutrition and surgical outcome in patients with inflammatory bowel disease. *Am J Surg*. 1982;143:139–143.

21. ASPEN Board of Directors and Clinical Guidelines Task Force. Guidelines for the use of parenteral and enteral nutrition in adult and pediatric patients. *JPEN*. 2002;26:76SA–77SA.

22. Scolapio JS, Fleming CR. Short bowel syndrome. *Gastroenterol Clin N Am*. 1998;27:467–479.

23. Jeejeebhoy KN. Short bowel syndrome. *CMAJ*. 2002;166:1297–1302.

24. Kern KA, Norton JA. Cancer cachexia. *JPEN*. 1988;12:286–298.

25. ASPEN Board of Directors and Clinical Guidelines Task Force. Guidelines for the use of parenteral and enteral nutrition in adult and pediatric patients. *JPEN*. 2002;26:82SA–83SA.

26. ASPEN Board of Directors and Clinical Guidelines Task Force. Guidelines for the use of parenteral and enteral nutrition in adult and pediatric patients. *JPEN*. 2002;26:95SA–96SA.

27. Klein S, Kinney J, Jeejeebhoy K, et al. Nutrition support in clinical practice: Review of published data and recommendations for future research directions. *JPEN*. 1997;21:133–157.

28. Torosian MJ. Perioperative nutrition support for patients undergoing gastrointestinal surgery: Critical analysis and recommendations. *World J Surgery*. 1999;23:565–569.

29. Braga M, Gianotti L, Vignali A, Carlo VD. Preoperative oral arginine and n-3 fatty acid supplementation improves the immunometabolic host response and outcome after colorectal resection for cancer. *Surgery*. 2002;132:805–814.

30. Gianotti L, Braga M, Nespoli L, Radaelli G, Beneduce A, Di Carlo V. A randomized controlled trial of preoperative oral supplementation with a specialized diet in patients with gastrointestinal cancer. *Gastroenterology*. 2002;122:1763–1770.

31. Moore FA, Feliciano DV, Andrassay RJ, et al. Early enteral feeding, compared with parenteral, reduces postoperative septic complications. The results of a meta-analysis. *Ann Surg*. 1992;216: 172–183.

32. Suchner U, Senftleben U, Eckart T, et al. Enteral versus parenteral nutrition: Effects on gastrointestinal function and metabolism. *Nutrition*. 1996;12:13–22.

33. Moore FA, Moore EE, Jones TN, et al. TEN versus parenteral nutrition following major abdominal trauma: Reduced septic morbidity. *J Trauma*. 1989;29:916–923.

34. Braunschweig CL, Levy P, Sheean PM, Wang X. Enteral compared with parenteral nutrition: A meta-analysis. *Am J Clin Nutr*. 2001;74:534–542.

35. Wolfe RR, O'Donnell TF, Stone MD, et al. Investigation of the factors determining the optimal glucose infusion rate in total parenteral nutrition. *Metabolism*. 1980;29:892–900.

36. Rosmarin, DK, Wardlaw GM, Mirtallo JA. Hyperglycemia associated with high, continuous infusion rates of total parenteral nutrition. *Nutr Clin Pract*.1996;11:151–156.

37. *Drug Facts and Comparisons, Facts and Comparisons 4.0*. http://online.factsandcomparisons.com/index.aspx. Accessed October 10, 2005.

38. Matarese LE. Rationale and efficacy of specialized enteral and parenteral formulas. In: Matarese LE, Gottschlich MM, eds. *Contemporary Nutrition Support Practice: A Clinical Guide*. 2nd ed. Philadelphia, Pa.: WB Saunders; 2003:263–275.

39. ASPEN Board of Directors and Clinical Guidelines Task Force. Guidelines for the use of parenteral and enteral nutrition in adult and pediatric patients. *JPEN*. 2002;26:65SA–68SA.

40. Jian ZM, Cao JD, Zhu XG, et al. The impact of alanyl-glutamine on clinical safety, nitrogen balance, intestinal permeability, and clinical outcome in postoperative patients: A randomized, double-blind, controlled study of 120 patients. *JPEN*. 1999;23(5 suppl):S62–S66.

41. Fuentes-Orozco C, Anaya-Prado R, Gonzalez-Ojeda A, et al. L-alanyl-L-glutamine-supplemented parenteral nutrition improves infectious morbidity in secondary peritonitis. *Clin Nutr*. 2004; 23(1):13–21.

42. Skipper A. Parenteral nutrition. In: Matarese LE, Gottschlich MM, eds. *Contemporary Nutrition Support Practice: A Clinical Guide*. 2nd ed. Philadelphia, Pa.: WB Saunders; 2003:227–241.

43. Covelli HD, Black JW, Olsen MS, et al. Respiratory failure precipitated by high carbohydrate load. *Ann Intern Med*. 1981;95:579–581.

44. Suchner U, Katz DP, Furst P, et al. Effects of intravenous fat emulsions on lung function in patients with acute respiratory distress syndrome or sepsis. *Crit Care Med*. 2001;29:1569–1574.

45. Lekka ME, Liokatas S, Nathanial C, et al. The impact of intravenous fat emulsion administration in acute lung injury. *Am J Respir Crit Care Med.* 2004;169:638–644.

46. Jensen GL, Mascioli EA, Seidner DL, et al. Parenteral infusion of long and medium chain triglycerides and reticuloendothelial system function in man. *JPEN.* 1990;14:467–471.

47. Malone AM, Ben-Avram D, eds. *Specialized Nutrition Support Tutorial: Writing Parenteral Nutrition Orders.* CD-ROM. ASPEN; 2005.

48. ASPEN Board of Directors and Clinical Guidelines Task Force. Guidelines for the use of parenteral and enteral nutrition in adult and pediatric patients. *JPEN.* 2002;26:38SA–39SA.

49. *Federal Register.* 2000;65:21200–21201.

50. CDC. Deaths associated with thiamine-deficient total parenteral nutrition. *Morbid Mortal Weekly Rep.* 1989;38:43–46.

51. Task Force for the Revisions of Safe Practices for Parenteral Nutrition. Safe practices for parenteral nutrition. *JPEN.* 2004;28:S39–S69.

52. Aluminum Task Force. ASPEN statement on aluminum in parenteral nutrition. *Nutr Clin Pract.* 2004;19:416–417.

53. Heyland DK, MacDonald S, Keefe L, et al. Total parenteral nutrition in the critically ill patient. A meta-analysis. *JAMA.* 1998;280:2013–2019.

54. Matarese LE. Metabolic complications of parenteral nutrition. In: Gottschlich MM, ed. *The Science and Practice of Nutrition Support: A Case-Based Core Curriculum.* Dubuque, Iowa: Kendall/Hunt Publishing; 2001:269–286.

55. Barber JR, Miller SJ, Sacks GS. Parenteral feeding formulations. In: Gottschlich MM, ed. *The Science and Practice of Nutrition Support: A Case-Based Core Curriculum.* Dubuque, Iowa: Kendall/Hunt Publishing; 2001:251–268.

56. McMahon MM. Management of hyperglycemia in hospitalized patients receiving parenteral nutrition. *Nutr Clin Pract.* 1997;12:35–38.

57. Van den Berghe G, Wouters P, Weekers F, et al. Intensive insulin therapy in critically ill patients. *N Eng J Med.* 2001;345:1359–1367.

58. McMahon MM. Management of parenteral nutrition in acutely ill patients with hyperglycemia. *Nutr Clin Pract.* 2004;19(2):120–128

59. Fuhrman MP. Management of complications of parenteral nutrition. In: Matarese LE, Gottschlich MM, eds. *Contemporary Nutrition Support Practice: A Clinical Guide.* 2nd ed. Philadelphia, Pa.: WB Saunders; 2003:243–263.

60. Speerhas RA, Wong J, Seidner D, Steiger E. Maintaining normal blood glucose concentrations with total parenteral nutrition: Is it necessary to taper total parenteral nutrition? *Nutr Clin Pract.* 2003;18(5):414–416.

61. Sachs GS. Is IV lipid emulsion safe in patients with hypertriglyceridemia? *Nutr Clin Pract.* 1997;12:120–123.

62. Knochel JP. The pathophysiology and clinical characteristics of severe hypophosphatemia. *Arch Intern Med.* 1977;137:203–220.

63. Crook MA, et al. The importance of the refeeding syndrome. *Nutrition.* 2001;17:632–637.

64. Brooks MJ, Melnik G. The refeeding syndrome: An approach to understanding its complications and preventing its occurrence. *Pharmacotherapy.* 1995;15(6):713–726.

65. Weinsier RL, Krumdieck CL. Death resulting from overzealous total parenteral nutrition: The refeeding syndrome revisited. *Am J Clin Nutr.* 1981;34:393–399.

66. Russell M, Cromer M, Grant J. Complications of enteral nutrition therapy. In: Gottschlich MM, ed. *The Science and Practice of Nutrition Support: A Case-Based Core Curriculum.* Dubuque, Iowa: Kendall/Hunt Publishers; 2001:189.

67. Soloman SM, Kirby DF. The refeeding syndrome: A review. *JPEN*. 1990;14(1):90–97.

68. Quigley EM, Marsh MN, Shaffer JL, et al. Hepatobiliary complications of total parenteral nutrients. *Gastroenterology*. 1994;104:286–301.

69. Pironi L, Labate A, Pertkiewicz M, et al. ESPEN-Home Artificial Nutrition Working Group. Prevalence of bone disease in patients on home parenteral nutrition. *Clin Nutr*. 2002;21:289–296.

70. Buchman AL, Moukarzel A. Metabolic bone disease associated with total parenteral nutrition. *Clin Nutr*. 2000;19:217–231.

71. Marik PE, Zaloga GP. Early enteral nutrition in acutely ill patients: A systematic review. *Crit Care Med*. 2001;29:2264–2270.

72. Minard G, Kudsk KA. Is early feeding beneficial? How early is early? *New Horiz*. 1994;2:156–163.

73. Alexander JW. Bacterial translocation during enteral and parenteral nutrition. *Proc Nutr Soc*. 1998;57:389–393.

74. Schroeder D, Gillanders L, Mahr K, et al. Effects of immediate post-operative enteral nutrition on body composition, muscle function and wound healing. *JPEN*. 1991;15:376–383.

75. Reynolds JV, Kanwar S, Welsh FK, et al. Does the route of feeding modify gut barrier function and clinical outcome in patients after major upper gastrointestinal surgery? *JPEN*. 1997;21:196–201.

76. Marian M, Charney P. Patient selection and indications for enteral feedings. In: Charney P, Malone A, eds. *A Pocket Guide to Enteral Nutrition*. Chicago, Ill.: American Dietetic Association; 2005: 1–25.

77. Lord L, Trumbore L, Zaloga G. Enteral nutrition implementation and management. In: Merritt RJ, ed. *ASPEN Nutrition Support Practice Manual*. Silver Spring, Md.: American Society of Parenteral and Enteral Nutrition; 1998:189.

78. Gottschlich MM. Early and perioperative nutrition support. In: Matarese LE, Gottschlich MM, eds. *Contemporary Nutrition Support Practice: A Clinical Guide*. 2nd ed. Philadelphia, Pa.: WB Saunders; 2003:276–289.

79. Baigrie RJ, Devitt PG, Watkins S. Enteral versus parenteral nutrition after esophagogastric surgery: A prospective randomized comparison. *Austral N Z J Surg*. 1996;66:668–670.

80. Baradi H, Walsh RM, Henderson JM, et al. Postoperative jejunal feeding and outcome of pancreaticoduodenostomy. *J Gastrointest Surg*. 2004;8:428–433.

81. Schunn CD, Daly JM. Small bowel necrosis associated with postoperative jejunal tube feeding. *J Am Coll Surg*. 1995;180:410–416.

82. Zaloga GP, Roberts PR, Marik P. Feeding the hemodynamically unstable patient: A critical evaluation of the evidence. *Nutr Clin Pract*. 2003;18:285–293.

83. McClave SA, Chang WK. Feeding the hypotensive patient: Does enteral feeding precipitate or protect against ischemic bowel? *Nutr Clin Pract*. 2003;18:279–284.

84. McClave SA, DeMeo MT, DeLegge MH, et al. North American summit on aspiration in the critically ill patient consensus statement. *JPEN*. 2002;26:S80–S85.

85. Malone AM. The role of specialized formulas in enteral formula selection. *Practical Gastroenterol*. 2005;29:44–74.

86. Marlett JA, McBurney MI, Slavin JL. Position of the American Dietetic Association: Health implications of dietary fiber. *J Am Diet Assoc*. 2002;102:993-1000.

87. Malone AM, The clinical benefits and efficacy in using specialized enteral feeding formulas. *Support Line*. 2002;24(1):3–11.

88. Malone AM. Enteral formula selection. In: Charney P, Malone A, eds. *A Pocket Guide to Enteral Nutrition*. Chicago, Ill.: The American Dietetic Association; 2005.

89. Cai B, Zhu Y, Ma Y, et al. Effect of supplementing a high-fat, low-carbohydrate enteral formula in COPD patients. *Nutrition*. 2003;19:229–232.

90. Al-Saady NM, Blackmore CM, Bennett ED. High fat, low carbohydrate, enteral feeding lowers PaCO$_2$ and reduces the period of ventilation in artificially ventilated patients. *Intensive Care Med.* 1989;15:290–295.

91. Malone AM. The use of specialized enteral formulas in pulmonary disease. *Nutr Clin Pract.* 2004;19:557–562.

92. van den Berg B, Bogaard JM, Hop WC. High fat, low carbohydrate, enteral feeding in patients weaning from the ventilator. *Intensive Care Med.* 1994;20:470–475.

93. Malone AM. The clinical benefits and efficacy in using specialized enteral feeding formulas. *Support Line*; 2002;24(1):3–11.

94. Gadek J, DeMichele S, Karlstad M, et al. Effect of enteral with eicosapentanoic acid, γ-linolenic acid, and antioxidants in patients with acute respiratory distress syndrome. *Crit Care Med.* 1999;27:1409–1420.

95. Tehila M, Gibstein L, Gordgi D, Cohen JD, Shapira M, Singer P. Enteral fish oil, borage oil and antioxidants in patients with acute lung injury (ALI). *Clin Nutr.* 2003;22:S1–S20.

96. Heyland DK, Novak F, Drover JW, et al. Should immunonutrition become routine in critically ill patients? A systematic review of the evidence. *JAMA.* 2001;286:944–953.

97. Heys SD, Walker LG, Smith I, Eremin O. Enteral nutritional supplementation with key nutrients in patients with critical illness and cancer. *Ann Surg.* 1999;329:467–477.

98. Burkovich G. Outcome studies using immune-enhancing diets: Blunt and penetrating torso trauma patients. *JPEN.* 2001;25:S14–S18.

99. Beale RJ, Bryg DJ, Bihari DJ. Immunonutrition in the critically Ill.: A systematic review of clinical outcome. *Crit Care Med.* 1999;27:2799–2805.

100. The American Dietetic Association Evidence Analysis Library. Available at: www.adaevidence library.com/topic.cfm?cat=1034. Accessed October 20, 2005.

101. Kudsk KA, Schloerb PR, DeLegge MH, et al. Consensus recommendations from the U.S. summit on immune-enhancing enteral therapy. *JPEN.* 2001;25:S61–S62.

102. Montejo JC. Enteral nutrition-related gastrointestinal complications in critically ill patients: A multicenter study. *Crit Care Med.* 1999;27:1447–1453.

103. Montejo JC, Grau T, Acosta J, et al. Multicenter, prospective, randomized, single-blind study comparing the efficacy and gastrointestinal complications of early jejunal feeding with early gastric feeding in critically ill patients. *Crit Care Med.* 2002;30:796–800.

104. Malone AM, Brewer CK. Monitoring for efficacy, complications and toxicity. In: Rolandelli RH, ed. *Clinical Nutrition: Enteral and Tube Feeding.* 4th ed. Philadelphia, Pa.: WB Saunders; 2005: 276–290.

105. Davies A, Prentice W. Fentanyl, morphine, and constipation. *J Pain and Symptom Management.* 1998;16:141–144.

106. Lin HC, Hasler WL. Disorders of gastric emptying. In: Yamada T, ed. *Textbook of Gastroenterology.* 2nd ed. Philadelphia, Pa.: JB Lippincott; 1995;1:1318.

107. McClave SA, Snider HL. Clinical use of gastric residual volumes as a monitor for patients on enteral tube feeding. *JPEN.* 2002;26:S43–S50.

108. Tarling MM, Toner CC, Worthington PS, et al. A model of gastric emptying using paracetamol absorption in intensive care patients. *Intens Care Med.* 1997;23:256–260.

109. McClave SA, Snider HL. Clinical use of gastric residual volumes as a monitor for patients on enteral tube feeding. *JPEN.* 2002;26:S43–S50.

110. McClave SA, Snider HL, Lowen CC, et al. Use of residual volume as a marker for enteral feeding intolerance: Prospective blinded comparison with physical examination and radiographic findings. *JPEN.* 1992;16:99–105.

111. Lefton J. Management of common gastrointestinal complications in tube-fed patients. *Support Line.* 2002;24:19–25.

112. Bliss DZ, Guenter PA, Settle RG. Defining and reporting diarrhea in tube-fed patients—What a mess! *Am J Clin Nutr.* 1992;16:488–489.

113. Beyer PL. Complications of enteral nutrition. In: Matarese LE, Gottschlich MM, eds. *Contemporary Nutrition Support Practice, A Clinical Guide.* Philadelphia, Pa.: WB Saunders Co; 1998:216.

CHAPTER 4

Cardiothoracic Nutrition

Roopa Vemulapalli, MD; and
Jennifer Tomesko, MS, RD, CNSD

INTRODUCTION

The thoracic cavity primarily contains the heart, lungs, esophagus, and thoracic duct. These organs are protected by bony structures: sternum anteriorly, ribs laterally, and vertebral column posteriorly. Cardiothoracic surgery focuses on treatment of the diseases involving these organs. Many cardiothoracic surgeries are preformed routinely, most of which require the usual pre- and postoperative nutrition management. However, several complex surgical procedures, such as antireflux repairs, coronary artery bypass grafts, esophagectomy, and heart/lung transplant, warrant specialized nutritional interventions for a successful outcome. This chapter discusses nutritional optimization and management during pre-, peri- and postoperative settings involving the previous mentioned disease states.

ESOPHAGEAL DISEASES

Gastroesophageal reflux disease (GERD) is defined as symptoms or mucosal damage produced by abnormal reflux of gastric contents into the esophagus (1). It is a common disorder of the western world with a prevalence of 10%–20% (2); it affects 5%–20% of the U.S. population at least once a week (3). Some degree of gastric reflux is physiologic which is usually postprandial, asymptomatic, and short lived. GERD is manifested by abnormal transient relaxation of the lower esophageal sphincter (4). It occurs with symptoms or mucosal damage, lasts longer periods of time, and occurs during sleep. A weak sphincter coupled with delayed return of the acidic contents to the stomach promotes increased esophageal erosion. Cardinal symptoms are heartburn and regurgitation, but other symptoms, such as water brash, globus sensation and nausea can also occur. Extraesophageal symptoms of GERD are asthma, laryngitis, and hoarseness of voice. Longstanding GERD can lead to complications such as esophagitis, peptic stricture, Barrett's esophagus, and adenocarcinoma, causing significant morbidity and negatively impacting quality of life. Esophagoscopy should be the initial evaluation for suspected GERD because it provides an opportunity for visualization, stratification, and management of esophageal manifestations. However, negative findings cannot necessarily preclude the diagnosis, because they can be manifested later. A 24-hour ambulatory pH monitoring is used for persistent symptoms (typical or atypical) and for monitoring adequacy of treatment in patients with persistent symptoms.

Treatment of GERD can be divided into three components: lifestyle modification, drug therapy, and surgical interventions. Lifestyle modifications alone often do not control symptoms, but can be beneficial in combination with medical therapy and/or surgery (5,6). Lifestyle modifications are aimed at reducing or eliminating behaviors that contribute to GERD by enhancing acid clearance and minimizing incidence of reflux events (see Table 4–1). Obesity is considered a risk factor for GERD by increasing lower esophageal sphincter (LES) gradient and intraabdominal pressure (7,8); bariatric surgery in morbid obesity has shown to decrease GERD (8). Acidic or spicy foods may exacerbate heartburn by direct irritation of already inflamed lower esophageal mucosa. Other foods such as citrus fruits, carbonated beverages, coffee, and chocolate may cause increased reflux by relaxing LES. Avoidance or limiting of these foods in the diet may lessen the symptoms of GERD. High-fat or large meals have been postulated to delay gastric emptying, which may lead to a greater incidence of reflux (9). A small recent study by Austin et al. of eight obese of individuals with a mean BMI of 43.5 showed that a very low carbohydrate diet (<20 gm/d) for 3 to 6 days decreased distal esophageal acid exposure with improved symptoms (10).

The American College of Gastroenterology recommends elevating the head of the bed; avoiding recumbent positions 3 hours after meals; avoiding alcohol and spicy foods; limiting the intake of fat, caffeine products, chocolate, and peppermint; and taking antireflux medications (1). Although recommendations are based on physiological evidence, there is conflicting data that lifestyle and dietary modifications, such as the cessation of tobacco and alcohol; avoidance of spicy and fatty foods, citrus fruits, peppermint, and chocolate and recumbent and left lateral po-

Table 4–1 Lifestyle Modifications for GERD

- Maintain a healthy weight.
- Limit high-fat foods.
- Avoid large and/or high-fat meals 3 hours before bedtime.
- Limit chocolate, peppermint, and coffee.
- Avoid alcohol.
- Quit smoking.
- Avoid acidic foods.
- Avoid beverages containing caffeine.
- Avoid recumbent positions for 3 hours after meals.
- Elevate the head end of the bed when sleeping.

sitions, improve GERD symptoms. A recent meta-analysis by Kaltenbach et al. shows that weight loss and elevation of head of the bed are the only effective lifestyle interventions that improve GERD (11). In addition to lifestyle modifications, medical management of GERD plays a role as first-line therapy.

Pharmacological therapy includes H_2 receptor blockers and proton pump inhibitors (PPIs). Strong inhibition of acid secretion provides the most reliable approach to symptom management. Symptoms of GERD resolve in days after starting a PPI. PPIs appear to provide the best symptom control in severe cases of GERD with 4-week healing rates approaching 90% (12). However, H_2-blockers may also be effective in less-severe GERD (5). Prokinetic agents improve LES pressure and peristalsis and enhance gastric emptying. They may be effective in conjunction with acid-suppressant medications, but these medications are rarely used due to their side effect profile. Prolonged use of PPIs can cause B_{12} deficiency. An acidic gastric environment is necessary for the release of B_{12} from the ingested dietary sources. PPIs create an alkaline environment and impair the release of B_{12}, resulting in decreased absorption (13). The recommended dietary allowance for B_{12} is 2 μg/day for adults, which can be achieved with the usual western diet containing 5 to 7 μg/day, but monitoring cyanocobalamin level in patients who are on long-term PPI therapy may be beneficial (13).

Surgical management is considered when symptoms persist after lifestyle and medical therapy. It is also indicated for severe esophagitis, Barrett's esophagus without dysplasia or carcinoma, and recurrent pulmonary symptoms in association with GERD. Because surgery in general poses additional risks of morbidity, it should be considered only after lifestyle modification and medical management have failed. However, there are no guidelines recommending specific antireflux surgeries tailored to different patient populations.

Fundoplication is considered the standard surgical treatment for GERD. By manipulating the proximal stomach and wrapping it around the lower esophagus, pressure is increased on the lower esophagus and reflux is prevented. Hiatal hernias, which can promote GERD, can also be repaired during fundoplication surgery. In general, laparoscopic Nissen fundoplication is comparable to open technique when done by an experienced surgeon. Transthoracic approach is used in shortened esophagus, morbid obesity, concomitant pulmonary issues requiring interventions, and extensive prior abdominal surgeries. Diet management in the postoperative period should begin with clear liquids and progress to a soft diet as tolerated. Soft foods cause less irritation to the surgical site (1). Perforation and obstruction can occur with hard, crispy, or crunchy foods during the early postoperative period. All meats with gristle should be avoided, as well as nuts, granola mixes, potato chips, and fruits with seeds. This diet should be followed for about 2–3 weeks postoperatively or until the follow-up visit with the surgeon (1). If dysphagia occurs due to the anastamosis being too tight, then this diet may be followed until the patient is able to safely swallow regular food. Dysphagia after fundoplication can be treated with dilation of the stricture.

ACHALASIA

Achalasia is a disorder of esophageal dysmotility of unknown etiology, where there is failure to relax the lower esophageal sphincter and absence of peristalsis in the distal esophagus. Although the etiology is still unclear, causes such as infections, autoimmunity, genetic mutations such as in Allgrove's syndrome, and neurotransmitters (nitric oxide) are postulated. Incidence is 1 in 100,000, occurring equally among men and women and those between 25 and 60 years of age (14).

Achalasia can be primary (idiopathic) or secondary. Secondary causes are infections (varicella, *Trypanosoma cruzi*), infiltration by carcinomas, amyloidosis, as a part of paraneoplastic syndrome, or vagal injury due to surgeries (14). Failure to relax the LES causes functional obstruction of the esophagus and may present with dysphagia to liquids and solids, regurgitation of retained food, failure to belch, noncardiac chest pain, weight loss, hiccups, and heartburn. Evaluation is initially by barium swallow, which shows a typically dilated esophagus with a beak-like narrowing. Esophageal manometry studies provide a definite diagnosis and reveal elevated LES pressures, incomplete relaxation, and absence of distal esophageal peristalsis.

Diet management should include small bites, chewing the food well, and eating slowly. The consistency or texture of food should be based on patient tolerance, but thin liquids and soft foods may pass more easily than thick liquids or crunchy foods. Surgical management includes endoscopic pneumatic dilation of the LES, surgical or endoscopic esophagomyotomy, and periodic botulinum toxin injections. Esophagomyotomy may be indicated for persons requiring frequent dilations or when dilations are ineffective in relieving the symptoms. Postmyotomy care must be taken to monitor for GERD symptoms due to decreased LES contractility. Postoperative diet management should initially consist of clear liquids and gradually progress to soft diet as tolerated, with resumption of regular diet after the inflammation from surgery has resolved.

ESOPHAGEAL CANCER

More than 14,550 people in the United States were expected to be diagnosed with esophageal carcinoma in 2006 according to American Cancer Society Facts and Figures Report. Esophagectomy or surgical resection of the tumor provides the best chance of disease-free survival. Proper nutrition support during chemotherapy, radiation therapy, and during the pre- and postoperative periods can improve the outcome and quality of life (15). Further discussion of the nutrition management of esophageal carcinoma and esophagectomy can be found in Chapter 8.

CARDIAC DISEASE

According to the American Heart Association, one out of every four Americans has some form of cardiovascular disease (CVD) such as hypertension, coronary artery disease (CAD), congestive heart failure, or stroke (16). As the prevalence of obesity and type 2 diabetes increases, associated complications such as CVD and hyperlipidemia have also increased. *Coronary artery disease* is an inflammatory state caused by the narrowing of the coronary vessels due to deposition of cholesterol plaques. Rupture of the plaque causes partial or complete occlusion of the coronary vasculature causing angina and ischemia. Extensive evidence cites inflammation as a key factor in promoting vascular endothelial dysfunction and insulin resistance leading to adverse cardiovascular events. Acute inflammatory markers such as C reactive protein (CRP), TNF-α, IL-6, and IL-18 not only increase the risk for ischemic events but also can contribute to their pathogenesis (17–19). Low plasma adiponectin levels are also an independent risk factor for the development of type 2 diabetes (20), and high levels are associated with a lower risk of myocardial infarction in men (21). Therefore, minimizing the proinflammatory milieu can reduce the risk of development and further progression of adverse cardiovascular events. Management of coronary heart disease encompasses lifestyle modifications alone or in combination with medical and surgical interventions.

The National Cholesterol Education Program (NCEP) issued its *Third Report on Detection, Evaluation and Treatment of High Blood Cholesterol in Adults*, also known as *ATP III*, in 2000. This report, like previous reports, identifies LDL cholesterol as the target lipoprotein marker for coronary heart disease (CHD) diagnosis and monitoring the treatment. The *ATP III* also advocates for therapeutic lifestyle changes (TLC) to decrease the risk of developing CHD. Statins are used for lowering LDL cholesterol and rising HDL cholesterol. They also stabilize the arterial plaque and prevent further ruptures. Blood lipid goals are better achieved when drug therapy is combined with a healthy diet (22) but diet and weight management alone often can allow patients to meet their cholesterol goals and should be attempted aggressively prior to initiation of drug therapy.

Coronary angioplasty or percutaneous transluminal coronary angioplasty (PTCA) and coronary artery bypass graft (CABG) are the surgical interventions used for reestablishing coronary flow. All surgical procedures for CHD are susceptible to restenosis of the arteries due to continued unhealthy lifestyle and diet. Postoperatively, diet management is imperative to achieve an acceptable cholesterol level and also to prevent disease in the grafted arteries. Several large clinical trials have demonstrated that further reduction of LDL cholesterol delays progression of atherosclerosis in saphenous vein grafts with a reduction in cardiac deaths and further need for bypass surgery (23,24). The American Heart Association and the American College of Cardiology have jointly issued management guidelines for patients with established CHD to minimize the risk of another cardiovascular event (see Table 4–2) (25). These guidelines are consistent with the TLC guidelines and also apply to diseases like diabetes and hypertension, which are strong risk factors for the development of CHD.

Lifestyle modifications should include a healthy diet and adequate physical exercise. The American Heart Association (AHA) released a scientific statement with updated guidelines in 2006 emphasizing dietary and lifestyle modifications for cardiovascular risk reduction (Table 4–3) (26).

Table 4–2 Guidelines for Secondary Prevention of CHD (25)

1. Quit smoking.
2. Control blood pressure to less than 140/90 or 130/85 if congestive heart failure, diabetes, or renal failure are present.
3. Maintain an LDL cholesterol level of <100mg/dL.
4. Exercise with moderate physical activity for 30 minutes 3 to 4 days each week.
5. Maintain a BMI of <25.
6. Keep the hemoglobin A1C below 7%.
7. Take 81 to 325 mg aspirin daily, if not contraindicated.
8. Take angiotensin-converting enzyme inhibitors (ACE) and β-blockers indefinitely after a myocardial infarction (MI) event.

Table 4–3 2006 American Heart Association Dietary Guidelines (26)

- **Consume an overall healthy diet.**
  Eat a diet rich in fruits and vegetables.
  Choose whole-grain, high-fiber foods.
  Eat fish, especially oily fish at least two times a week.
  Minimize the intake of food and drinks with added sugars.
  Choose and prepare foods with little or no added salt.
  Limit saturated fat to <7% of energy, trans fat to <1% of energy, and cholesterol to <300 mg /day.
  Consume alcohol in moderation.
- **Maintain a healthy body weight (BMI between 18.5–24.9 kg/m².**
- **Be physically active at least 30 minutes every day.**
- **Avoid the use of and exposure to tobacco products.**
- **Maintain recommended lipid levels.**
  LDL cholesterol <100 mg/dL, if at high risk
  LDL cholesterol <130 mg/dL, if at moderate risk
  LDL cholesterol <160 mg/dL, if at low risk
  HDL >50 mg/dL in women, >40 mg /dL in men
  Triglycerides <150 mg /dL
- **Maintain a blood pressure of <120/80 mm Hg.**
- **Fasting blood glucose should be <100 mg/dL.**

DIET

A diet high in refined starches, sugars, saturated and trans fatty acids, and poor in natural antioxidants and fiber from fruits, vegetables, and whole grains may cause an imbalance between proinflammatory and anti-inflammatory cytokines, favoring a proinflammatory milieu. This can predispose susceptible individuals to coronary events. The TLC diet emphasizes increased consumption of omega-3 fatty acids, substitution of nonhydrogenated unsaturated fats for saturated and trans fats, and a diet that is high in fruits, vegetables, nuts, and whole grains and is low in refined carbohydrates, such as sugars (27) (see Table 4–4).

Table 4–4 TLC Diet

Food Group	Allow	Limit
Lean meat, poultry, fish ≤5 oz per day	Lean, well-trimmed, loin, or round cuts; fish; cold cuts made with lean meat; soy; poultry without skin	Other higher fat cuts of meat, bacon, sausage, hot dogs, organ meat; any fried meat
Dairy products 2–3 servings per day	Low-fat milk, yogurt, cheese, ice cream, cottage cheese, fat-free sour cream, fat-free coffee creamer	Whole milk, evaporated whole milk, full fat ice cream, yogurt, cheeses, half and half milk, whipping cream, regular sour cream
Eggs ≤2 egg yolks per week	Egg white, egg substitutes made with egg whites	Whole eggs, egg yolks; eggs used in cooking or baking
Breads and cereals ≥6 servings per day; adjusted for caloric intake	Whole-grain breads, English muffins, bagels; pasta, rice, dried beans, peas; whole-grain cereals (oats, barley, bran, corn, multigrain); low-fat crackers (graham, animal)	Biscuits, donuts, cheese puffs, croissants, sweet rolls, potato or corn chips; Danish and other high-fat bakery products
Vegetables 3–5 servings per day	All fresh, frozen, or canned without added fat or salt	Fried vegetables, those prepared with butter, cheese, or cream sauce
Fruits 2–4 servings per day	All fresh, frozen or canned	Any fried or served with cream
Fats and oils Adjust intake to caloric level	Unsaturated oils (olive, safflower, sunflower, canola, peanut); margarine made with unsaturated oils or vegetable oil spreads; salad dressing made with unsaturated oils, seeds, and nuts	Butter, shortening, stick margarine, saturated oils (coconut, palm, palm kernel), lard; salad dressings made with eggs, whole milk, or sour cream

Omega-3 fatty acids, eicosapentaenoic acid (EPA), and decosahexaenoic acid (DHA) found in fatty fish such as mackerel, lake trout, herring, sardines, albacore tuna, and salmon, have proven to reduce sudden cardiac death and decrease serum triglyceride levels and the progression of atherosclerotic plaques in several epidemiological and clinical trials. Intake of omega-3 fatty acids is also inversely related to levels of proinflammatory cytokine markers, C-reactive protein (CRP), IL-1, TNF α; a higher effect was observed if taken in combination with a reduction in omega-6 fatty acids intake (28,29). In a population-based cohort study in the province of Attica, Greece, consumption of at least 300 grams of fish per week caused a 33% reduction in CRP levels (30). However, using fish oil or pure omega-3 fatty acid supplements has failed to show any effect on CRP levels, unless fish-oil supplementation was taken in high doses (14 grams/day) (31). Intake of more than 3 grams/day from capsules can cause bleeding in some patients, so this should be done only on a physician's advice. Further randomized, placebo-controlled studies are required to document the efficacy and safety of omega-3 fatty supplements in high-risk individuals (those with type 2 diabetes, dyslipidemia, or hypertension, or those who smoke). Mercury contamination of fish is a concern and caution must be exercised before consuming certain types of fish (e.g., shark, tilefish, swordfish, and mackerel). A detailed list of mercury content of commercial fish and shellfish can be found at *www.cfsan.fda.gov/~frf/sea-mehg.html*. Alpha linolenic acid (ALA)—found in tofu, soybeans, canola oil, walnuts, flaxseeds, and their oils—can convert into omega-3 fatty acids in the body and was also shown to decrease CRP levels (32). More studies are required to show a cause-and-effect relationship between ALA and heart disease. The AHA recommendations for consumption of omega-3 fatty acids for cardiovascular protection are as follows:

1. Patients without documented CHD:
   - Eat a variety of fish (fatty fish) at least twice a week.
   - Include oils and food rich in ALA (flaxseed, canola, and soybean oils; flaxseed and walnuts).
2. Patients with documented CHD:
   - Consume 1 gram/d of EPA+DHA, preferably from fatty fish; consult a physician if required in a capsule form.
3. Patients with high triglyceride levels:
   - 2 to 4 grams of EPA+DHA per day, provided in capsules under physician's care.

A decreased consumption of saturated and trans fats is the primary focus of the TLC diet. A diet with high-saturated fat, trans fat, and cholesterol has been shown to increase inflammatory markers in observational and interventional studies (33,34). A long-term vegetarian diet that is low in saturated and trans fat is associated with high antioxidant levels, better CHD profile, and reduced CRP levels compared to people eating an omnivore diet (35). The majority of saturated fats and cholesterol in the American diet are found in animal products. Therefore, lean meats should be limited to 5 ounces per day, eggs yolks to two per week, and whole-fat dairy products should be avoided. Total fat intake need not be restricted, but should be based on required energy intake. Studies have shown that isocaloric substitution of fat for carbohydrate does not cause weight gain (36). Fat intake should be proportionate to total caloric intake to achieve a healthy weight, because fats are concentrated sources of calories.

Fruits, vegetables, and low-fat whole-grain breads and cereals should make up the majority of caloric intake. An inverse relationship was found between fruits and vegetable consumption and CVD risks. These foods also lower inflammatory markers, CRP, and homocysteine (37). Anti-inflammatory effects may be due to their antioxidants, vitamins, and flavonoid properties (38). These foods also provide a variety of nutrients and soluble fiber.

Soluble fiber plays a role in reducing LDL cholesterol and CRP levels (39). Good sources of soluble fiber are barley, oatmeal, citrus fruits, pears, dried beans, and brussels sprouts. At least 5–10 grams of soluble fiber daily should be consumed; higher intakes may be even more beneficial. Plant stanols/sterols also have demonstrated LDL cholesterol–lowering effect. They are found in soybeans, tall pine-tree oils, and in special cholesterol-lowering margarines. The presence of plant stanols/sterols is listed on the food labels.

Nuts are also a source of healthy fat. They are palatable and rich in monounsaturated and polyunsaturated fatty acids. Nuts can have a cardioprotective effect by lowering serum cholesterol; this may be due to their high arginine content, since consumption of arginine-rich food lowered CRP levels (40).

Refined starches are highly processed resulting in the removal of vitamins, essential fatty acids, fiber, minerals, and phytonutrients. High intake of these refined starches can cause rapid fluctuations in blood glucose and insulin levels, with elevation of free fatty acids, which in turn release free radicals and proinflammatory cytokines (41,42). To avoid these deleterious metabolic consequences, consumption of these foods should be avoided.

Salt intake should also be monitored with the goal of ≤2400 mg per day. This can be difficult because salt is added for palatability in many low-fat or fat-free foods. Closely monitoring food labels and learning how to season foods without added salt will allow for better achievement of this goal.

There is no definite data for the beneficial role of nondietary antioxidant supplements in the primary prevention of a cardiovascular event. On the contrary, supplementation with 50 IU vitamin E and 20 mg of β-carotene for 5 to 8 years caused an unexpected increased in mortality from hemorrhagic stroke, lung cancer, and ischemic heart disease, respectively (43). In another study conducted over 12 years, neither a beneficial nor a harmful effect was found due to β-carotene intake (44). However, in secondary prevention trials, a beneficial effect of supplementation with vitamin E was associated with a 38% reduction in nonfatal myocardial ischemia, but β-carotene intake caused an increased risk in fatal coronary end points (45). The AHA recommends an intake of antioxidants, β-carotene, and vitamins C and E, in the form of dietary sources instead of vitamin supplements. β-Carotene is found in yellow-orange fruits such as cantaloupe and vegetables such as carrots and in green, leafy vegetables. Citrus fruits and vegetables including red and green peppers, potatoes, tomatoes, and green, leafy vegetables are rich sources of vitamin C. Vitamin E is found in vegetable oils (soybean, corn, and safflower), vegetable oil products (e.g., margarine), whole grains, wheat germ, nuts, seeds, and green, leafy vegetables.

High-serum homocysteine levels are considered a moderate risk factor for coronary atherogenesis (46). Dietary supplementation with folate and fortified grain products decreases homocysteine levels but there is no clear evidence that lowering their levels by vitamin supplementation causes a decrease in cardiovascular events (47). Prior studies suggested beneficial effects of folate supplementation in reducing the risk of restenosis after percutaneous intervention, especially balloon angioplasty (48). However, in a recent study by Lange et al., oral supplementation with vitamin B_6, B_{12}, and folic acid after an initial intravenous bolus significantly increased the risk of restenosis in patients who received bar metal stents (49). The AHA recommendations emphasize meeting the current recommended dietary allowances (RDA) for folate, B_6, and B_{12} by consuming good dietary sources of folate including dark-green leafy vegetables, fruits, legumes, meats, fish, fortified grains, and cereals. It does not recommend use of herbal or botanical supplements for cardiovascular risk reduction due to lack of controlled clinical trials for efficacy, long-term safety, and drug interactions.

Physical inactivity and obesity are major risk factors for CHD. These factors enhance the risk by increasing serum lipid levels and also the nonlipid risk factors of metabolic syndrome. Regular physical activity increases HDL and lowers LDL cholesterol, blood pressure, and insulin resistance. A reduction in weight, as seen after bariatric surgery, can decrease the levels of the proinflammatory markers CRP, IL-6, and IL-18, and raise adiponectin levels (50–52).

TLC should be a slow, step-wise process in order to reduce the overwhelming feeling that some individuals might have, with a number of suggested dietary and lifestyle changes all at once (53). Table 4–5 outlines these steps. Consultation with a dietitian should be encouraged. Dietitians can provide individualized nutrition counseling and help with compliance to lifestyle changes.

CARDIAC CACHEXIA

Cardiac cachexia (*CC*) is defined as a nonedematous weight loss of 6% or more over a 6-month period in congestive heart failure (CHF) patients (54). About 12%–16% of CHF patients with New York Heart Association (NYHA) classification 1 and 2 and 50% with NYHA 3 and 4 have CC. CC carries a poor prognosis and is an independent risk factor for increased mortality (54,55). Preoperative nutritional therapy in CHF patients with cachexia is associated with improved postoperative survival rates (56). Hence, identifying susceptible patients and intervening prior to development of cardiac cachexia is necessary.

Cardiac cachexia is a multifactorial neurohumoral and metabolic disorder characterized by the wasting of lean-muscle mass, resulting in skeletal atrophy, the severe loss of fat stores, and decreased bone mineral density (57). Several mechanisms have been proposed for cardiac cachexia. Elderly patients have a high incidence of inadequate nutritional intake due to a number of reasons including anorexia of aging, dysgeusia, dysphagia, side effects such as nausea from medications, depression, and isolation. Micronutrient and antioxidant deficiencies from diuretic therapy can also precipitate malnutrition. Other mechanisms such as decreased exercise capacity, increased resting energy expenditure, oxidative stress from neu-

Table 4–5 Steps in TLC

Visit 1
Obtain a baseline LDL level.
Emphasize a decrease in saturated fat and cholesterol intake.
Encourage a gradual increase in physical activity.
Consider a referral to a dietitian.

Visit 2
If the goal LDL is not reached, intensify diet and physical activity management.
Reinforce the need to decrease the intake of saturated fat and cholesterol.
Consider adding plant stanols/sterols.
Encourage a gradual increase in soluble fiber intake.
Consider a referral to a dietitian.

Visit 3
If the LDL goal is still not reached, consider adding drug therapy.
Intensify the weight management and physical activity.
Continue to reinforce diet principles.
Consider a referral to a dietitian.

Visit N*
Monitor compliance with TLC.

Note: Visits 1, 2, and 3 should be scheduled approximately 6 weeks apart.
*Visit N should be conducted every 4 to 6 months after the goal LDL is achieved.

---

rohumoral, inflammatory cytokine activation, and endotoxinemia from bowel wall edema are also implicated. Neurohumoral activation with high renin, aldosterone, cortisol, catecholamine, and insulin-like growth factor (IGF 1) in heart failure promote oxidative stress. This results in the activation of proinflammatory cytokines such as tumor necrosis factor-alpha (TNF-α), interleukin 1(IL-1), IL-6, and gamma interferon (γ-IGN), which play an important role in the tissue catabolism (58). Deficiencies of antioxidants like selenium, copper, zinc, and magnesium, and calcium losses from diuretic treatment accelerate the oxidative stress. Elevated catecholamine levels result in hyperinsulinemia and stimulate lipolysis, leading to muscle wasting. The role of leptin has also been studied. Leptin released by the hypothalamus suppresses appetite and increases resting energy levels. Higher leptin levels have been found in heart failure patients (59), but in a retrospective study, they were inappropriately low. Therefore, further research is necessary to understand the role of leptin in the development of cardiac cachexia.

Cardiac cachexia is a poor prognosticator and should be recognized early. Treatment options include nutritional optimization, pharmacological intervention, exercise, ventricular assist devices, and cardiac transplantation. Cardiac rehabilitation plays an important role with improvement in oxygen consumption and exercise capacity. Micronutrient deficiencies should be recognized and repleted promptly.

PHARMACOLOGIC MANAGEMENT

Fish oils with omega-3 fatty acids have been shown to decrease TNF-α and IL-1 level, and improved cachexia in animal studies, thus supplementation may be beneficial. Beta blockers and ACE inhibitors can prevent development of cachexia in CHF (60). Beta-blocker therapy with carvedilol or metoprolol showed a significantly greater weight gain compared with noncachectic CHF patients (60). Angiotensin-converting enzymes inhibitors (ACEI) have been shown to improve mortality, increase lean body mass, and decrease proinflammatory cytokines. Enalapril decreased the risk of weight loss in heart failure (61), while fondopril and lisinopril were shown to inhibit the renin-angiotensin aldosterone activation and decrease both the levels of proinflammatory cytokines and resting energy expenditure. Statins have also been found to decrease TNF-α, IL-6, and IL-10 levels. Simvastatin has been shown to affect the myocardial remodeling following oxidative stress and may be beneficial (62). Anabolic steroids increase muscle mass but their side effects generally limit their use on a widespread basis. In two case reports, short periods of high-dose recombinant growth hormone, 70–98 IU per week, were shown to increase lean body mass and exercise capacity without side effects in three cachectic patients (63). A recently discovered hormone, ghrelin, is an appetite stimulant that is another promising option on the horizon. It has been shown to inhibit myocyte apoptosis and improve ventricular function and body weight in animal models (64). More research is needed to determine its efficacy in cardiac cachexia.

LOW CARDIAC FLOW STATES

Cardiac function can be compromised due to structural abnormalities, perfusion defects, and reduced contractile function, causing a decrease in systemic blood pressure or in critical illness leading to cardiogenic shock. Typically, after a meal, mucosal energy expenditure and oxygen requirements increase, leading to a 40% increase in splanchnic circulation. Thus, in low cardiac flow states, enteral feeding can cause a "steal" effect on the already compromised hemodymanic function, further leading to hypotension. The small bowel is most susceptible to ischemia; ischemic bowel is a rare but severe complication carrying a mortality rate of 100%. Ischemic bowel is manifested by abdominal distension, increased gastric residuals, and diarrhea. Formulas high in fat, fiber, and complex foods tend to increase the energy expenditure and decreased gut perfusion. Thus, the dilemma arises whether to initiate feeds or to hold them in the setting of hemodynamic instability. Enteral feeds are always recommended when compared with parenteral nutrition in critical illnesses, especially sepsis, if the gut is functioning. Mucosal stimulation helps decrease bacterial translocation into the bloodstream. Isoosmolar, low-fiber formulations should be utilized initially while monitoring for signs of small bowel ischemia (65). Warning signs such as a sudden increase in nasogastric output, abdominal distention, new onset of abdominal pain, or decreased stool output and/or flatus should prompt holding the enteral feeds until bowel ischemia is ruled out. Feeds should also be held if blood pressure is below 70 mm Hg, and with increased requirements for pressors and ventilatory support (65). A question often asked with the hypotensive patient on pressors is: "Can enteral feedings be initiated? If so, when?" In patients receiving stable doses of pressor agents, enteral nutrition can be initiated as long as the patient is volume repleted and the mean arterial blood pressure can be sustained >70 mm Hg (65). Specialized nutrition support with parenteral nutrition may be necessary in patients who are unable to tolerate enteral nutrition. These patients can have multisystem organ failure involving the heart, lungs, kidneys, and gut. In these scenarios, caution should be exercised with the total volume of PN and/or EN, rate of administration, and composition. The total volume should be adjusted according to the urinary output. Renal failure patients requiring dialysis have increased protein and energy requirements, similar to the patients who experience serious infections or acute inflammation. It is important to obtain a positive energy balance along with an even or positive nitrogen balance for these patients. By providing sufficient nutrition, the degree of protein catabolism, as well as the severity of negative nitrogen balance may decrease. In patients with renal failure not receiving dialysis, the provision of protein may need to be restricted. Tight glycemic control with blood sugar levels between 80 and 110 mg/dL should also be achieved to prevent adverse outcomes (66).

PULMONARY DISEASE

Pulmonary disease encompasses a wide array of medical conditions such as tuberculosis, asthma, cancer, cystic fibrosis, emphysema, chronic obstructive pulmonary disease, and the like. Cough, early satiety, anorexia, and dyspnea during food preparation and consumption are all symptoms of pulmonary disease that can affect nutritional status. As the pulmonary disease progresses, these symptoms may be more pronounced and have a greater effect on oral intake and nutrition status (see Table 4–6).

Table 4–6 Lung Disease Symptoms Affecting Oral Intake

- Cough, dyspnea, tachypnea.
- Early satiety, anorexia, nausea, vomiting, altered taste
- Weight loss
- Fatigue
- Depression

Surgical management of pulmonary disease involves lobectomy, pneumonectomy, or lung transplantation. Poor nutrition status is known to play an important role in determining outcomes after surgical procedures; hence, adequate measures should be implemented to optimize pre-, peri- and postoperative nutrition (67). Preoperative nutrition support of the pulmonary patient focuses on counteracting the effect disease symptoms have on nutrition intake.

Table 4–7 lists the management strategies for common symptoms affecting nutrition intake. Most strategies aim to increase consumption of nutrient-dense foods (i.e., fortified oral nutrition beverages, high-calorie/nutritious meals, use of fats and protein supplements to increase the caloric or protein content of foods).

Table 4–8 shows how to "power pack" or increase the nutrition density of foods. Postoperative nutrition with a focus on appropriate dietary intake to maximize wound healing is discussed in detail in Chapter 14.

LUNG CANCER

The American Cancer Society estimated that over 174,470 people would be diagnosed with lung cancer in 2006, making it the second most common newly diag-

Table 4–7 Nutrition Strategies for Pulmonary Disease

Barrier to Optimal Nutrition Intake	Suggestions to Eliminate Barrier
Difficulty in preparing food due to fatigue	Energy Conservation • Frozen, ready-to-eat meals • Prepare double recipes and freeze leftovers in single servings • Have friends/family help with food preparation • Home delivery of groceries • Take-out or carry-out meals
Decreased intake due to early satiety, dyspnea, and fatigue at meals	• Small, frequent meals (6–8 small meals/snacks daily)* • "Power-pack" foods to increase nutritional value (see Table 4–8) • Fortified oral nutrition beverages between meals or in addition to a meal • Soft or pureed foods • Keep snacks at bedside or within reach at all times

*Consume fluids between meals

Table 4–8 "Power-Pack" Foods

- Butter or margarine, cream cheese, sour cream
- Half and half or whole milk, coffee creamer
- Mayonnaise or salad dressing
- Dried fruits, nuts, granola
- Peanut butter, jams, and jellies
- Gravies and sauces
- Fortified oral nutrition beverages in place of low-calorie beverages

High-Protein Food
- Low-fat dry milk powder, milk or cream, yogurt, eggs, cheese, cottage cheese
- Peanut butter, seeds, nuts, beans, and legumes
- Fortified oral nutrition beverages (powder or liquid)
- Tofu
- Cooked meats, poultry, and fish

---

nosed cancer for both men and women. Cancer of the lung is usually due to prolonged tobacco smoking. Environmental pollutants may also play a role in the initiation of the malignant process. Symptoms previously discussed for pulmonary disease can also occur with lung cancer. The nutritional management is similar to other recommendations described previously. In addition, nutritional status in patients with lung cancer is often impacted by the side effects of chemotherapy and radiotherapy. Chemotherapy can have gastrointestinal side effects such as nausea, vomiting, diarrhea, anorexia, mucositis, and altered taste. Radiotherapy, depending on the site radiated, may cause dysphagia, mucositis, and esophagitis. Management of these side effects is discussed in greater detail in Chapter 8. As with all pulmonary disease, nutrition management of lung cancer focuses on maintaining adequate protein and calorie intake in the setting of treatment side effects. Weight loss and decline in other nutritional anthropometrics and laboratory values is likely to be consistent with a decline in prognosis (67). Nutrition status should be optimized prior to surgery to allow for the best outcome (68).

Chronic and Acute Lung Disease

Patients with underlying malnutrition are at risk of poor outcomes due to the combined effect of altered pulmonary and immune system function. Alterations in pulmonary function in malnourished individuals includes reduced respiratory muscle strength, reduced alveolar ventilation, and altered surfactant production. Pulmonary defense mechanisms can become impaired, which can also result in an increased risk of pneumonia.

COPD

Chronic obstructive pulmonary disease (COPD) is a chronic lung disease that has a high incidence of malnutrition. It is defined as weight loss of 5%–10% of current weight or <90% IBW, and occurs in ≥35% of patients with COPD (69). Malnutrition has been shown to be an independent predictor of mortality and can lead to an increased need for mechanical ventilation. Mechanisms are elevated resting energy expenditure (REE), a decreased food intake as compared to REE, an accelerated nitrogen imbalance, medication effects, and systemic inflammatory responses. Patients with COPD have a tendency to lose fat-free mass, even in the absence of weight loss. Clinical trials have shown that oral nutritional supplementation can result in increase in body weight and muscle strength (70). However, the effect of nutritional supplementation alone on clinically significant outcomes such as pulmonary function and exercise capacity is minimal (70). Utilizing indirect calorimetry may be beneficial for the measurement of energy requirements to avoid overfeeding. An initial caloric goal of REE × 1.3 is suggested for initiation of enteral nutrition support (70,71). Protein provisions starting at 1.5 gm/kg/day are recommended but can vary depending on the catabolic state of the disease (71). Hence, measurement of urinary urea nitrogen can be used to adequately meet protein requirements. Frequent calculation of protein requirements should be done to prevent further weight and lean body mass loss.

It has been hypothesized that diet consisting of a higher proportion of nonprotein calories as fat instead of carbohydrate may be optimal because of the higher CO_2 production and ventilatory load from the carbohydrate metabolism. However, there is no significant evidence to support their use (72). Delayed gastric emptying occurred in patients receiving the high-fat, low-carbohydrate formulas (73). When providing nutrition support to the patient with COPD, it is the total caloric load provided to the patient that is of benefit to avoid overfeeding, rather than the alteration in macronutrient composition. Currently, there is no significant data on the use of parenteral nutrition in COPD patients.

ARDS

Acute respiratory distress syndrome (ARDS) is an acute diffuse inflammatory process in the lungs due to a variety of infectious and noninfectious conditions. It is characterized by damage to pulmonary epithelial cells, with subsequent alveolar capillary leak and exudative pulmonary edema. The main clinical features include rapid onset of dyspnea, severe defects in gas exchange, and imaging studies demonstrating diffuse pulmonary infiltrates. Patients with ARDS are at increased nutritional risk secondary to the catabolic state from proinflammatory mediators affecting the disease course. Patients with ARDS require prolonged mechanical ventilation and specialized nutrition support. The use of enteral nutrition is recommended unless gastrointestinal dysfunction is present. Detailed discussion of nutritional management in ARDS can be found in Chapter 3.

CHYLOTHORAX

Chylothorax is accumulation of chyle in the pleural space from injury to the lymphatic system (74). Causes of chylothorax include a congenital defect, malignancy obstructing lymphatic drainage, lymphangiomatosis, Kaposi's sarcoma, abdominal processes that produce chylous ascites, or traumatic injury during a surgical procedure. Close proximity of the lymphatic system vessels to the heart, lungs, esophagus, and other organs in the thoracic cavity makes traumatic injury to the vessels the second most common cause of chylothorax, besides lymphoma. Worldwide, the incidence of chylothorax following cardiothoracic surgery is 0.2%–1% (75).

Chyle is a milky, white, odorless liquid rich in protein and lipids. About 2–4 liters of chyle flow through the thoracic duct daily and empty back into venous circulation. Chyle is a rich source pf lymphocytes, and also provides about 200 kcal/liter, greater than 30 gm protein/L and 4–40 gm lipid/L (76). Due to its contents, continued chyle leak can lead to rapid malnutrition. Diagnosis of chylothorax can be made from milky output from the drains or by restricting oral intake and monitoring if drain output becomes clear and decreases in volume. Several laboratory tests including triglyceride levels of chylous fluid provide a more objective way to diagnose chylothorax. To better understand the nutrition management of chylothorax, metabolism and absorption of triglycerides will be briefly reviewed.

Long-chain triglycerides (LCT) are the primary fat component in the diet contributing to chyle formation. Once ingested, LCTs are converted into water soluble micelles by bile salts in the proximal small bowel. Micelles also provide a greater surface area for pancreatic enzymes to break down the LCT. The byproducts of triglyceride breakdown, monoglycerides (MCT) and free fatty acids (FFA), are then transported across the bowel mucosa for absorption. They are reesterified into triglycerides and packaged with proteins and cholesterol to chylomicrons. Chylomicrons, as chyle, enter the lymphatic system via the lacteals. The chyle is then returned to venous circulation via the thoracic duct. MCT are primarily absorbed across the gastrointestinal mucosa directly into the portal vein. Up to 20% of triglyceride fatty acids in lymph may be medium chain (77), and as the intake of LCT increases along with the MCT, a higher percentage of MCT is absorbed via the lymphatic system.

The goals of management of chylothorax are to decrease chylous output, replace fluid and electrolytes, and maintain nutrition status (77). No prospective, randomized, controlled trials address the treatment of chyle leaks. There is also no standardized definition of an acceptable volume of chylous drainage per 24 hours. Therefore, the efficacy of nutrition support can be assessed by decrease in chyle output, improvement of effusions on serial chest X-rays, or a decrease in the need for serial thoracenteses.

Conservative nutrition management focuses on limiting the amount of ingested fat, specifically LCT. It is suggested, if oral intake is possible, a fat-free diet be prescribed, although it is almost impossible to eliminate all the fat from the diet due to traces of fat in many fruits, vegetables, and fat-free products. This diet can be difficult for a person to maintain due to limited food choices. It also has the potential to be inadequate in protein, essential fatty acids, and fat-soluble vitamins. However, careful diet planning can prevent any nutrient deficiencies. Fat-free oral supplements such as Resource Breeze, Enlive, or Resource Fruit Beverage will help to meet caloric, protein, and vitamin needs. Other fat-free protein sources include egg whites, fat-free milk, nonfat cheese, or nonfat dry milk powder. There are also a variety of nutritional supplement protein powders available in the market that can be added to foods as needed. A daily multivitamin with minerals is suggested to prevent vitamin and mineral deficiencies.

MCT-based formulas are high in MCT and low in LCT. Very low fat formulas tend to be low in both LCT and MCT; however, all enteral formulas provide adequate EFA and fat-soluble vitamins to meet a person's daily requirement. These formulas are more expensive than standard enteral formulas, but they are much less expensive than and do not carry the same risks as parenteral nutrition (PN). Table 4–9 details the nutritional composition of some commonly available very low fat enteral formulas.

Table 4–9 Nutritional Composition of Enteral Formulas for Use in Chylothorax

Formula	% Total Calories as Fat	Total Fat (g/L)	MCT (g/L)	LCT (g/L)	Form	Manufacturer
AlitraQ®	13.2	15.5	8.2	7.3	Powder	Ross
F.A.A.	10	11.2	2.8	8.4	Liquid	Nestle Nutrition
Peptinex DT®	15	17.4	8.7	8.7	Liquid	Novartis Medical Nutrition
Tolerex®	1	1.5	0	1.5	Powder	Novartis Medical Nutrition
Vital HN®	9.5	10.8	6.0	4.8	Powder	Ross
Vivonex Plus®	6	6.7	0	6.7	Powder	Novartis Medical Nutrition
Vivonex RTF®	10	12	0	12	Liquid	Novartis Medical Nutrition

Sources: Information gathered from individual manufacturer's Web sites.

PN should only be considered when a fat-free oral diet or very low fat enteral feedings fail to decrease the amount of chyle output. Disadvantages of PN include increased cost, atrophy of the gastrointestinal tract, and an increased risk of infection. Essential fatty acid deficiency (EFAD) will not be a concern with PN, because parenteral lipid formulations are composed of phospholipids and directly enter the bloodstream, bypassing the lymphatic system (78). Therefore, lipids can be used safely with PN.

A suggested progression for diet management of chylothorax is as follows:

1. Nothing by mouth for 24 hours for baseline volume of chylous output.
2. Begin fat-free diet, encouraging adequate intake of fat-free protein sources and a multivitamin with minerals or enteral feedings.
3. Monitor chylous output and adjust oral/enteral intake as necessary. If on fat-free diet for greater than 5 to 7 days, consider small amount of safflower oil daily to prevent EFAD.
4. If chylous output increases or does not decrease, consider PN.

In many patients, medical management with a low-fat diet or PN is effective in decreasing chyle sufficiently to allow for spontaneous closure of the leak. If medical management fails, surgical ligation of the leak may be considered. The literature does not offer a clear idea on duration of medical management before surgery becomes the next option.

CONCLUSION

Nutritional management plays a key role in the outcome of medical and surgical interventions involving the structures in the cardiothoracic cavity. Surgical intervention can place patients at increased nutritional risk, especially if newly diagnosed, or they are not in compliance with previous medical advice. In circumstances when specialized nutrition support is indicated, it can aid in improving a patient's nutritional status. Emphasis should be placed on nutritional optimization in susceptible individuals for primary prevention of adverse events. This can be accomplished collectively, by increasing awareness of a healthy lifestyle, working with nutrition professionals, and maintaining compliance with medications and physician advice.

REFERENCES

1. DeVault KR, Castell DO. Updated guidelines for the diagnosis and treatment of gastroesophageal reflux disease. *Am J Gastro.* 2005;100:190–200.
2. Dent J, El-Serag HB, Wallander MA, Johansson S. Epidemiology of gastroesophageal reflux disease. A systematic review. *Gut.* 2005;54(5):710–717.
3. Locke GR, Talley NJ, Fett SL, Zinsmeister AR, Melton LJ. Risk factors associated with symptoms of gastroesophageal reflux. *Am J Med.* 1999;106:642–649.

4. Nandurkar S, Talley NJ. Epidemiology and natural history of reflux disease. *Baillieres Best Pract Res Clin Gastroenterol.* 2000;14:743–757.

5. Holtmann G. Understanding GERD symptoms in the clinical setting. *Drugs Today.* 2005;41 (suppl B):13–17.

6. Poelmans J, Tack J. Extraoesophageal manifestations of gastro-oesophageal reflux. *Gut.* 2005; 54:1492–1499.

7. Murray L, Johnston B, Lane A, et al. Relationship between body mass and gastro-esophageal reflux symptoms: The Bristol Helicobacter Project. *Int J Epidemiol.* 2003;32:645–650.

8. Smith SC, Edwards CB, Goodman GN. Symptomatic and clinical improvement in morbidly obese patients with gastroesophageal reflux disease following Roux-en-Y gastric bypass. *Obes Surg.* 1997;7:479–484.

9. Penagini R. Fat and gastro-oesphageal reflux disease. *Eur J Gastroenterol Hepatol.* 2000; 12:1343–1345.

10. Austin GL, Thiny MT, Westman EC, Yancy WS Jr, Shaheen NJ. A very low carbohydrate diet improves gastroesophageal reflux and its symptoms. *Dig Dis Sci.* 2006;51:1307–1312.

11. Kaltenbach TS, Crockett S, Gerson LB. Are lifestyle measures effective in patients with gastroesophageal reflux disease? An evidence-based approach. *Arch Intern Med.* 2006;166:965–971.

12. Holtmann G, Adam B, Liebregts T. Review article: The patient with gastro-oesophageal reflux disease lifestyle advice and medication. *Aliment Pharmacol Ther.* 2004;20S8:24–27.

13. Sharma N, Trope B, Lipman T. Vitamin supplementation: What the gastroenterologist needs to know. *J Clin Gastroenterol* 2004;30:844–854.

14. Kraichely RE, Farrugia G. Achalasia: Physiology and etiopathogenesis. *Dis Esophagus.* 2006; 19:213–223.

15. Peltz G. Nutrition support in cancer patients: A brief review and suggestion for standard indications criteria. *Nutr J.* 2002;1:1–5.

16. Cobb LA, Eliastam M, Kerber RE, et al. Report of the American Heart Association Task Force on the future of cardiopulmonary resuscitation. *Circulation.* 1992;85:2346–2355.

17. Libby P, Ridker PM, Maseri A. Inflammation and atherosclerosis. *Circulation.* 2002;105: 1135–1143.

18. Ridker PM, Rifai N, Pfeffer M, Sacks F, Lepage S, Braunwald E. Elevation of tumor necrosis factor-alpha and increased risk of recurrent coronary events after myocardial infarction. *Circulation.* 2000;101:2149–2153.

19. Blankenberg S, Tiret L, Bickel C, et al. Interleukin-18 is a strong predictor of cardiovascular death in stable and unstable angina. *Circulation.* 2002;106:24–30.

20. Lindsay RS, Funahashi T, Hanson RL, et al. Adiponectin and development of type 2 diabetes in the Pima Indian population. *Lancet.* 2002;360:57–58.

21. Pischon T, Girman CJ, Hotamisligil GS, et al. Plasma adiponectin levels and risk of myocardial infarction in men. *JAMA.* 2004;291:1730–1737.

22. Krummel T, Dervaux T, Parves-Braun L, Hannedouche T. Why and how to measure cardiovascular risk? *Rev Prat.* 2004;54:615–617,619,621–625.

23. Cashin-Hemphill L, Mack WJ, Pogoda JM, Sanmarco ME, Azen SP, Blankenhorn DH. Beneficial effects of colestipol-niacin on coronary atherosclerosis. A 4-year follow-up. *JAMA.* 1990; 264:3013–3017.

24. Campeau L, Knatterud G, Hunninghake B, Domanski M. Optimizing cholesterol lowering therapy: Contribution of the Post Coronary Artery Bypass Graft Trial. *Eur Heart J.* 1997;18:1683–1685.

25. Smith SC Jr, Blair SL, Bonow RO, et al. AHA/ACC scientific statement: AHA/ACC guidelines for preventing heart attack and death in patients with atherosclerotic cardiovascular disease: 2001 update: A statement for healthcare professionals from the American Heart Association and the American College of Cardiology. *Circulation.* 2001;104:1577–1579.

26. Lichtenstein AH, Appel LJ, Brands M, et al. Diet and lifestyle recommendations revision 2006. A scientific statement from the American Heart Association Nutrition Committee. *Circulation.* 2006;114:82–96.

27. Hu FB, Willett WC. Optimal diets for prevention of coronary heart disease. *JAMA.* 2002; 288:2569–2578.

28. Pischon T, Hankinson SE, Hotamisligil GS, Rifai N, Willet WC, Rimm EB. Habitual dietary intake of n-3 and n-6 fatty acids in relation to inflammatory markers among U.S. men and women. *Circulation.* 2003;108:155–160.

29. Ciubotaru I, Lee YS, Wander RC. Dietary fish oil decreases C-reactive protein, interleukin-6, and triacylglycerol to HDL-cholesterol ratio in postmenopausal women on HRT. *J Nutr Biochem.* 2003;14:513–521.

30. Zampelas A, Panagiotakos DB, Pitsavos C, et al. Fish consumption among healthy adults is associated with decreased levels of inflammatory markers related to cardiovascular disease the AT-TICA study. *J Am Coll Cardiol.* 2005;46:120–124.

31. Giugliano D, Ceriello A, Esposito K. The effects of diet on inflammation: Emphasis on metabolic syndrome. *J Am Coll Cardiol.* 2006;48:677–685.

32. Bemelmans WJ, Lefrandt JD, Feskens EJ, et al. Increased alpha-linolenic acid intake lowers C-reactive protein, but has no effect on markers of atherosclerosis. *Eur J Clin Nutr.* 2004; 58:1083–1089.

33. Hu FB, Stampfer MJ, Manson JE, et al. Dietary fat intake and the risk of coronary heart disease in women. *N Engl J Med.* 1997;337:1491–1499.

34. Mozaffarian D, Pischon T, Hankinson SE, et al. Dietary intake of trans fatty acids and systemic inflammation in women. *Am J Clin Nutr.* 2004;79:606–612.

35. Szeto YT, Kwok TC, Benzie IF. Effects of long-term vegetarian diet on biomarkers of antioxidant status and cardiovascular disease risk. *Nutrition.* 2004;20:863–866.

36. Leibel RL, Hirsch J, Appel BE, Checani GC. Energy intake required to maintain body weight is not affected by wide variation in diet composition. *Am J Clin Nutr.* 1992;55(2):350–355.

37. Gao X, Bermudez OI, Tucker KL. Plasma C-reactive protein and homocysteine concentrations are related to frequent fruit and vegetable intake in Hispanic and non-Hispanic white elders. *J Nutr.* 2004;134:913–918.

38. Maron DJ. Flavonoids for reduction of atherosclerotic risk. *Curr Atheroscler.* 2004;6:73–78.

39. Ajani UA, Ford ES, Mokdad AL. Dietary fiber and C-reactive protein findings from National Health and Nutrition Examination Survey data. *J Nutr.* 2004;134:1181–1185.

40. Wells BJ, Mainous AG, Everett CJ. Association between dietary arginine and C-reactive protein. *Nutrition.* 2005;21:125–130.

41. Kris-Etherton PM. AHA science advisory. Monounsaturated fatty acids and risk of cardiovascular disease. *Circulation.* 1999;100:1253–1258.

42. Williams SB, Goldfine AB, Timimi F, et al. Acute hyperglycemia attenuates endothelium-dependent vasodilation in humans in vivo. *Circulation.* 1998;97:1695–1701.

43. The Alpha-Tocopherol, Beta-Carotene Cancer Prevention Study Group. The effect of vitamin E and beta-carotene on the incidence of lung cancer and other cancers in male smokers. *N Engl J Med.* 1994;330:1029–1035.

44. Hennekens CH, Buring JE, Manson JE, Stampfer M, et al. Lack of effect of long-term supplementation with beta carotene on the incidence of malignant neoplasms and cardiovascular disease. *N Engl J Med.* 1996;334:1145–1149.

45. Rapola JM, Virtamo J, Ripatti S, et al. Randomised trial of α–tocopherol and ß-carotene supplements on incidence of major coronary events in men with previous myocardial infarction. *Lancet.* 1997;349:1715–1720.

46. Homocysteine Studies Collaboration. Homocysteine and risk of ischemic heart disease and stroke: A meta-analysis. *JAMA.* 2002;288:2015–2023.

47. Nygard O, Nordrehaug JE, Refsum H, Ueland PM, Farstad M, Vollset SE. Plasma homocysteine levels and mortality in patients with coronary artery disease. *N Engl J Med.* 1997;337:230–236.

48. Schnyder G, Roffi M, Pin R, et al. Decreased rate of coronary restenosis after lowering of plasma homocysteine levels. *N Engl J Med.* 2001;345:1593–1600.

49. Lange H, Suryapranata H, De Luca G, et al. Folate therapy and in-stent restenosis after coronary stenting. *N Engl J Med.* 2004;350:2673–2681.

50. Oberbach A, Tonjes A, Kloting N, et al. Effect of a 4 week physical training program on plasma concentrations of inflammatory markers in patients with abnormal glucose tolerance. *Eur J Endocrinol.* 2006;154(4):577–585.

51. Park HS, Park JY, Yu R. Relationship of obesity and visceral adiposity with serum concentrations of CRP, TNF alpha, IL-6. *Diabetes Res Clin Pract.* 2005;69(1):29–35.

52. Sattar N, Wannamethee G, Sarwar N, et al. Adiponectin and coronary heart disease. A prospective study and meta-analysis. *Circulation.* 2006;114(7):623–629.

53. Karner A, Tingstrom P, Abrandt-Dahlgren M, Bergdahl B. Incentives for lifestyle changes in patients with coronary heart disease. *J Adv Nurs.* 2005;51(3):261–275.

54. Anker SD, Ponikowski M, Varney S, et al. Wasting as independent risk factor for mortality in chronic heart failure. *Lancet.* 1997;349:1050–1053.

55. Cicoira M, Davos CH, Francis DP, et al. Prediction of mortality in chronic heart failure from peak oxygen consumption adjusted for either body weight or lean tissue. *J Card Fail.* 2004;10(5):421–426.

56. Otaki M. Surgical treatment of patients with cardiac cachexia. An analysis of factors affecting operative mortality. *Chest.* 1994;105(5):1347–1351.

57. Anker SD, Clark AL, Teixeira MM, Hellewell PG, Coats JC. Loss of bone mineral in patients with cachexia due to chronic heart failure. *Am J Cardiol.* 1999;83(4):612–615.

58. Anker SD, Sharma R. The syndrome of cardiac cachexia. *Int J Cardiol.* 2002;85(1):51–66.

59. Leyva F, Anker SD, Egerer K, Stevenson JC, Kox WJ, Coats AJ. Hyperleptinaemia in chronic heart failure. Relationships with insulin. *Eur Heart J.* 1998;19(10):1547–1551.

60. Springer J, Filippatos G, Akashi YJ, Anker SD. Prognosis and therapy approaches of cardiac cachexia. *Curr Opin Cardiol.* 2006;21(3):229-233

61. Anker SD, Negessa A, Coats AL, et al. Prognostic importance of weight loss in chronic heart failure and the effect of treatment with angiotensin-converting-enzyme inhibitors: An observational study. *Lancet.* 2003;361(9363):1077–1083.

62. Anker SD, Clark AL, Winkler R, et al. Statin use and survival in patients with chronic heart failure—Results from two observational studies with 5200 patients. *Int J Cardio.* 2006;112(2):234–242.

63. Cuneo RC, Wilmshurst P, Lowy C, McGauley G, Sonksen PH. Cardiac failure responding to growth hormone. *Lancet.* 1989;1(8642):838–839.

64. Cicoira M, Kalra PR, Anker SD. Growth hormone resistance in chronic heart failure and its therapeutic implications. *J Card Fail.* 2003;9(3):219–226.

65. McClave SA, Chang WK. Feeding the hypotensive patient: Does enteral feeding precipitate or protect against ischemic bowel? *Nutr Clin Pract.* 2003;18(4):279–284.

66. Van den Berghe G, Wouters P, Weekers F, et al. Intensive insulin therapy in critically ill patients. *N Engl J Med.* 2001;345:1359–1367.

67. Jagoe RT, Goodship TH, Gibson GJ. Nutritional status of patients undergoing lung cancer operations. *Ann Thorac Surg.* 2001;71(3):929–935.

68. Chlebowski RT, Palomares MR, Lillington L, Grosvenor M. Recent implications of weight loss in lung cancer management. *Nutrition.* 1996;12(1S):S43–S47.

69. Mallampalli A. Nutritional management of the patient with chronic obstructive pulmonary disease. *Nutr Clin Pract.* 2004;19(6):550–556.

70. Shoup R, Dalsky G, Warner S, et al. Body composition and health-related quality of life in patients with obstructive airways disease. *Eur Respir J.* 1997;10(7):1576–1580.

71. Donahoe M. Nutritional support in advanced lung disease. The pulmonary cachexia syndrome. *Clin Chest Med.* 1997;18(3):547–551.

72. Schols A. Nutritional modulation as part of the integrated management of chronic obstructive pulmonary disease. *Proc Nutr Soc.* 2003;62(4):783–791.

73. Akrabawi SS, Mobarhan S, Stoltz RR, Ferguson PW. Gastric emptying, pulmonary function, gas exchange, and respiratory quotient after feeding a moderate versus high fat enteral formula meal in chronic obstructive pulmonary disease patients. *Nutrition.* 1996;12(4):260–265.

74. Kozar R, Adams SD, Cipolla J. Chylothorax. Available online at: www.emedicine.com/med/topic381.htm. Accessed October 3, 2005.

75. De Beer G, Mol MJ, Janssen JP. Chylothorax. *Neth J Med.* 2000;56(1):25–31.

76. Jensen GL, Mascioli EA, Meyer LP, et al. Dietary modification of chyle composition in chylothorax. *Gastroenterol.* 1989;97(3):761–765.

77. Parrish CR, McCray S. When chyle leaks: Nutrition management options. *Prac Gastroenterol.* 2004;28:60–76.

78. Hehar SS, Bradley PJ. Management of chyle leaks. *Current Opin Otolaryngol Head Neck Surg.* 2001;9:120–125.

CHAPTER 5

Surgical Nutrition for General Gastrointestinal and Vascular Surgery Patients

David August, MD; and Maureen Huhmann, MS, RD

INTRODUCTION

Nutrition support is an integral component of the care of surgical patients. Understanding of the metabolic changes associated with surgery, stress, and infection has increased dramatically over the past few decades. The importance of the timing, composition, and route of administration of nutrition support to surgical patients has been explored in many clinical studies. This chapter presents a review of the nutritional physiology of gastrointestinal (GI) and vascular surgical procedures, the perioperative impact of these procedures on nutrition status, nutrition management considerations in perioperative patients, and the long-term digestive and nutritional consequences of these procedures.

NUTRITIONAL PHYSIOLOGY

Topologically, the GI tract is in continuity with the body's external environment. The mucosal lining of the GI tract has functions analogous to the skin, including maintenance of a functional barrier to protect the body's internal milieu from mechanical, chemical, and microbial insults originating in the external environment. Strikingly, however, and in contrast to the skin, the GI mucosa must fulfill these functions while allowing selective movement of nutrients across the barrier and into the internal milieu. The GI tract is comprised of four layers: the mucosa, submucosa, muscularis propria, and serosa (except the mouth, esophagus, and rectum, which are not serosalized). The mouth and esophagus are lined by squamous mucosae. The mucosae of the stomach, small bowel, and colon are composed of cuboidal glandular epithelium.

Blood is supplied to the intraabdominal GI tract via the celiac axis and the superior and inferior mesenteric arteries. These arteries receive one sixth of the cardiac output. Although there are many areas of the GI tract in which blood supply is redundant, injury or occlusion of the superior mesenteric artery is devastating. The blood flow in this complex system is regulated both longitudinally (segmentally) along the lumen and between segment layers (transmural). The blood flow is dynamic, adjusting to changes in supply and demand. Blood supply is affected by the presence of food in and distention of the GI tract, the buildup of metabolic end products (e.g., CO_2, lactate), and sympathetic stimulation (α-adrenergic). Animal research indicates that the reactivation of the gut and expansion of the villi after hibernation is due to rapid influx of blood into the villi and not an increase in number of cells (1). Although the dramatic increase in blood flow to the gut in response to a meal in a snake (tenfold) is exaggerated in comparison to humans (50%), the mechanisms appear similar (1). The portal system drains nutrient-rich venous blood from the small and large intestine to the liver, and from there to the systemic circulation. The first pass access of the liver to splanchnic blood is trophic for the liver and necessary for normal liver function and for hepatocyte regeneration (2).

The lymphatic system of the intestines originates as lacteals in the mucosal wall, which drain into local lymph nodes and lymphatic channels, ultimately leading to the thoracic duct. The small bowel lymphatics play an important role in the absorption and transport of ingested fats.

The autonomic nervous system provides most of the innervation to the GI tract. This innervation is both vagotonic and sympathomimetic. The autonomic ganglia, located both outside and inside the walls of the GI tract, are integral to the motility of the stomach and intestines.

Peritoneal Cavity

The serosal surface covering the outer surface of the stomach and intestines is continuous with the peritoneum. The portion of the peritoneum coating the intraabdominal organs is referred to as the visceral peritoneum, whereas the parietal peritoneum covers the wall of the abdominal cavity. The peritoneum is comprised of a single layer of fluid-producing serous cells. The peritoneal cavity, or the space between the two layers, is filled with a small amount (about 50 mL) of slippery fluid that allows the two layers to slide freely over each other. The peritoneum both supports the abdominal organs and serves as a conduit for blood and lymphatic vessels and nerves. It can also serve as an absorptive surface (3). Intraperitoneal nutrition has been used to effectively augment dietary intake in patients receiving peritoneal dialysis (3). In some situations, the inability of peritoneal absorption to keep up with net fluid entry into the peritoneal cavity can lead to the development of ascites.

Mouth

The mouth is the initial point of entry to the GI tract. Saliva, produced by the salivary glands, contains enzymes (especially amylase) and microorganisms important to digestion. There are over 700 species of microorganisms found in the oral cavity (4). The mouth contains both beneficial and pathogenic bacteria. The "good" bacteria and microbes found in the mouth compete with pathogenic bacteria, keeping them in check. One of the primary functions of saliva is moistening food to enable formation of a food bolus. The teeth and tongue are also vital to the process of digestion, assisting with mastication and movement of the food bolus to the pharynx for transport to the esophagus, respectively.

Esophagus

The esophagus transports food and saliva from the mouth to the stomach. Peristaltic waves move the food bolus down the squamous mucosa-lined, 25-centimeter tube to the lower esophageal sphincter (LES). The LES, the primary function of which is to prevent gastroesophageal reflux, opens in response to the presence of food to allow passage into the stomach.

Stomach

The stomach is a circular muscle, which churns and combines food with gastric juices. The stomach mucosa marks an abrupt transition from the stratified squamous epithelium of the esophagus to a columnar epithelium dedicated to secretion. Four major types of secretory epithelial cells cover the surface of the stomach: mucous cells, parietal cells, chief cells, and G cells. Table 5–1 provides a description of the secretions of these cells and their roles in digestion. The stomach has very little absorptive capacity; however, small amounts of aspirin, other nonsteroidal anti-inflammatory drugs, and ethanol are absorbed in the stomach. The primary functions of the stomach are: protection from microbes by virtue of its antimicrobial acid environment; reservoir, to allow the consumption of large meals with subsequent delayed entry to the duodenum and small bowel; and secretion of intrinsic factor by the parietal cells to permit vitamin B_{12} absorption in the terminal ileum.

Gastric function is regulated by vagal stimulation and gastric distention, both of which stimulate acid secretion and gastric peristalsis. Gastric function is also regulated by hormones; whereby the entry of food into the stomach stimulates a series of hormonal reactions. Gastrin, a peptide synthesized in gastric G-cells, stimulates gastric acid secretion and increases gastric motility. The acidic food mixture moves into the small intestine and stimulates the release of secretin. Secretin release, triggered by an acidic environment in the small intestine, inhibits gastric acid secretion and gastric emptying and stimulates the release of pancreatic bicarbonate. The return of the small intestine lumen to a neutral pH signals the release

Table 5–1 Exocrine and Endocrine Secretions of the Gastrointestinal Tract

Organ of Secretion	Secretory Product	Function
Mouth		
Acinar cells	Salivary alpha amylase (ptyalin)	Hydrolysis of starch
Stomach		
Chief cells	Pepsin	Active form of pepsinogen; hydrolysis of the interior peptide bonds
	Gastric lipase	Hydrolysis of fat
G cells	Gastrin	Stimulates the secretion of hydrochloric acid
Parietal cells	Hydrochloric acid	Denatures protein, kills bacteria, activates pepsinogen
	Intrinsic factor	Mediates the absorption of vitamin B_{12} in the intestine
Mucus cells	Mucin	Protects mucosa
Duodenum		
S cells	Secretin	Triggered by HCl in the duodenum; inhibits gastric acid secretion and gastric emptying; stimulates secretion of pancreatic bicarbonate
Brunner's glands and pancreatic ducal cells	Bicarbonate	Raises the pH of the chyme entering the duodenum
Paneth cells	Enteropeptidase (enterokinase)	Activates pancreatic enzymes
I cells	Cholecystokinin (CCK)	Stimulates gallbladder contraction; stimulates secretion of bicarbonates
Liver	Bile	Emulsification of lipid; formation of micelles for absorption
Pancreatic ascinar cells	Trypsinogen/trypsin	Hydrolysis of peptide bonds at carboxyl end of basic AA
	Chymotrypsinogen/ chymotrypsin	Hydrolysis of interior peptide bonds of aromatic AA, MET, ASN, HIS

Table 5–1 Continued

Organ of Secretion	Secretory Product	Function
	Pancreatic alpha amylase	Hydrolysis of starch α 1–4 bonds
	Pancreatic lipase	Hydrolysis of triacylglycerols
	Carboxypeptidase A	Hydrolysis of carboxyterminal neutral AA
	Carboxypeptidase B	Hydrolysis of carboxyterminal basic AA
	Elastase	Hydrolysis of fibrous peptides
	Collagenase	Hydrolysis of collagen
	Phosopholipase A1 and A2	Hydrolysis of phospholipids
	Cholesterol esterase	Hydrolysis of cholesterol and triacylglycerols
Jejunum		
Endocrine cells of the crypt of lieberkühn	Aminopeptidases	Hydrolysis of N-terminal AA
	Tripeptidases	Hydrolysis of tripeptides
	Dipeptidases	Hydrolysis of dipeptides
	Nucleases	Hydrolysis of DNA and RNA
	Isomaltase	Hydrolysis of starch α 1–6 bonds
	Glucoamylase	Hydrolysis of starch α 1–4 bonds
	Glucosidase	Hydrolysis of starch α 1–4 bonds
	Maltase	Hydrolysis of maltose
	Lactase	Hydrolysis of lactose
	Sucrase	Hydrolysis of sucrose
	Lecithinase	Hydrolysis of lecithin
Ileum		
Epithelial goblet cells	Mucus	Protection
Colon		
Epithelial goblet cells	Mucus Bicarbonate	Protection

HCl, hydrochloric acid; AA, amino acid; MET, methionine; ASN, asparagine; HIS, histidine; DNA, deoxyribonucleic acid; RNA, ribonucleic acid of more gastric contents into the small intestine (Table 5–2). Cholecystokinin (CCK), expressed in the duodenum and jejunum, is secreted into circulation to signal satiety. CCK also stimulates the release of enzymes from the pancreas and gallbladder, inhibits gastric emptying, and increases intestinal motility (5).

Small Bowel

The small bowel is about 7 meters long and consists of three subdivisions: the duodenum, jejunum, and ileum. The villi of the small bowel increase the absorptive surface area dramatically. If the intestine were simply a tube, the absorptive area would be approximately 1 square meter; the intestinal villi increase this surface to 250 square meters. The duodenum is the primary site of absorption for calcium and magnesium. The jejunum is responsible for absorption of carbohydrate, protein, water-soluble vitamins, and iron. Lipid, fat-soluble vitamins, cholesterol, bile salts, and vitamin B_{12} are absorbed in the ileum.

The gut has a highly active immune system that is regulated to prevent augmented response to food and microorganisms. The primary cellular barrier to antigens is a single layer of gut epithelium, which can detect commensal bacteria and pathogens (6). Disruptions in epithelial homeostasis lead to shifts in the activity of the commensal flora to a pathogenic nature. This barrier is not impervious to all luminal antigens; therefore some intact food proteins can be found in the plasma (6). Every day, intestinal plasma cells produce more antibodies than do all other lymphoid organs combined (7). Immunoglobulin-A (IgA), secreted in large quantities in intestinal fluid, inhibits the absorption of antigens, neutralizes toxins, interferes with mucosal adherence of pathogenic organisms, and acts as an anti-inflammatory agent. Commensal organisms are also coated with IgA but are able to resist its bactericidal actions, unlike pathogenic organisms (7). Tight junctions in the gut epithelium prevent the leakage of these pathogenic organisms into lymphatics, the blood stream, and the peritoneal cavity, thereby preventing systemic

Table 5–2 Gastrointestinal Tract Secretion Volumes

Secretion	Volume, mL/d	Na, mEq/L	K, mEq/L	Cl, mEq/L	HCO₃-, mEq/L
Saliva	1500	9	26	10	10–15
Gastric secretions	2500	60	9	84	0
Bile	500	149	5	101	40
Pancreatic juices	700	141	5	77	121
Small intestine	3000	111	5	104	31

Source: Adapted with permission from: Barrocas A, Foss L, Jastram C. Critical care. In: Miller R, Kirby R, Schwinn D, et al. eds. *Atlas of Anesthesia.* New York: Elsevier; 1999.

infection (8). In fact, epithelial dysfunction may contribute to the organ dysfunction that occurs in sepsis (8).

Colon

The colon is approximately 5 feet in length and is responsible for absorption of water, sodium, chloride, and potassium. In the distal colon, bacterial concentrations may rise as high as 10^{11} per gram of stool. Bacteria within the colon produce vitamin K and deconjugate bile salts (9). The colon also functions in the formation and storage of waste.

Pancreas

The pancreas, located in the retroperitoneal space of the upper abdomen, contains both exocrine and endocrine tissues. More than 98% of the pancreas is exocrine tissue which is responsible for the production of digestive enzymes. The endocrine tissue, found in the islets of Langerhans, secretes hormones such as insulin, glucagon, and somatostatin. The islets of Langerhans are scattered throughout the pancreas, but are most prominent in the tail of the pancreas. Pancreatic digestive enzymes are delivered to the duodenum via the main pancreatic duct, which shares its entry into the intestine with the common bile duct through the ampula of Vater. The secretion of enzymes by the pancreas is controlled by cholecystokinin, secretin, and vagal nerve impulses.

Liver

The liver, located in the right upper quadrant, is attached to the gallbladder and the extrahepatic bile ducts. These ducts connect the liver to the duodenum. Hepatocytes comprise 90% of the total mass of the liver. The liver has four major functions: excretory, metabolic, storage, and synthetic. Bile is the main excretory product, and the liver is the primary storage site for carbohydrate and lipid. All major plasma proteins, except immunoglobulins, are produced in the liver. The liver is the predominant site of cytochrome P450 activity in the body, and it therefore plays a central role in drug metabolism and detoxication. Arterial blood arrives at the liver via the hepatic artery, which branches off of the abdominal aorta. Nutrient-rich blood is delivered from the intestine through the portal vein. While portal blood flow supplies approximately 70% of the hepatic inflow, roughly two thirds of oxygen delivery is via the hepatic arteries. The hepatic veins drain blood that has circulated through the liver into the inferior vena cava just below the diaphragm.

Abdominal Aorta

The abdominal aorta is the main arterial blood supply to the abdominal and pelvic organs and the legs. It begins at the diaphragm and bifurcates at approximately the level of the third lumbar vertebra (near the level of the umbilicus) to form the common iliac arteries.

NUTRITIONAL PATHOPHYSIOLOGY

Various diseases and conditions can greatly impact an individual's ability to ingest and absorb nutrients. Nutrient deficiencies may in themselves cause GI dysfunction. Examples include gut mucosal atrophy that occurs during prolonged bowel rest, and hypoalbuminemia, which has been linked to small bowel dysmotility (10,11).

Peritoneal Cavity

Due to the proximity of the peritoneum to the organs of the GI system, infections, cancers, and other abnormalities that involve the peritoneum have the potential to disrupt normal GI function (12). *Peritonitis*, or inflammation of the peritoneum, due to intestinal perforation, intraabdominal infections, or chemical irritation (such as bile peritonitis) can cause ileus and impaired gut absorption. Malnutrition has been implicated as a predisposing factor for peritonitis (13). Maintenance of adequate energy, protein, and micronutrient intake is vital to recovery. In the setting of peritonitis, perioperative nutrition is necessary to promote wound healing and preserve gut function (12). It has been suggested that a feeding tube should be placed at the time of surgery in patients with complicated peritoneal infections (12). Often, however, specialized nutrition support (SNS) in patients with peritonitis must be initiated via the parenteral route because of the profound ileus that usually accompanies peritonitis. As the peritonitis and ileus resolve, the feeding tube may then be used to initiate enteral nutrition support.

Ascites reflects an imbalance between lymph transudation and lymph absorption within the peritoneal cavity. Causes of ascites include cirrhosis, cancer, congestive heart failure, and mycobacterium tuberculosis. Cirrhotic ascites or chylous ascites and ascitic leaks can cause hypoalbuminemia and malnutrition. Repeated paracentesis of the protein-rich ascitic fluid may lead to hypoalbuminemia and acute fluid shifts between body compartments. Gross ascites often leads to anorexia and poor oral intake because of the pressure the fluid exerts upon intraabdominal organs, the abdominal wall, and the retroperitoneum (14). Operative or endoscopic placement of feeding tubes in patients with ascites is contraindicated because the gastrointestinal serosal surface is unlikely to adhere to the abdominal wall peritoneum leading to leakage of gastrointestinal contents into the peritoneal cavity.

Mouth

Americans spend more than $60 billion per year to treat tooth decay and 3 out of 10 people over 65 have lost all their teeth (4). Tooth loss often leads to dietary modifications that are nutritionally incomplete or unpalatable. *Xerostomia*, or dry mouth, as a result of Sjogren's syndrome, medication, or radiation therapy, predisposes teeth to decay and oral infection. Xerostomia causes difficulty in bolus formation and swallowing as well as taste alterations. Management of xerostomia includes modification of the diet to include primarily soft, moist, sometimes blenderized foods to meet nutrition requirements. Liquid nutrition supplements are often utilized to supplement dietary intake. Use of saliva substitutes is also indicated; however poor compliance limits the applicability of use. *Stomatitis*, or inflammation of the oral mucosa, can range from mild, requiring food consistency alterations, to severe, requiring SNS. Stomatitis is caused by oral infection, mouth injury, xerostomia, allergic response, chemical irritation, vitamin deficiency, or certain toxins.

Esophagus

Although the sole function of the esophagus is to transport food from the mouth to the stomach, there may be significant nutritional consequences that result from esophageal resections. Esophagectomy can contribute to malnutrition from reflux (the lower esophageal sphincter is generally sacrificed with the resection), dysmotility of the remaining esophagus, gastric dysmotility secondary to resection of the vagus nerves with the esophagus, and dumping syndrome. A feeding jejunostomy tube is often placed at the time of esophageal surgery to allow enteral SNS while healing takes place. Stricture may occur after esophagectomy as a result of decreased vascularization and late ischemia in response to a decrease in blood supply to the stomach (15). Stricture often requires dilation to allow for normal oral intake. Sensation in the stomach often is altered during esophageal surgery due to disruption in normal vagal nerve function. This denervation may lead to inability to detect feelings of fullness (15). As a result overeating occurs, leading to food regurgitation.

Esophagitis, or inflammation of the esophagus, can be caused by infection, reflux of gastric acid or bile, or exogenous irritants. Esophageal reflux with aspiration can lead to chronic pulmonary infection. Elevation of the head of the bed at night and maintenance of upright posture for at least 2 hours after eating help manage esophageal reflux. If the reflux is acidic, the use of H_2-blockers or proton pump inhibitors and enhancement of gastric emptying with promotility agents are important. Nissen fundoplication, a surgical procedure in which the fundus of the stomach is wrapped around the inferior section of the esophagus, may be performed if medical management has failed.

Stomach

Reservoir Function

Gastric resection leads to a decrease in stomach capacitance with resultant compromise of reservoir function. The capacity of the GI tract to store food following gastrectomy can vary greatly. This can lead to unintentional food regurgitation (16). Gastric resections that include removal of either the pylorus or LES may also be problematic. Removal of the LES promotes reflux; if the procedure also includes disruption of pyloric function or a gastrojejunostomy, bile reflux into the esophagus can occur. This is particularly difficult to manage because, unlike acid, there are no drugs available to neutralize the irritant effects of bile on the esophageal squamous epithelium. The cytoprotective and bile absorptive effects of sucralfate sometimes remediate symptoms of bile reflux. Postgastrectomy, the absence of the lower esophageal sphincter eliminates the barrier for the reflux of food and digestive juices. This is observed in as many as 58% of patients who undergo esophagectomy (17) and 80% of patients who undergo a total gastrectomy (16).

Disruption of the pyloric sphincter and gastrojejunostomy may lead to dumping syndrome. This occurs with rapid passage of hyperosmotic undigested food into the small bowel with secondary hypersecretion of succus and extracellular fluid into the bowel lumen. This may cause hypotension and flushing, as well as cramps secondary to rapid distention of the bowel. Untreated, these problems can lead to weight loss, malnutrition, and increased mortality (18). Management of dumping syndrome should include small, frequent meals with limitation of portion sizes and separation of foods and fluids to prevent regurgitation. Elimination of simple carbohydrates and concentrated fats from the diet may also be helpful.

B_{12} Absorption

The acidic environment of the stomach assists in the release of vitamin B_{12} from food. The stomach is responsible for the release of intrinsic factor by parietal cells to permit the absorption of vitamin B_{12}. Intrinsic factor binds to vitamin B_{12} in the duodenum. The complex of vitamin B_{12} and intrinsic factor aids in the absorption of vitamin B_{12} in the terminal ileum (19). Chronic gastritis induces gastric mucosal atrophy and achlorhydria. Resultant loss of intrinsic factor may result in vitamin B_{12} malabsorption. Chronic gastritis may result from chronic infection with *helicobacter pylori*. Loss of intrinsic factor also occurs with proximal gastric resection. B_{12} deficiency induced by a lack of intrinsic factor can lead to megaloblastic anemia, and dementia (20). B_{12} deficiency can develop as early as 1 year after total gastrectomy (21). Deficiency is often diagnosed through measurement of serum vitamin B_{12} levels (<200 pg/mL). Metabolites of vitamin B_{12}, such as methylmalonic acid and homocysteine, may often be utilized to diagnose deficiency (19). Patients in whom all of the proximal stomach is removed should be evaluated for the need for vitamin B_{12} replacement. Vitamin B_{12} supplementation is available in enteral and parenteral formulations (19). Enterally supplemented B_{12} treatment has been found to increase serum B_{12} concentration and routine prescription has been recommended to patients undergoing total gastrectomy (19,21).

Antimicrobial Function

Achlorhydria may allow bacterial and fungal overgrowth (22,23). This can cause pain when eating, leading to suboptimal intake. Chronic gastritis also predisposes to cancer development (24,25).

Small Bowel

Nutrient Absorption

The major role of the small bowel is nutrient absorption. Resection of any significant portion of the small bowel can result in decreased transit time, thereby producing malabsorption. As previously mentioned, hormones released in response to the entry of food into the small intestine affect pancreatic and gallbladder function as well as gastric emptying and feelings of satiety. The loss of portions of the jejunum can result in inappropriate secretion of digestive enzymes and accelerated gastric emptying. Significant resection of the lower jejunum and ileum can cause reduced intestinal absorption secondary to the loss of absorptive surface, or short bowel syndrome. Occasionally, fluid and electrolyte needs cannot be met with standard oral feedings alone and require SNS (26). Short bowel syndrome is discussed in depth in Chapter 13.

Bacterial Homeostasis

An acidic environment in the small bowel lumen deactivates digestive enzymes and deconjugates bile acids. This may occur with increased gastric acid secretion and decreased transit time that are seen following small bowel resection. This leads to further malabsorption. The malabsorbed food moves into the colon where carbohydrate is fermented by bacteria into D-lactic acid. Buildup of D-lactic acid can cause metabolic acidosis. D-lactic acidosis is managed with carbohydrate restriction, antibiotics, and probiotics (27). Additionally, massive bowel resection frequently leads to bacterial overgrowth, increasing the risk of bacterial translocation. Bacterial overgrowth is commonly treated with antibiotics and probiotics (28,29). Probiotics are live microorganisms such as *lactobacillus* or *bifidobacterium,* that may produce beneficial health effects in humans (30). Probiotics are available in food and pharmaceutical preparations

Colon

Fluid Balance

A major function of the colon is fluid resorption and electrolyte absorption. Resections of the terminal ileum and colon and creation of ileostomy and colostomy can have a significant impact on electrolyte and fluid balance. After resection, the remaining intestine undergoes structural and functional adaptation to increase fluid and nutrient absorption. However, this process can take 2 years or more (26). Patients with an ileostomy are at an increased risk for dehydration and electrolyte abnormalities (31). There is an above-average need for sodium and water to balance increased losses in the stool. Patients are commonly instructed to consume at least 1 liter more fluid than their ostomy output (32).

Bacterial Homeostasis

As discussed earlier, bacteria in the colon serve a host of functions including vitamin K and short-chain fatty acid production as well as defense against pathogenic microorganisms. The colon can contain up to 10^{11} or 10^{12} bacterial cells/gram luminal contents (33). Following surgery, bacterial overgrowth can occur as the result of impaired intestinal peristalsis or anatomical abnormalities that alter luminal flow (34). Dysfunction of the gut barrier following colon resection can lead to translocation of microorganisms, sepsis, shock, multisystem organ failure, and even death (33). Ileocolectomy has been associated with a significant increase in ileal and colonic bacterial counts (35). Bacterial overgrowth in the terminal ileum following ileocecal valve resection can adversely impact the specialized absorptive functions of the ileum.

Pancreas

Pancreatic Exocrine Function

Pancreatic enzymes play a role in the digestion of starches, proteins, and lipids. Procedures, both directly to the pancreas and to the GI tract, can affect pancreatic enzyme secretion. Impaired pancreatic enzyme function resulting from pancreatic duct obstruction, resection, or dysregulation can be compensated for, to some extent, by oral administration of pancreatic enzymes, diet modification, and a physiologic shift of the site of digestion to the distal small intestine. Partial enzyme compensation by other extrapancreatic sites (such as gastric lipase) may also occur (36). In general, derangements in postoperative pancreatic exocrine function are determined by type of resection, resection of adjacent organs, the underlying disease, and preoperative pancreatic function. After major pancreatic surgery, enzyme replacement is usually required. Pancreatic enzyme supplementation starts with 40,000–120,000 IU of lipase and is titrated according to patient response (36). The addition of a proton pump inhibitor assists in the prevention of early activation of enzymes by gastric acid (36). Pancreaticocibal asynchrony occurs when pancreatic enzyme secretion is mistimed, resulting in malabsorption. This occurs in 16%–43% of gastrectomy patients (16). Oral pancreatic enzyme replacement in this setting is helpful.

Pancreatic Endocrine Function

The type of pancreatic resection affects the extent of endocrine insufficiency. After a Whipple procedure, 20%–50% of patients develop diabetes mellitus. In some patients, hypoglycemia occurs due to postoperative insulin sensitivity in the presence of decreased glucagon secretion (36). Pylorus-preserving Whipple seems to impair endocrine function more than a traditional Whipple procedure (37). In some cases, such as in chronic pancreatitis, pancreatic head resection can improve endocrine secretion (36). Functional islet cell, or *neuroendocrine*, tumors such as insulinomas, gastrinomas, glucagonomas, and VIPomas, are a relatively rare indication for pancreatic surgery. Insulinomas cause fasting hypoglycemia. Gastrinomas are associated with recurrent ulcers, diarrhea, and gastroesophageal reflux. Glucagonomas cause erythema and diabetes (38). VIPomas secrete excessive amounts of vasoactive intestinal peptide, which causes a clinical syndrome characterized by secretory diarrhea, hypokalemia, and achlorhydria (39). Drugs such as octreotide assist in palliation with these tumors; however, the only curative option is surgery (38). Fortunately, surgery corrects most symptoms.

Liver and Gallbladder

Hepatic Protein Synthesis

The liver has important roles in protein synthesis, glucose homeostasis, bilirubin excretion, and detoxication, among other functions. Hepatic proteins are commonly categorized as positive acute-phase proteins (i.e., complement system, transport proteins, and antiproteases) or negative acute-phase proteins (i.e., albumin, prealbumin, and transferrin) (40). Positive acute-phase protein levels rise in the face of stress, and negative acute-phase protein levels decrease. These proteins are synthesized in hepatocytes and released into circulation. Albumin is the hepatic protein synthesized in the largest quantity, 12–25 grams per day, making up 40% of total hepatic protein synthesis (40). There is little storage of hepatic proteins in the liver. When protein requirements exceed availability, muscle tissue is catabolized.

Profound changes in hepatic protein synthesis occur in response to trauma and critical illness (41). Whole-body protein synthesis is modified after surgery of moderate severity (41). Mediators of inflammation, including cytokines, seem to affect serum protein levels through both alteration of normal synthesis and catabolism, and induction of capillary leak (40).

Hepatic Metabolism

The varied, complex functions of the liver include synthesis and degradation of glucose and glycogen, fatty acid metabolism, synthesis and degradation of serum proteins, detoxification of lipid soluble toxins, and metabolism of bilirubin (42). This central role of liver functions in nutrient metabolism highlights the risk of severe metabolic derangement after liver surgery. Preoperative liver disease may produce hypoalbuminemia, hyperglucagonemia, increased energy expenditure, depleted skeletal muscle mass, and anorexia prior to surgery (43). Postoperative tolerance of the liver resection as well as the liver's ability to regenerate and regain function after liver surgery varies greatly. The presence of malnutrition impacts the return of liver function and regeneration, as well as morbidity and mortality (26). Surgical techniques such as portal vein embolization can assist in preserving functional liver volume by inducing preoperative hepatic hypertrophy (42). Symptoms that limit food intake before and after liver surgery include altered taste due to zinc and magnesium deficiency, early satiety due to ascites, steatorrhea due to bile salt deficiency, anorexia, nausea, and vomiting (26).

The use of branched chain amino acids (BCAA) to treat hepatic encephalopathy and to improve liver function has been explored (43). A Cochrane review indicates little benefit and great expense associated with the use of BCAA in patients with liver disease (44). It has been suggested that patients with chronic liver disease should receive less-expensive, standard amino acid formulae when nutrition support is required, reserving the use of BCAA for patients with severe hepatic encephalopathy (45).

Abdominal Aorta

Nutrient Provision

The abdominal aorta provides blood to intestinal anatomy via the celiac trunk, the superior mesenteric artery, the inferior mesenteric artery, and the internal iliac artery (Table 5–3). Adequate blood flow is vital to the preservation of bowel integrity. Lack of adequate circulation can lead to inadequate nutrient absorption and threat to intestinal viability. Visceral ischemia/reperfusion syndrome can cause the breakdown of GI integrity. This can lead to increased gut permeability and microbial translocation (46). Mesenteric angina can lead to chronic malnutrition secondary to pain, anorexia, and altered postprandial motility. Elemental feedings, very low fat, and enteral formulas containing free amino acids provide some palliation of symptoms associated with food-induced ischemic pain (47). Adequate blood flow is also important in postoperative anastomotic healing, return of gut function, and gut hypertrophy.

Table 5–3 Structures Supplied by the Abdominal Aortic Branches

Branch	Structures Supplied
Celiac trunk	Abdominal esophagus
	Stomach
	Liver
	Gallbladder
	Duodenum (partial)
	Pancreas (partial)
Superior mesenteric artery	Pancreas (partial)
	Duodenum (partial)
	Ileum
	Jejunum
	Cecum
	Appendix
	Ascending colon
	Transverse colon (partial)
Inferior mesenteric artery	Transverse colon (partial)
	Descending colon
	Sigmoid colon
	Rectum
Internal iliac artery	Perineum

IMPACT OF MALNUTRITION ON GI AND VASCULAR SURGERY OUTCOMES

Nutrition status is an important determinant of uneventful recovery following surgery. There is a highly significant correlation between preoperative malnutrition and postoperative morbidity (48). Inadequate nutrient intake leads to changes in intermediary metabolism, tissue function, and body composition (49). Major surgery itself is linked with deterioration in nutrition status (48). Patients with more invasive surgical procedures experience higher incidence of complications, longer hospital stays, prolonged anorexia, and protein calorie malnutrition (48,50).

What is the relationship between a nutrition assessment, nutrition status, malnutrition, and severity of disease? It may be that a formal nutrition assessment does not define the presence and extent of malnutrition, but rather identifies metabolic consequences of an underlying disease that happen to coincide with derangements seen in pure starvation. In reality, it is likely that the information provided by a formal nutrition assessment reflects the metabolic consequences of *both* malnutrition and the underlying disease state. Several indices have been explored as indicators of nutrition status. Decreased albumin is associated with increased surgical mortality and morbidity, especially sepsis and healing complications (51). However, the interaction between malnutrition and the acute phase response limits the use of nutrition indicators such as albumin and prealbumin. It has been suggested that neither albumin nor weight loss in isolation are specific predictors of complications (48), but they are strong predictors within multivariable models (see Table 5–4).

Table 5–4 Relationship between Nutrition Assessment Measures and Risk of Complications

	Odds Ratio	95% Confidence Interval	P Value
BMI	1.001	1.000–1.002	0.89
Albumin	0.919	0.845–1.000	0.05
Cancer	4.232	1.317–13.594	0.015
SGA-B	3.308	1.283–8.528	0.013
SGA-C	4.410	1.293–15.042	0.018
NRI mild	1.926	0.274–13.513	0.51
NRI moderate	3.525	1.071–11.599	0.038
NRI severe	9.854	1.768–54.922	0.009

BMI, body mass index; SGA, subjective global assessment; NRI, nutrition risk index

Source: Reprinted with permission from: Sungurtekin H, Sungurtekin U, Balci C, Zencir M, Erdem E. The influence of nutritional status on complications after major intraabdominal surgery. *J Am Coll Nutr.* 2004;23(3):227–232.

Many formulae have been developed to predict the impact of nutrition status on morbidity and mortality in surgical patients. The predictive value of these formulae varies (50). Table 5–5 reviews some of these methods.

Accurate nutrition assessment of preoperative patients should include both subjective and objective data (48). The Subjective Global Assessment (SGA) is an example of an effective tool for assessment of nutrition status in hospitalized patients. The SGA utilizes physical assessment in combination with subjective assessment to predict nutrition related complications. It compares favorably with objective nutrition assessment tools (52).

NUTRITIONAL CONSIDERATIONS IN OPERATIVE PLANNING

Historically, oral and enteral tube feeding have been discouraged following GI and abdominal vascular surgical procedures. Bowel rest was thought to promote anastomotic healing and prevent nausea and vomiting (53). More recently, it has become clear that GI function returns rapidly postoperatively in most patients, and intraluminal nutrients promote bowel hypertrophy and anastomotic healing (53). The small intestine regains the ability to absorb nutrients quickly after surgery, even in the absence of peristalsis. Early enteral nutrition in surgical patients is associated with improved wound healing, maintenance of gut function, and improved gut immune function. It is also associated with decreased length of stay in intensive care (53–55). Furthermore, early resumption of oral/enteral feeding is only occasionally associated with unwanted side effects such as nausea, vomiting, colic, and anorexia. Maintenance of nutrition status perioperatively can be facilitated by careful preoperative planning and creation of a postoperative nutrition care plan (56). Failure to consider nutrition and diet issues perioperatively can result in lost opportunities to maintain nutrition status and to avoid nutrition-related complications. The following issues should be considered prior to surgery to facilitate the smoothest transition back to oral feeding.

Feeding Access

The postoperative nutrition care plan should be determined and discussed with the patient prior to surgery. It has become commonplace to establish enteral feeding access during major gastrointestinal procedures (57,58). Facilitation of early enteral feeding in patients with moderate or severe preoperative malnutrition can improve surgical outcomes (26,59,60). In these circumstances, the benefits of access outweigh the risks of access-related complications (61). In patients who are malnourished preoperatively or in whom a prolonged period of poor oral intake is anticipated (7–14 days), intraoperative placement of a feeding tube for enteral access should be strongly considered. This can take the form of a gastrostomy or jejunostomy tube, depending on the particular clinical circumstances. Situations in which the risks of establishment of enteral access may outweigh the benefits include the

Table 5–5 Nutritional Assessment Formulae/Methods in Gastrointestinal Surgery

	History/Uses	Formula
Subjective Global Assessment (SGA) (98)	Validated in a number of diverse patient populations (62)	Utilizes physical assessment, weight change, change in intake, GI symptoms, and functional capacity to assign a score of: SGA-A—well nourished SGA-B—moderately malnourished SGA-C—severely malnourished
Prognostic Nutritional Index (PNI) (63)	Validated prospectively Calculates percentage risk of an operative complication occurring in an individual Can distinguish patients at low risk for nutrition related complications (<10%) from those at high risk (>50%)	Percentage risk of complication = $158 - 16.6$ (s. albumin; g/dL) $- 0.78$ (TSF; mm) $- 0.20$ (s. transferrin; g/dL) $- 5.8$ (delayed hypersensitivity reaction)
Nutrition Risk Index (NRI) (51, 64)	Used to stratify nutrition risk in the Veterans Affairs Total Parenteral Nutrition Cooperative Study Group trial of perioperative PN Classifies individuals as either well nourished or malnourished	NRI = 1.519 (s. albumin; g/dL) + 41.7 (current weight/usual weight)
Hospital Prognostic Index (HPI) (65)	Identifies high risk patients and evaluates the efficacy of hospital therapy	HPI = 0.91(s. albumin; g/dL) $- 1.0$ (delayed hypersensitivity reaction) $- 1.44$ (sepsis rating) + 0.98 (diagnosis rating) -1.09

SGA, subjective global assessment; PNI, prognostic nutritional index; TSF, triceps skin fold; delayed hypersensitivity reaction, 0=nonreactive, 1=5 mm induration, 2= >5 mm induration; NRI, nutrition risk index; PN, total parenteral nutrition; HPI, hospital prognostic index; sepsis Rating, 1 = present, 2 = absent; diagnosis rating, 1 = cancer present, 2 = cancer not present

Source: Adapted with permission from: August DA, Huhmann MB. Nutritional care of cancer patients. In: Norton J, Barie P, Bollinger R, et al., eds. *Surgery: Basic Science and Clinical Evidence.* 2nd ed. New York: Springer Publishing; 2006.

presence of ascites, peritoneal carcinomatosis, or inoperable bowel obstruction. In the latter situation, tube placement for drainage may assist palliation.

Preoperative Education

Upper GI surgical resection is associated with significant postoperative morbidity, including dumping syndrome, delayed gastric emptying, outlet obstruction, gastroesophageal reflux, and postgastrectomy syndrome (dumping, fat maldigestion, gastric stasis, and lactose maldigestion) (52,66). Manifestation of these complications can lead to weight loss, malnutrition, and increased mortality (18). Preoperative education to inform patients of normal and abnormal postoperative events can allow them to playing an active role in their recovery, identifying signs of complications, and anticipating normal physiologic responses to GI surgery that, left untreated, can compromise nutrition status.

Nutrition education by a registered dietitian has become commonplace in many settings, including diabetes clinics and even some doctor's offices. For example, the dramatic incidence of malnutrition in bariatric surgery patients (67) has prompted many insurance companies to require preoperative nutrition education by a registered dietitian (68,69). Unfortunately, there are few data on the role of nutrition education in patients undergoing GI surgery. Several studies indicate that patients who receive preoperative education regarding expectations and pain management (70) experience less anxiety (71,72) and pain (73,74), have improved outcomes (63,75), and have increased satisfaction (76,77).

Transit Time

The most common problems related to surgery of the GI tract result from alterations in transit time. These problems may occur because of transit of solids and liquids that is too fast, too slow, or occurring in the wrong direction (16). Clinical manifestations include dumping syndrome, heartburn, feelings of fullness, pain, meteorism, abdominal distention, dysphagia, constipation, or diarrhea (16). Denervation (15,78) is one of the many causes of chronic dysmotility. Dysmotility may cause any or all of these symptoms (16).

Gastric Emptying

Delayed gastric emptying is associated with early satiety, postprandial fullness, heartburn, dysphagia, aspiration, and pneumonia. Accelerated transit of hypertonic solutions in the small intestine causes dumping syndrome, which can manifest as diarrhea (early dumping syndrome) or hypoglycemic symptoms (late dumping syndrome).

Decreased Transit Time/Malabsorption

Decreased transit time frequently occurs with removal of a large section of bowel, inflammatory bowel disease, radiation to the abdomen or pelvis, ileocecal valve resection, and ileostomy. Postoperative nutrition interventions such as limiting dietary insoluble fiber intake; small, frequent meals; and specific food elimination play a role in palliation of symptoms. However, the most effective approach is the intraoperative preservation of bowel length and LES, pylorus, and ileocecal sphincter integrity.

PERIOPERATIVE FEEDING

The indications for surgical resections of the GI tract are inherently associated with conditions that lead to malnutrition. Thus, many patients are malnourished prior to surgery. Preoperative malnutrition is associated with increased morbidity and mortality. Compounding this are the surgical effects of increased catabolism and nutrient losses. Operative trauma, in combination with anesthesia, can cause intestinal dysfunction, impairment of bowel permeability, and changes in gut-associated lymphoid tissue (53). Early initiation of SNS in the postoperative period is vital. Nutrition therapy should focus on preserving gut integrity, maintaining or even improving nutrition status, and decreasing complications.

Route of Administration

In the 1980s and 1990s, numerous studies examined the impact of route of administration on outcome (see Table 5–6). Specifically of interest were the relative

Table 5–6 Route of Nutrition Administration (26)

Route	Risks/Benefits
Enteral	Requires functioning GI tract
	Reduced cost
	Better maintenance of gut integrity; prevention of bacterial translocation
	Earlier return of bowel function postoperatively
	Reduced infection rate
	Shorter LOS
Parenteral	Should be avoided with functioning GI tract
	Invasive therapy
	Increased cost
	Increased risk of infection
	Decreased incidence of gastrointestinal upset (e.g., nausea, diarrhea)

GI, gastrointestinal; LOS, length of stay

Source: A.S.P.E.N. Board of Directors and Clinical Guidelines Task Force. Guidelines for the use of parenteral and enteral nutrition in adult and pediatric patients. *JPEN.* 2002;26(1 suppl):1SA–138SA.

benefits of enteral nutrition (EN) versus parenteral nutrition (PN) and vice versa. The majority of these studies were performed in cancer patients undergoing elective surgical resections with curative intent.

Oral Nutrition

Most patients resume oral intake within 6–9 days postoperatively (79). The American Society for Enteral and Parenteral Nutrition (ASPEN) guidelines suggest that SNS is indicated only in individuals anticipated to require support for more that 7–10 days (26), unless the patient is malnourished. Research suggests that early oral intake, in combination with epidural analgesia, and mobilization facilitate faster recovery and discharge (80,81).

Enteral Nutrition

Many trials have attempted to assess the efficacy of EN in perioperative care (60). Unfortunately, these trials are difficult to compare because of differing definitions of malnutrition and study designs. Enteral administration of nutrients postoperatively is generally acknowledged as the first choice (79). The rationale for this is that EN is theoretically more physiologic in nature, may be associated with fewer complications, and is less expensive (55). Arguments against EN include increased risk of gastrointestinal side effects. EN is generally well tolerated postoperatively. Complications of enteral feeding, such as diarrhea and nausea, can usually be corrected with temporary decreases in infusion rate.

Studies suggest EN has advantages over PN. An early meta-analysis indicated cost benefits of EN over PN (82). Subsequent meta-analyses confirmed this economic advantage and also implied a decreased risk of infection associated with EN in comparison to PN (26,56). Studies also point to decreased intestinal permeability and lower incidence of hyperglycemia in comparison to PN (83). ASPEN guidelines recommend that perioperative EN is indicated in patients anticipated to be unable to meet nutritional needs orally for a period of 7 to 10 days and whose GI tract is functional (26).

Parenteral Administration

Multiple studies have been undertaken to assess the risks and benefits of PN in surgical patients. Before drawing conclusions from these studies, it is important to understand that the studies involved heterogeneous populations. Many, but not all, included cancer patients. Some studies excluded severely malnourished patients from randomization for fear of depriving them of nutrition support, thus excluding those who might be expected to benefit most from PN. PN composition and route of administration varied widely between studies, and in many studies, the SNS regimen would today be considered suboptimal because of overfeeding and inappropriate substrate composition (60,84).

Routine administration of perioperative PN does not benefit well-nourished or mildly malnourished patients undergoing major thoracic or GI surgery (55). The large Veterans Affairs Cooperative Study Group trial of perioperative PN in 395 patients undergoing major abdominal or thoracic procedures failed to demonstrate benefit to PN given 7 to 15 days preoperatively and for at least 3 days postoperatively, except in severely malnourished patients. In fact, PN increased the risk of perioperative infectious complications, primarily pneumonia and bacteremia. However, PN did reduce the incidence of healing complications, including anastomotic dehiscence. This healing benefit balanced the increased risk of infection in moderately malnourished patients, and provided net benefit in severely malnourished patients (51). A major meta-analysis of perioperative nutrition support in surgical patients indicated early postoperative PN was associated with a 10% increased risk in postsurgical complications, and a possible benefit of 7–10 days of preoperative PN on complications (84). It is generally agreed that PN should be reserved for those patients who cannot tolerate oral or enteral tube feedings, and who are either severely malnourished or who are anticipated to tolerate adequate oral or enteral tube feedings for at least 7–10 days (26).

Timing

Following major abdominal surgery, the small bowel regains function almost immediately. Therefore, jejunal feedings are recommended for the immediate postoperative period in severely malnourished patients or those in whom a prolonged period of inadequate oral intake is expected (55). With proper planning, jejunostomy tubes can be placed intraoperatively, preventing the need for nasojejunal feeding tubes.

The results of two well-designed, prospective randomized trials of postoperative PN versus standard oral diet (SOD) (85) and of postoperative EN versus SOD (86) indicate that routine use (in all patients, including those who are *not* malnourished) of nutrition support is not indicated. Neither study showed a benefit to routine use of nutrition support, true for both EN and PN. This is in agreement with ASPEN guidelines that state SNS should be avoided unless anticipated needs exceed 7–10 days (26).

Duration

In patients in whom SNS is initiated, support should continue until oral intake meets 50% of energy requirements on several consecutive days. When intake reaches 50% of needs, SNS should be progressively weaned (87).

Composition of Feeding

There are many options for parenteral and enteral feeding formulations. The composition of the feeding can impact patient tolerance and response.

PARENTERAL FEEDING FORMULATIONS

Glutamine

Glutamine (GLN), the most abundant amino acid in the human body, is an important substrate for rapidly proliferating cells such as lymphocytes, macrophages, enterocytes, fibroblasts, and renal epithelium (88). GLN is a precursor for the synthesis of purines, pyrimidines, and amino acids and acts as a nitrogen shuttle between tissues (89). Standard PN does not contain GLN due to instability in its free form. When used in PN, GLN is provided as a dipeptide. Common GLN dipeptides that are stable in an aqueous solution are alanyl-glutamine and glycyl-glutamine (90).

Arginine

In animal models, arginine (ARG) affects nitrogen metabolism, wound healing, immunocompetence, and tumor metabolism. It is a nonessential amino acid that may become conditionally essential during periods of physiological stress. ARG is a substrate in the urea cycle and plays a role in protein, creatinine, and polyamine synthesis (89). Perioperative parenteral ARG supplementation in patients receiving colon resection produced enhanced immune responsiveness when compared to controls (91). Despite this, ARG is not commonly supplemented in PN.

ENTERAL FEEDING FORMULATIONS

Immune-Enhancing Formulae

Several studies have investigated the impact of "immunonutrition" or nutritional supplementation with micro- or macronutrients with the intent of preserving or improving immune status. Examples of immune-enhancing nutrients, presented in Table 5–7, include omega-3 fatty acids (ω-3), GLN and ARG, nucleic acids, and combinations of these nutrients. The n-3 fatty acids are essential in the diet. Omega-3 fatty acids are essential and therefore must be obtained from the diet. Additionally, ω-3 fatty acids favor production of prostaglandins in the 3-series (PGE3) and leukotrienes in the 5-series. These cytokines are associated with improved immunocompetence and reduced inflammatory responses. Omega-3 fatty acids also promote reduced levels of the PGE2 and leukotrienes in the 4-series, which are known to be immunosuppressive and proinflammatory (92,93). The n-3 fatty acids have been provided in a variety of forms, including enterally in pill form and in liquid nutrition supplements, as well as parenterally. Studies of ARG in combination with other immunonutrients indicate improved immune parameters and decreased incidence of infection. Enterally supplemented ARG alone had little impact on morbidity and mortality in two studies; however both studies were flawed (94,95). Nucleotides, administered in the form of nucleic acids, seem to stimulate nonspecific parameters of immune function, but the mechanism of action is not understood (89).

Table 5–7 Substrates with Potential Beneficial Effects for Use as Nutritional Pharmacological Agents

Substrate	Metabolic Activities	Clinical Use
Glutamine	Most abundant amino acid in the human body; nonessential Important substrate for rapidly proliferating cells such as lymphocytes, macrophages, enterocytes, fibroblasts, and renal epithelium Nitrogen shuttle between tissues Precursor for the synthesis of purines, pyrimidines, and amino acids	Potentially beneficial in stimulating postoperative return of gastrointestinal function and decrease in permeability (96); may reverse postoperative immunodepression (97)
Arginine	Nonessential amino acid, may become conditionally essential during periods of physiologic stress Substrate in the urea cycle, roles in protein, creatinine, and polyamine synthesis Effects nitrogen metabolism, wound healing, immune competence, and tumor metabolism	May improve immunologic indices postoperatively (91); Decreased incidence of postoperative fistula (95)
Nucleic acids	Stimulatory effects on nonspecific parameters of immune function Mechanism of action not understood	No clinical studies performed
Essential fatty acids	n-3 polyunsaturated fatty acids (PUFAs) favor production of 3-series prostaglandins (PGE3) and 5-series leukotrienes (immune-enhancing and anti-inflammatory) n-3 PUFAs reduce production of 2-series prostaglandins (PGE2) and 4-series leukotrienes (immunosuppressive and proinflammatory)	May improve postoperative inflammatory and immune response (98); may decrease need for ventilator and LOS in patients with major abdominal surgery (99)

PUFA, polyunsaturated fatty acids; PGE3, prostaglandin E3; PGE2, prostaglandin E2; LOS, length of stay

Source: Adapted with permission from: August DA, Huhmann MB. Nutritional Care of Cancer Patients. In: Norton J, Barie P, Bollinger R, et al., eds. *Surgery: Basic Science and Clinical Evidence.* 2nd ed. New York: Springer Publishing; 2006.

The immune-enhancing product most extensively studied contains a combination of ω-3 fatty acids, ARG, and nucleic acids. Several meta-analyses have explored the benefits of immune-enhancing EN above that of standard EN (80,100, 101). These studies indicate reduction in postoperative infections and LOS in comparison with standard feeding formulae. Although these studies are limited by the inclusion of heterogeneous patient populations and unequal provision of nutrients among groups, there appears to be a trend toward decreased infectious complications with the use of immune-enhancing EN, especially with those formulas that were high in ARG. This benefit was more significant in surgical patients as opposed to critically ill patients (101).

LONG-TERM FEEDING ISSUES

The long-term complications of upper GI resections can be placed into the following categories: abnormal transit, malassimilation, and obstruction. Table 5–8 provides a description of the manifestations of these complications as well as suggestions for dietary interventions. The long-term presence of these complications has a deleterious effect on the quality of life (102).

The success of nutrition preservation in upper GI resections often depends on patient management of eating restrictions. This includes food choices, eating habits, and quantity consumed. Rapid intake of food and inadequate mastication after major upper abdominal surgery induces symptoms of heartburn, pain, regurgitation, and vomiting (67). Preoperative and postoperative education can assist in facilitating patient compliance with dietary modifications (67,103,104).

CONCLUSION

GI resections as well as vascular surgical interventions have the potential to greatly impact the nutrition status of patients. Postoperative choice of feeding type and regimen are of the utmost importance. Preoperative planning and the development of a nutrition care plan can help to ensure immediate nutrition initiation postoperatively with rapid attainment of feeding goals. Enteral feedings should be given preference over parenteral feedings to promote gut integrity. Long-term complications should be anticipated and patients should be instructed about the dietary management of these issues.

REFERENCES

1. Pennisi E. The dynamic gut. *Science.* 2005;307:1896–1899.
2. Wanless I. Physioanatomic considerations. In: Schiff E, Sorrell M, Maddrey W, eds. *Schiff's Diseases of the Liver.* 9th ed. New York, NY: Lippincott Williams & Wilkins; 2003.
3. Canepa A, Carrea A, Menoni S, et al. Acute effects of simultaneous intraperitoneal infusion of glucose and amino acids. *Kidney Int.* 2001;59:1967–1973.
4. Pennisi E. A mouthful of microbes. *Science.* 2005;307:1899–1901.

Table 5–8 Long-Term Feeding Issues

Category	Issue	Manifestation	Nutrition Intervention
Abnormal transit	Dumping syndrome	Early: Diarrhea, bloating, nausea, tachycardia immediately—thirty minutes after a meal Late: Hypoglycemic symptoms, dizziness—90–180 minutes after a meal	Small, frequent meals Separation of solids and fluids at meals Reduction in simple carbohydrate and concentrated fat intake Increase in soluble fiber intake (16)
	Reflux esophagitis	Regurgitation of food and digestive juices causing heartburn, nausea, or vomiting	Small, frequent meals Use of antacids or sucralfate (16)
	Delayed gastric emptying/gastric stasis	Early satiety, post-prandial fullness, heartburn, dysphagia, aspiration (15)	Small frequent meals Prokinetic agents (66)
	Pancreaticocibal aschrony	Steatorrhea, frequent light, greasy stools	Addition of pancreatic enzymes at meals and snacks
Malassimilation	Reduced intake, impaired absorption, disturbed metabolism, increased loss (16)	Micronutrient deficiencies	Enteral or parenteral replacement
Obstruction	Stricture, gastric outlet obstruction	Vomiting, constipation	Enteral or parenteral nutrition support depending upon extent, Endoscopic balloon dilation or surgical stenting Promotility agent (15)
Pancreatic insufficiency	Pancreatic enzyme insufficiency	Steatorrhea, bloating	Pancreatic enzyme replacement (36)

5. Stanley S, Wynne K, McGowan B, Bloom S. Hormonal regulation of food intake. *Physiol Rev.* 2005;85:1131–1158.

6. Macdonald TT, Monteleone G. Immunity, inflammation, and allergy in the gut. *Science.* 2005;307:1920–1925.

7. Mestecky J, Russell MW, Elson CO. Intestinal IgA: Novel views on its function in the defence of the largest mucosal surface. *Gut.* 1999;44:2–5.

8. Fink MP. Intestinal epithelial hyperpermeability: Update on the pathogenesis of gut mucosal barrier dysfunction in critical illness. *Curr Opin Crit Care.* 2003;9:143–151.

9. Gilliland SE, Speck ML. Deconjugation of bile acids by intestinal lactobacilli. *Appl Environ Microbiol.* 1977;33:15–18.

10. Saitoh O, Sugi K, Lojima K, et al. Increased prevalence of intestinal inflammation in patients with liver cirrhosis. *World J Gastroenterol.* 1999;5:391–396.

11. Sun Z, Wang X, Andersson R. Role of intestinal permeability in monitoring mucosal barrier function. History, methodology, and significance of pathophysiology. *Dig Surg.* 1998;15:386–397.

12. Genuit T, Napolitano L. Peritonitis and abdominal sepsis. Available at: www.emedicine.com/med/topic2737.htm. Accessed September 15, 2005.

13. Alden SM, Frank E, Flancbaum L. Abdominal candidiasis in surgical patients. *Am Surg.* 1989;55:45–49.

14. Allard JP, Chau J, Sandokji K, Blendis LM, Wong F. Effects of ascites resolution after successful TIPS on nutrition in cirrhotic patients with refractory ascites. *Am J Gastroenterol.* 2001;96:2442–2447.

15. Lerut TE, van Lanschot JJ. Chronic symptoms after subtotal or partial oesophagectomy: Diagnosis and treatment. *Best Pract Res Clin Gastroenterol.* 2004;18:901–915.

16. Scholmerich J. Postgastrectomy syndromes—Diagnosis and treatment. *Best Pract Res Clin Gastroenterol.* 2004;18:917–933.

17. Shibuya S, Fukudo S, Shineha R, et al. High incidence of reflux esophagitis observed by routine endoscopic examination after gastric pull-up esophagectomy. *World J Surg.* 2003;27:580–583.

18. Rey-Ferro M, Castano R, Orozco O, Serna A, Moreno A. Nutritional and immunologic evaluation of patients with gastric cancer before and after surgery. *Nutrition.* 1997;13:878–881.

19. Oh R, Brown DL. Vitamin B_{12} deficiency. *Am Fam Physician.* 2003;67:979–986.

20. Malouf M, Grimley EJ, Areosa SA. Folic acid with or without vitamin B_{12} for cognition and dementia. *Cochrane Database Syst Rev.* 2003:CD004514.

21. Adachi S, Kawamoto T, Otsuka M, Todoroki T, Fukao K. Enteral vitamin B_{12} supplements reverse postgastrectomy B_{12} deficiency. *Ann Surg.* 2000;232:199–201.

22. Pereira SP, Gainsborough N, Dowling RH. Drug-induced hypochlorhydria causes high duodenal bacterial counts in the elderly. *Aliment Pharmacol Ther.* 1998;12:99–104.

23. Williams C. Occurrence and significance of gastric colonization during acid-inhibitory therapy. *Best Pract Res Clin Gastroenterol.* 2001;15:511–521.

24. Houben GM, Stockbrugger RW. Bacteria in the aetio-pathogenesis of gastric cancer: A review. *Scand J Gastroenterol Suppl.* 1995;212:13–18.

25. Lahner E, Bordi C, Cattaruzza MS, et al. Long-term follow-up in atrophic body gastritis patients: Atrophy and intestinal metaplasia are persistent lesions irrespective of Helicobacter pylori infection. *Aliment Pharmacol Ther.* 2005;22:471–481.

26. Directors ASPEN. Guidelines for the use of parenteral and enteral nutrition in adult and pediatric patients. *JPEN.* 2002;26(1 suppl):1SA–138SA.

27. Uchida H, Yamamoto H, Kisaki Y, Fujino J, Ishimaru Y, Ikeda H. D-lactic acidosis in short-bowel syndrome managed with antibiotics and probiotics. *J Pediatr Surg.* 2004;39:634–636.

28. De Groote MA, Frank DN, Dowell E, Glode MP, Pace NR. Lactobacillus rhamnosus GG bacteremia associated with probiotic use in a child with short gut syndrome. *Pediatr Infect Dis J.* 2005;24:278–280.

29. Ziegler TR, Evans ME, Fernandez-Estivariz C, Jones DP. Trophic and cytoprotective nutrition for intestinal adaptation, mucosal repair, and barrier function. *Annu Rev Nutr.* 2003;23:229–261.

30. Salminen S, von Wright A, Morelli L, et al. Demonstration of safety of probiotics—A review. *Int J Food Microbiol.* 1998;44:93–106.

31. Phang PT, Hain JM, Perez-Ramirez JJ, Madoff RD, Gemlo BT. Techniques and complications of ileostomy takedown. *Am J Surg.* 1999;177:463–466.

32. Beyer P. Medical nutrition therapy for lower gastrointestinal tract disorders. In: Maham L, Escott-Stump S, eds. *Krause's Food, Nutrition, and Diet Therapy.* 11th ed. New York, NY: Elsevier; 2004:705–737.

33. Guarner F, Malagelada JR. Gut flora in health and disease. *Lancet.* 2003;361:512–519.

34. Husebye E. The pathogenesis of gastrointestinal bacterial overgrowth. *Chemotherapy.* 2005;51 (suppl 1):1–22.

35. Neut C, Bulois P, Desreumaux P, et al. Changes in the bacterial flora of the neoterminal ileum after ileocolonic resection for Crohn's disease. *Am J Gastroenterol.* 2002;97:939–946.

36. Kahl S, Malfertheiner P. Exocrine and endocrine pancreatic insufficiency after pancreatic surgery. *Best Pract Res Clin Gastroenterol.* 2004;18:947–955.

37. Buchler MW, Friess H, Muller MW, Wheatley AM, Beger HG. Randomized trial of duodenum-preserving pancreatic head resection versus pylorus-preserving Whipple in chronic pancreatitis. *Am J Surg.* 1995;169:65–69; discussion 69–70.

38. Pereira PL, Wiskirchen J. Morphological and functional investigations of neuroendocrine tumors of the pancreas. *Eur Radiol.* 2003;13:2133–2146.

39. Nikou GC, Toubanakis C, Nikolaou P, et al. VIPomas: An update in diagnosis and management in a series of 11 patients. *Hepatogastroenterology.* 2005;52:1259–1265.

40. Fuhrman MP, Charney P, Mueller CM. Hepatic proteins and nutrition assessment. *J Am Diet Assoc.* 2004;104:1258–1264.

41. Barle H, Nyberg B, Essen P, et al. The synthesis rates of total liver protein and plasma albumin determined simultaneously in vivo in humans. *Hepatology.* 1997;25:154–158.

42. Schneider PD. Preoperative assessment of liver function. *Surg Clin North Am.* 2004;84:355–373.

43. Marchesini G, Marzocchi R, Noia M, Bianchi G. Branched-chain amino acid supplementation in patients with liver diseases. *J Nutr.* 2005;135(6 suppl):1596S–1601S.

44. Als-Nielson B, Koretz R, Kjaergard L, Gluud C. Branched-chain amino acids for hepatic encephalopathy. *Cochrane Database of Systematic Reviews.* 2005.

45. Poon RT, Fan ST. Perioperative nutritional support in liver surgery. *Nutrition.* 2000;16:75–76.

46. Karwowska KA, Dworacki G, Trybus M, Zeromski J, Szulc R. Influence of glutamine-enriched parenteral nutrition on nitrogen balance and immunologic status in patients undergoing elective aortic aneurysm repair. *Nutrition.* 2001;17:475–478.

47. El-Matary W, Sharples P, Sandhu B. Use of elemental feed in mesenteric ischemia. *J Pediatr Gastroenterol Nutr.* 2003;37:85–86.

48. Dannhauser A, Van Zyl JM, Nel CJ. Preoperative nutritional status and prognostic nutritional index in patients with benign disease undergoing abdominal operations—Part I. *J Am Coll Nutr.* 1995;14:80–90.

49. Sungurtekin H, Sungurtekin U, Balci C, Zencir M, Erdem E. The influence of nutritional status on complications after major intraabdominal surgery. *J Am Coll Nutr.* 2004;23:227–232.

50. Hirsch S, de Obaldia N, Petermann M, et al. Nutritional status of surgical patients and the relationship of nutrition to postoperative outcome. *J Am Coll Nutr.* 1992;11:21–24.

51. The Veterans Affairs Total Parenteral Nutrition Cooperative Study Group. Perioperative total parenteral nutrition in surgical patients. *N Engl J Med.* 1991;325:525–532.

52. Gupta D, Lammersfeld CA, Vashi PG, Burrows J, Lis CG, Grutsch JF. Prognostic significance of Subjective Global Assessment (SGA) in advanced colorectal cancer. *Eur J Clin Nutr.* 2005;59:35–40.

53. Gabor S, Renner H, Matzi V, et al. Early enteral feeding compared with parenteral nutrition after oesophageal or oesophagogastric resection and reconstruction. *Br J Nutr.* 2005;93:509–513.

54. Andersen H, Lewis S, Thomas S. Early enteral nutrition within 24h of colorectal surgery versus later commencement of feeding for postoperative complications. *Cochrane Database of Systematic Reviews.* Vol. 4. Cochrane Database of Systematic Reviews; 2005.

55. Fearon KC, Luff R. The nutritional management of surgical patients: Enhanced recovery after surgery. *Proc Nutr Soc.* 2003;62:807–811.

56. Braunschweig CL, Levy P, Sheean PM, Wang X. Enteral compared with parenteral nutrition: A meta-analysis. *Am J Clin Nutr.* 2001;74:534–542.

57. Date RS, Clements WD, Gilliland R. Feeding jejunostomy: Is there enough evidence to justify its routine use? *Dig Surg.* 2004;21:142–145.

58. Jensen GL, Sporay G, Whitmire S, Taraszewski R, Reed MJ. Intraoperative placement of the nasoenteric feeding tube: A practical alternative? *JPEN.* 1995;19:244–247.

59. Klein S, Koretz RL. Nutrition support in patients with cancer: What do the data really show? *Nutr Clin Pract.* 1994;9:91–100.

60. August D, Huhmann M. Nutritional care of cancer patients. In: Norton J, Barie P, Bollinger R, et al., eds. *Surgery: Basic Science and Clinical Evidence.* 2nd ed. New York, NY: Springer Publishing; 2006.

61. Gerndt SJ, Orringer MB. Tube jejunostomy as an adjunct to esophagectomy. *Surgery.* 1994;115: 164–169.

62. Detsky AS, McLaughlin JR, Baker JP, et al. What is subjective global assessment of nutritional status? *JPEN.* 1987;11:8–13.

63. Buzby GP, Mullen JL, Matthews DC, Hobbs CL, Rosato EF. Prognostic nutritional index in gastrointestinal surgery. *Am J Surg.* 1980;139:160–167.

64. Franch-Arcas G. The meaning of hypoalbuminaemia in clinical practice. *Clin Nutr.* 2001;20:265–269.

65. Harvey KB, Moldawer LL, Bistrian BR, Blackburn GL. Biological measures for the formulation of a hospital prognostic index. *Am J Clin Nutr.* 1981;34:2013–2022.

66. Radigan A. Post-gastrectomy: Managing the nutrition fall-out. *Practical Gastroenterol.* 2004;28:63–75.

67. Israel A, Sebbag G, Fraser D, Levy I. Nutritional behavior as a predictor of early success after vertical gastroplasty. *Obes Surg.* 2005;15:88–94.

68. Madan AK, Tichansky DS. Patients postoperatively forget aspects of preoperative patient education. *Obes Surg.* 2005;15:1066–1069.

69. Garza SF. Bariatric weight loss surgery: Patient education, preparation, and follow-up. *Crit Care Nurs Q.* 2003;26:101–104.

70. Watt-Watson J, Stevens B, Katz J, Costello J, Reid GJ, David T. Impact of preoperative education on pain outcomes after coronary artery bypass graft surgery. *Pain.* 2004;109:73–85.

71. Danino AM, Chahraoui K, Frachebois L, et al. Effects of an informational CD-ROM on anxiety and knowledge before aesthetic surgery: A randomised trial. *Br J Plast Surg.* 2005;58:379–383.

72. Pager CK. Randomised controlled trial of preoperative information to improve satisfaction with cataract surgery. *Br J Ophthalmol.* 2005;89:10–13.

73. Sjoling M, Nordahl G, Olofsson N, Asplund K. The impact of preoperative information on state anxiety, postoperative pain and satisfaction with pain management. *Patient Educ Couns.* 2003;51:169–176.

74. Ratanalert S, Soontrapornchai P, Ovartlarnporn B. Preoperative education improves quality of patient care for endoscopic retrograde cholangiopancreatography. *Gastroenterol Nurs.* 2003;26: 21–25.

75. Giraudet-Le Quintrec JS, Coste J, Vastel L, et al. Positive effect of patient education for hip surgery: A randomized trial. *Clin Orthop Relat Res.* 2003:112–120.

76. Snyder-Ramos SA, Seintsch H, Bottiger BW, Motsch J, Martin E, Bauer M. Patient satisfaction and information gain after the preanesthetic visit: A comparison of face-to-face interview, brochure, and video. *Anesth Analg.* 2005;100:1753–1758.

77. Asilioglu K, Celik SS. The effect of preoperative education on anxiety of open cardiac surgery patients. *Patient Educ Couns.* 2004;53:65–70.

78. Koda K, Saito N, Seike K, Shimizu K, Kosugi C, Miyazaki M. Denervation of the neorectum as a potential cause of defecatory disorder following low anterior resection for rectal cancer. *Dis Colon Rectum.* 2005;48:210–217.

79. Huckleberry Y. Nutritional support and the surgical patient. *Am J Health Syst Pharm.* 2004;61: 671–682.

80. Heys SD, Walker LG, Smith I, Eremin O. Enteral nutritional supplementation with key nutrients in patients with critical illness and cancer: A meta-analysis of randomized controlled clinical trials. *Ann Surg.* 1999;229:467–477.

81. Holte K, Kehlet H. Epidural anaesthesia and analgesia—Effects on surgical stress responses and implications for postoperative nutrition. *Clin Nutr.* 2002;21:199–206.

82. Lipman TO. Grains or veins: Is enteral nutrition really better than parenteral nutrition? A look at the evidence. *JPEN.* 1998;22:167–182.

83. Heys SD, Ogston KN. Peri-operative nutritional support: Controversies and debates. *Int J Surg Investig.* 2000;2:107–115.

84. Klein S, Kinney J, Jeejeebhoy K, et al. Nutrition support in clinical practice: Review of published data and recommendations for future research directions. *JPEN.* 1997;21:133–156.

85. Brennan MF, Pisters PW, Posner M, Quesada O, Shike M. A prospective randomized trial of total parenteral nutrition after major pancreatic resection for malignancy. *Ann Surg.* 1994;220:436–441; discussion 441–434.

86. Heslin MJ, Latkany L, Leung D, et al. A prospective, randomized trial of early enteral feeding after resection of upper gastrointestinal malignancy. *Ann Surg.* 1997;226:567–577; discussion 577–580.

87. Charney P. Enteral nutrition: Indications, options, and formulations. In: Gottschlich M, ed. *The Science and Practice of Nutrition Support.* Dubuque, Iowa: Kendall/Hunt Publishing; 2001:141–166.

88. Savarese DM, Savy G, Vahdat L, Wischmeyer PE, Corey B. Prevention of chemotherapy and radiation toxicity with glutamine. *Cancer Treat Rev.* 2003;29:501–513.

89. Heys SD, Gough DB, Khan L, Eremin O. Nutritional pharmacology and malignant disease: A therapeutic modality in patients with cancer. *Br J Surg.* 1996;83:608–619.

90. Scheid C, Hermann K, Kremer G, et al. Randomized, double-blind, controlled study of glycyl-glutamine-dipeptide in the parenteral nutrition of patients with acute leukemia undergoing intensive chemotherapy. *Nutrition.* 2004;20:249–254.

91. Song JX, Qing SH, Huang XC, Qi DL. Effect of parenteral nutrition with L-arginine supplementation on postoperative immune function in patients with colorectal cancer. *Di Yi Jun Yi Da Xue Xue Bao.* 2002;22:545–547.

92. Jho DH, Cole SM, Lee EM, Espat NJ. Role of omega-3 fatty acid supplementation in inflammation and malignancy. *Integr Cancer Ther.* 2004;3:98–111.

93. Hardman WE. Omega-3 fatty acids to augment cancer therapy. *J Nutr.* 2002;132(11 suppl): 3508S–3512S.

94. van Bokhorst-De Van Der Schueren MA, Quak JJ, von Blomberg-van der Flier BM, et al. Effect of perioperative nutrition, with and without arginine supplementation, on nutritional status, immune function, postoperative morbidity, and survival in severely malnourished head and neck cancer patients. *Am J Clin Nutr.* 2001;73:323–332.

95. de Luis DA, Izaola O, Cuellar L, Terroba MC, Aller R. Randomized clinical trial with an enteral arginine-enhanced formula in early postsurgical head and neck cancer patients. *Eur J Clin Nutr.* 2004;58:1505–1508.

96. De-Souza DA, Greene LJ. Intestinal permeability and systemic infections in critically ill patients: Effect of glutamine. *Crit Care Med.* 2005;33:1125–1135.

97. Yao GX, Xue XB, Jiang ZM, Yang NF, Wilmore DW. Effects of perioperative parenteral glutamine-dipeptide supplementation on plasma endotoxin level, plasma endotoxin inactivation capacity and clinical outcome. *Clin Nutr.* 2005;24:510–515.

98. Nakamura K, Kariyazono H, Komokata T, Hamada N, Sakata R, Yamada K. Influence of preoperative administration of omega-3 fatty acid-enriched supplement on inflammatory and immune responses in patients undergoing major surgery for cancer. *Nutrition.* 2005;21:639–649.

99. Tsekos E, Reuter C, Stehle P, Boeden G. Perioperative administration of parenteral fish oil supplements in a routine clinical setting improves patient outcome after major abdominal surgery. *Clin Nutr.* 2004;23:325–330.

100. Beale RJ, Bryg DJ, Bihari DJ. Immunonutrition in the critically ill: A systematic review of clinical outcome. *Crit Care Med.* 1999;27:2799–2805.

101. Heyland DK, Novak F, Drover JW, Jain M, Su X, Suchner U. Should immunonutrition become routine in critically ill patients? A systematic review of the evidence. *JAMA.* 2001;286 944–953.

102. McLarty AJ, Deschamps C, Trastek VF, Allen MS, Pairolero PC, Harmsen WS. Esophageal resection for cancer of the esophagus: Long-term function and quality of life. *Ann Thorac Surg.* 1997;63:1568–1572.

103. Chaudhri S, Brown L, Hassan I, Horgan AF. Preoperative intensive, community-based vs. traditional stoma education: A randomized, controlled trial. *Dis Colon Rectum.* 2005;48:504–509.

104. Ikeuchi H, Yamamura T, Nakano H, Kosaka T, Shimoyama T, Fukuda Y. Efficacy of nutritional therapy for perforating and non-perforating Crohn's disease. *Hepatogastroenterology.* 2004;51: 1050–1052.

CHAPTER 6

Bariatric Surgery

Scott A. Shikora, MD, FACS; Leonardo Claros, MD;
and Margaret Furtado, MS, RD, LD/N

INTRODUCTION

Bariatric surgery can achieve significant and sustainable weight loss. However, the current operative procedures alter gastrointestinal (GI) anatomy and/or physiology and may radically change dietary habits. For these reasons, nutritional complications may develop. Therefore, a thorough understanding of the potential long-term consequences, lifelong patient surveillance, and the appropriate intervention are important to maximize the likelihood of a successful outcome.

Each year, more than 300,000 deaths are attributed to obesity in the United States, making obesity the second leading cause of preventable death behind tobacco (1,2). Four of five obese people have at least one debilitating illness associated with underlying obesity. Bariatric surgery has been recognized as the only treatment for morbid obesity that can achieve meaningful and sustainable weight loss. The introduction of minimally invasive surgical approaches to treat obesity and the very public experience with surgery of a few celebrities have led to a tremendous interest in bariatric operations. As a result, bariatric surgery is currently the most rapidly growing field of surgery. Therefore, a larger number of patients (approximately 190,000 for 2006) are having surgery and are in great need of careful and meticulous long-term follow-up in order to prevent them from developing nutritional complications. All clinicians, the vast majority of whom are not directly involved in bariatric surgery, will be/are caring for patients who have had weight-loss surgery.

It is well known that the currently performed bariatric procedures result in dramatic changes in GI anatomy, physiology, and/or dietary habits and that good surgical results do not ensure a successful outcome. Additionally, these anatomic and physiologic changes could result in devastating complications. Therefore, bariatric patients require close and detailed follow-up. The long-term consequences of bariatric surgery will vary according to the procedure performed. Some complications are common to all procedures while others may be specific to one operative procedure. For the nutritional derangements, the etiology may be multifactorial, i.e., secondary to the dramatic reduction of macro- and micronutrient intake, altered dietary choices, and/or nutrient malabsorption. The degree of the deficiencies will be determined not only by the specific operative procedure, but also by the dietary habits of the individual patient. Some deficiencies may develop quickly, while others develop slowly and in an insidious manner. For nutritional complications, a misdiagnosis, an inability to diagnose, or a delay in diagnosis may all have severe consequences. Therefore, a solid knowledge of these issues and an understanding of the treatments are necessary to minimize their impact and achieve the best outcomes.

COMMONLY PERFORMED BARIATRIC PROCEDURES

In order to better understand the potential long-term consequences of bariatric surgery, it is imperative to become familiar with the most commonly performed procedures. For the sake of this chapter, we will limit discussion to the most commonly performed operative procedures, roux-en-Y gastric bypass (RYGBP), laparoscopic adjustable gastric band (LAGB), and the biliopancreatic diversion with or without duodenal switch (BPD+/-DS) (see Figures 6–1 through 6–4). A variety

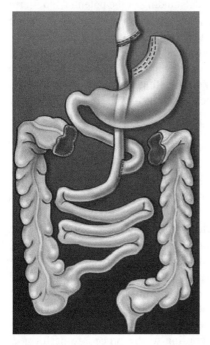

Figure 6–1 Roux-en-Y Gastric Bypass

Source: Reprinted with permission from the American Society for Bariatric Surgery.

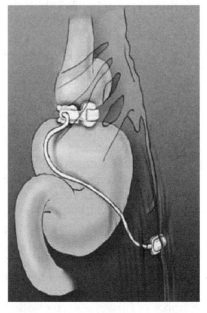

Figure 6–2 Adjustable Gastric Bypass

Source: Reprinted with permission from the American Society for Bariatric Surgery.

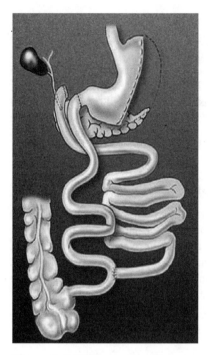

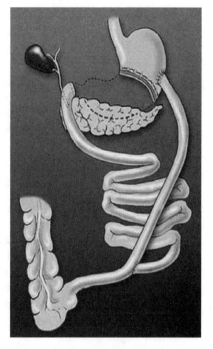

Figure 6–3 Biliopancreatic Diversion with Duodenal Switch

Source: Reprinted with permission from the American Society for Bariatric Surgery.

Figure 6–4 Biliopancreatic Diversion without Duodenal Switch

Source: Reprinted with permission from the American Society for Bariatric Surgery.

of these procedures are available; essentially, the mechanism by which weight loss occurs is either through restriction of food intake (restrictive procedures), the limiting of nutrient absorption (malabsorptive procedures), or a combination of both.

The LAGB is a restrictive procedure in which an adjustable silicone band connected to a subcutaneous saline port is placed encircling the proximal portion of the stomach, creating a small pouch of 15–30 cc. The absence of a staple line and of the associated risk of staple line dehiscence is a theoretical advantage of this procedure, dramatically reducing the operative and long-term complications. The mortality is reported to be a mere 0.1% (3).

Gastric bypass was first developed by Edward Mason from the observation that patients with a small gastric remnant after subtotal gastrectomy experienced significant weight loss. The RYGBP also relies on a small gastric pouch reservoir of 15–30 cc, which is created by surgical stapling devices. The pouch drains through a narrow anastomosis into a roux limb of jejunum. Weight loss is due predominantly to nutrient restriction. However, the bypass of the fundus, duodenum, and proximal jejunum may contribute to the weight loss by influencing gut hormones, such as ghrelin, and by causing aversions to high sugar food with the dumping syndrome.

The principle mechanism for weight loss of the BPD+/-DS is the malabsorption of the ingested nutrients. The biliary and pancreatic secretions are diverted into the distal 50 cm of the ileum, thereby preventing them from exposure to the nutrient stream in most of the small intestine. A small degree of gastric restriction is also added by performing a partial gastrectomy. This is done to mildly reduce the gastric reservoir volume. Subsequently, an anastomosis is created between the distal ileum to the stomach pouch or duodenum. Nutrients bypass the majority of the small bowel. Weight loss is mainly due to the limited intestinal absorptive capacity in the terminal ileum.

THE SIGNIFICANCE OF LONG-TERM FOLLOW-UP

There is generally believed to be a close correlation between weight-loss success and patient well-being with aggressive follow-up, especially during the first year when patient monitoring is most critical. At these visits, weight loss is monitored, and patients are evaluated for overall health, vitamin levels, medication titration, activity level, dietary habits, bowel function, and hydration status. After the first postoperative year, patients are seen less frequently, generally once or twice yearly. However, at these visits, patients should be assessed for nutritional deficiencies, appropriateness of their diet, weight maintenance, the presence of symptoms, and for overall health.

NUTRITIONAL DEFICIENCIES

In order to better understand the potential deficiencies that can develop after surgery, it is also important to know where along the gastrointestinal tract that the macro- and micronutrients are absorbed (Figure 6–5). Procedures that reroute the nutrient stream away from the gastric acid and/or the proximal small intestine can be assumed to put patients at risk for developing deficiencies, such as iron, vitamin B_{12}, folic acid, and calcium. Some nutrients are preferentially absorbed more proximally in the GI tract and others more distally. In addition, certain nutrients require specialized mixing for maximal absorption. For example, iron represents both. It is preferentially absorbed in the proximal small intestine and is best absorbed after contact with an acid environment. Therefore, the type and severity of nutrient deficiency will vary according to the operative procedure performed (see Table 6–1).

PROTEIN-CALORIE MALNUTRITION

The gastric restrictive procedures, including the RYGBP, rarely cause protein-calorie malnutrition. The weight loss seen is predominantly from fat with only minimal changes in lean body tissue (4,5). However, in patients with dysfunctional eating habits such as anorexia or the avoidance of protein food sources and in patients with protracted vomiting, protein malnutrition can occur. For the malab-

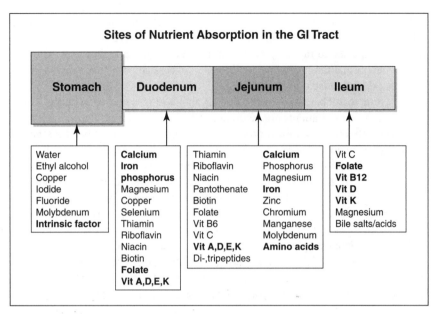

Figure 6–5 Nutrient Absorption and the GI Tract

sorptive procedures, such as the distal gastric bypass and the BPD+/-DS, malnutrition is not uncommon because ingested protein may also be lost in the stool. The incidence has been reported to be approximately 7%–21% (6). With these procedures, hypoalbuminemia is commonly seen within 6 months after surgery but gradually returns to preoperative levels. Tacchino et al. studied changes in total and segmental body composition at 2, 6, 12, and 24 months postoperative BPD. They discovered that weight loss after BPD was achieved with an appropriate decline of lean body mass and all parameters reaching at stable weight, values similar to weight-matched controls (7). However, the yearly hospitalization rate for protein deficiency after BPD is reported to be 1%. Persistent hypoalbuminemia and its associated complications led to revisional surgery in 1%–2% of patients who underwent BPD with duodenal switch (8).

Table 6–1 Likelihood of Vitamin/Mineral Deficiencies after Bariatric Procedures

Procedure	Iron	Folate	Vitamin B_{12}	Calcium	Vitamin D	Thiamine
LapBand/VBG	**	**	*	*	*	*
RYGBP	***	**	***	**	**	*
BPD	***	**	***	**	**	*

Note: * = Not very likely; ** = Somewhat likely; *** = Highly likely

Unfortunately, diagnosing protein malnutrition may be challenging. Although clinical signs of protein malnutrition can be seen even in overweight patients, patients are expected to rapidly lose weight and thus serum protein levels will often stay in the normal range (9–11). Additionally, excess adipose tissue masks visible signs of skeletal muscle wasting.

Therefore, for all bariatric patients, dietary monitoring is important during weight loss and long term. Patients are instructed to follow a high-protein diet to include approximately 60–80 grams of protein daily. Higher intake may be necessary for those patients who underwent the malabsorptive procedures. Protein-intake guidance should be guided not only by serum protein levels but also by diet and bowel habit activity. In the most extreme or intractable cases, common channel limb lengthening, or even reversal, may be necessary to improve protein absorption.

Severe calorie deficiency (*cachexia*) is also unusual after bariatric surgery but may be seen in patients with protracted vomiting, diarrhea, or anorexia. Treatment includes nutritional supplementation (even involuntary, if necessary), correction of any underlying anatomical abnormalities (i.e., stricture, obstruction), and/or psychologic intervention as indicated. In the most extreme or intractable cases, common channel limb lengthening, or even reversal, may also be necessary.

DEHYDRATION

Mild dehydration is commonly seen in the early postoperative period in patients who have had any of the bariatric procedures (as in any other surgical patient), mainly due to decreased fluid intake. Patients who have had restrictive procedures have difficulty drinking the necessary amount of fluid as they adapt to very small gastric capacities. Additionally, with the malabsorptive procedures, frequent watery stools are a source of significant fluid loss. Vomiting or diarrhea may also exacerbate fluid losses. On the basis of body weight, obese patients require a greater amount of fluid per day to maintain normal fluid balance than their lean counterparts. This volume is obtained directly from the liquid consumed and indirectly from the water in the food eaten. Standard fluid recommendations are impossible, given the heterogeneity of the patients. In addition, there are no mathematical equations that accurately estimate fluid needs in the obese. Patients are instructed to use thirst and urine concentration as a guide for fluid intake and to monitor their hydration status via awareness of potential signs of dehydration, such as dizziness and dry skin. Fluid status can be managed by encouraging patients to travel with a fluid source (e.g., water bottle) and to drink continuously throughout the day, one swallow at a time, until the symptoms of dehydration are relieved. If dehydration occurs, these patients have great difficulty catching up because they cannot drink fluid quickly. For those patients with vomiting and an inability to tolerate oral intake, intravenous fluids may be necessary to restore intravascular volume. Dehydration may also cause nausea, which may exacerbate intolerance to the diet or fluids. Therefore, it is critical that patients drink enough fluid postoperatively to prevent dehydration. Intake of 64 ounces of fluid per day is recommended. However, some patients may even require more, especially if they are extremely heavy, physically active, or live in a humid climate.

Patients should be frequently reminded that meeting their fluid goal takes precedence over food, including protein intake. Whenever possible, postoperative patients suffering from dehydration who are unable to ingest adequate protein from solid foods alone should include high-protein, low-carbohydrate liquid supplements in their diet. In order to minimize the risk of dumping syndrome, patients are often advised to select supplements 13 grams (or less) of sugars per serving.

NAUSEA AND VOMITING

Nausea and vomiting are common after gastric restrictive surgery. In many cases, dysfunctional eating habits (such as overeating, eating too fast, or not chewing food well) cause these symptoms. However, other causes, including dumping syndrome, medication intolerance, anastomotic strictures, and marginal ulcers, must be ruled out. A thorough history may help differentiate causes. For example, a patient who develops solid food intolerance approximately 4–6 weeks after surgery, which necessitates a change in diet to only liquids, may have an anastomotic stricture. On the other hand, a patient who becomes nauseated or vomits only occasionally and without any obvious pattern is most likely to be eating incorrectly (e.g., too quickly, excessive volume of food).

VITAMIN/MINERAL DEFICIENCIES

Vitamin and/or mineral deficiencies are prevalent after all bariatric procedures and in particular after gastric bypass and biliopancreatic diversion (11–28). After surgery, all patients may be at risk for an array of dietary vitamin and/or mineral deficiencies and therefore should comply with lifelong supplementation. Of note, micronutrient deficiencies may develop slowly and not become evident until years after surgery (see Table 6–2). Therefore, patients need to be seen annually.

The gastric restrictive procedures generally cause few micronutrient deficiencies (14). This is presumably because nutrients aren't diverted from the duodenum and gastric mixing is essentially normal. However, deficiencies may develop in those patients with intractable vomiting or among those with suboptimal nutrient intake. Intake may be inadequate because the meal size is dramatically reduced, and because many patients change their dietary choices. For example, many of these patients do not tolerate red meat, so they may avoid it altogether. Gastric bypass patients are at additional risk due to the fact that the nutrient stream bypasses the fundus, duodenum, and proximal jejunum, causing malabsorption of iron, folate, calcium, and vitamin B_{12}.

The malabsorptive procedures such as the BPD+/-DS place patients at even greater risk for deficiencies of the noted vitamins and calcium, as well as for the fat-soluble vitamins (A, D, E, and K); electrolytes such as sodium, potassium, chloride, phosphorus, magnesium; and possibly even zinc (18,25). For all bariatric

Table 6–2 Nutritional Deficiencies Can Be Seen Months after Gastric Bypass Surgery

Laboratory Value	% Abnormal Values Preoperatively	Mean Abnormal Value	Month First Observed
Potassium	56 (7)	3.2+0.1 mEq/L	6+10
Magnesium	. 34 (4)	1.3+0.1 mEq/L	15+16
Albumin	0 (5)		
Vitamin A	10 (5)	11+6 ug/dl	31+22
Vitamin B_{12}	64 (3)	166+27 pg/ml	28+18
Folate	38 (11)	1.8+0.6 ng/ml	15+11
Iron	49 (4)	43+11 ug/dl	27+12

Source: Adapted from Halverson JD. Micronutrient deficiencies after gastric bypass for morbid obesity. *Am Surg.* 1986;52:594–598.

patients, serum levels need to be aggressively followed annually, and supplementation should be prescribed judiciously. Because many bariatric programs rely on different supplementation protocols, there is no consensus as to what represents the optimal regimen. However, there is general agreement concerning the importance of lifelong surveillance of patients' vitamin/mineral status. Table 6–3 presents the specific vitamin and mineral supplementation protocol for the Obesity Consult Center at Tufts-New England Medical Center in Boston.

Iron

Iron deficiency is commonly found in bariatric patients, and in particular, in premenopausal women (16,19,24,27,28). Among super-obese patients undergoing RYGBP, iron deficiency was discovered in 49% to 52% and anemia in 35% to 74% after 3 years, depending on the Roux limb length (29). Microcytosis was not observed in approximately one third of the iron-deficient women, so this may not be a reliable marker. The etiology for iron deficiency is multifactorial. It is partly due to the nutrient restriction that limits intake of dietary iron. In addition, after RYGBP and the BPD, malabsorption of iron also occurs. Iron absorption is facilitated by gastric acid. After RYGBP, gastric acid production is dramatically reduced in the small gastric pouch (15). In addition, iron is predominantly absorbed in the duodenum and proximal jejunum. Both RYGBP and BPD reroute the nutrient stream from the upper stomach pouch directly into the jejunum or ileum, thereby avoiding the duodenum altogether. Therefore, patients are unlikely to maintain normal serum levels of iron or iron saturation after these procedures. The BPD+/-DS keeps the duodenum in the nutrient circuit but bypasses all of the jejunum. Finally, patients who do not tolerate or avoid meat in their diet will be more likely to be iron deficient (10).

Table 6–3 Vitamin/Mineral Supplementation Protocols for Treating Deficiencies

All Patients Postoperatively
Complete MVI with iron P.O. qd.
Calcium with vitamin D 1200–1500 mg P.O. qd.
Patients should be advised against taking a calcium supplement that does not
include vitamin D.

Specific Vitamin/Mineral

Iron
Fe sat <10% and ferritin <10 ng/ml or Fe sat <7% (regardless of ferritin)
Supplement with $FeSO_4$ 325 mg plus 250 mg vitamin C P.O. qd
Increase to TID as tolerated; patient is instructed to take with orange
juice.

Folate
If red blood cell (RBC) folate level is low:
First replete vitamin B_{12}
1 mg of folate P.O. qd × 3 months

Vitamin B_{12}
If neurologic symptoms (regardless of level) or if level is <100 mcg/dl:
Vitamin B_{12} 1000 mcg IM q week × 4 weeks, then 1000 mcg IM q month ×
4 months and recheck.
If level is 100–150 pg/dl:
Vitamin B_{12} 1000 mcg IM q month, and recheck in 3–4 months.
If level is 150–250 pg/dl:
Vitamin B_{12} 1000 mcg P.O. qd, and recheck in 3–4 months.
Vitamin B_{12} can also be administered sublingually or by nasal spray.

Vitamin D
If low-serum vitamin D level:
Vitamin D 50,000 IU P.O. q week for 6–8 weeks; recheck level in 3–6
months.
If vitamin D level in 3–6 months is normal, go back to baseline
postoperative supplements, and recheck in 3 months.

Ensure that the patient takes 1200–1500 mg elemental calcium per day.

Key: P.O. = Per os (oral); qd = once daily; ng = nanograms; mg = milligrams; mcg = micrograms; IM = intramuscular; IU = international units

Source: Obesity Consult Center Guidelines, Tufts-NEMC, Boston, MA.

Oral iron supplementation may be warranted when diet and multivitamin/mineral supplementation alone is not enough to maintain acceptable iron levels. Supplemental iron is available in two forms: ferrous and ferric. Ferrous iron salts (ferrous fumarate, ferrous sulfate, and ferrous gluconate) are the best-absorbed forms of iron supplements (30). A multivitamin with iron was not found to prevent deficiency, while ferrous sulfate (640 mg/day or 100 mg elemental iron/day) was found to be preventive of deficiency over 2 years after RYGBP among menstruating women who adhered with the regimen (22,29,31).

Although physicians evaluate each patient individually when prescribing oral iron therapy, the CDC recommends 50–60 mg of oral elemental iron (the approximate amount of elemental iron in one 300 mg tablet of ferrous sulfate) twice daily for 3 months for the therapeutic treatment of iron-deficiency anemia. The patient should be made aware that these supplements may cause gastrointestinal side effects such as nausea, vomiting, constipation, dark-colored stools, and/or abdominal distress (32). Starting with half the recommended dosage (e.g., once per day for at least 1 week before increasing) may help minimize these symptoms. Iron from enteric-coated or delayed-release preparations may have minimal side effects, but may also not be as well absorbed, and are therefore not recommended (33). If oral iron repletion is unsuccessful or poorly tolerated, parenteral iron infusions may be required.

Folic Acid

Folic acid deficiency is also a potential complication following bariatric surgery. It can manifest as macrocytic anemia, leukopenia, thrombocytopenia, glossitis, or megaloblastic marrow. For the most part, folate deficiency is thought to be predominantly due to decreased intake and not to malabsorption, and is easily corrected by oral vitamin supplementation (12). It has also been shown to be less likely in meat eaters than meat avoiders (10). Vitamin B_{12} is also necessary for the conversion of methyltetrahydrofolic acid to tetrahydrofolic acid; therefore, a B_{12} deficiency may result in a folate deficiency. Unfortunately, serum folate levels are more indicative of acute dietary insufficiency of folate than more chronic tissue levels (11). Red blood cell folate levels change more gradually and are thought to be more predictive of tissue levels. However, the significance of lower red blood cell folate levels is questioned because few patients actually develop megaloblastic anemia. Folic acid absorption, which occurs preferentially in the proximal portion of the small intestine, can take place along the entire small bowel with adaptation after RYGBP surgery (34). Therefore, folic acid deficiency may be preventable and promptly corrected with supplementation of 1 mg of folate daily (34).

Vitamin B_{12}

Deficiencies of vitamin B_{12} have been reported to commonly occur following RYGBP (16,20,24,27). Some reports describe the incidence of low-serum vitamin

B_{12} levels to occur in 26%–70% of RYGBP patients. Significant deficiencies can lead to macrocytic anemia, megaloblastosis of the bone marrow, leukopenia, thrombocytopenia, glossitis, or neurologic derangements. However, despite the high incidence of low-serum levels, few patients develop these sequelae. The normal absorption of vitamin B_{12} is a complex process. The vitamin must first be freed from the food source, particularly meat protein. This is facilitated by gastric acid. The free B_{12} is then bound to R-protein in the stomach. Within the duodenum, R-protein is cleaved from the vitamin, which then binds to intrinsic factor (IF). The B_{12}-IF complex then travels intact through the intestinal tract and is absorbed into the circulation in the distal ileum.

As with iron and folate, B_{12} intake is diminished after bariatric surgery. Absorption of available B_{12} may also be compromised. The gastric pouch produces little acid, thereby preventing the normal cleavage of B_{12} from its food source (15). Several studies have reported that oral crystalline B_{12} can be absorbed and normal serum levels maintained in RYGBP patients (13,5). Some researchers have suggested that a significant etiology for the B_{12} deficiency after RYGBP is the decrease in IF (34,35). Marcuard et al. demonstrated low IF levels in 53% of RYGBP patients with B_{12} deficiency (36). However, some of these patients had low levels of B_{12} and IF prior to surgery. In addition, other studies reported normal Schilling tests on RYGBP patients, suggesting that the IF mixing is adequate despite the bypass of the duodenum.

There is a general consensus that few RYGBP patients can adequately maintain normal serum B_{12} levels from diet alone (12,13). Interestingly, Avinoah et al. found better B_{12} (as well as iron and folate) levels in patients who were able to tolerate meat compared to those who could not (10). In many patients, acceptable vitamin B_{12} serum levels can be obtained if the vitamin is provided orally. Several of the studies recommend 500–600 mcg daily. If a mild or moderate deficiency is identified, our practice is to orally supplement with 1000 mcg daily. If oral supplementation does not replete the deficiency, or if it is severe, an intramuscular injection (1000 mcg) may be administered monthly.

Vitamin B_{12} deficiency should be much less likely after LAGB procedures where the nutrient stream is not diverted and after BPD+/-DS where gastric acid production is less altered than RYGBP and the terminal ileum is kept intact. If a deficiency is identified, poor dietary choices, suboptimal intake and/or nonadherence with vitamin supplementation may be implicated.

Vitamin D and Calcium

RYGBP and BPD patients may be at increased risk for vitamin D deficiency, suboptimal calcium absorption, osteopenia, and elevated markers of bone turnover (38–40). In addition, there may be a higher risk for bone mass abnormalities among these patients (37–43). Possible etiologies for this include restriction of calcium intake due to the malabsorption of calcium and vitamin D. Decreased calcium absorption is related to the fact that the site where calcium is maximally absorbed, the duodenum and proximal jejunum, is no longer present among RYGBP patients. In addition, vitamin D is preferentially absorbed in the jejunum and ileum. The overall decrease in calcium absorption may stimulate the production of parathyroid hormone (PTH), which may then result in increased production of 1,25 dihydroxyvitamin D, then causing the subsequent release of calcium from the bone. The possible result of these events may be a long-term risk for osteoporosis (38).

Thiamine

Thiamine deficiency is generally uncommon after bariatric surgery; however, it must always be considered for any patient who presents with intractable vomiting and dehydration. Thiamine depletion and/or deficiency may be seen among RYGBP patients due to a combination of reduction in acid production by the gastric pouch, decreased food intake, and frequent vomiting, in some cases even inducing Wernicke-Korsakoff syndrome (44–47). Rehydration with a glucose-based intravenous fluid without the supplementation of thiamine may also be a factor in Wernicke-Korsakoff syndrome among these patients (45–47). In patients with persistent vomiting after any bariatric procedure, parenteral administration of thiamine for 6 weeks should prevent this deficiency (38).

Patients who have undergone gastric banding may also exhibit thiamine deficiency, though certainly it is less common than with RYGBP patients (48). In a case report, a patient presented with severe vomiting 1 week after the gastric band was placed. Physical examination showed no abnormalities except for neurological signs (ataxia, disorientation, and diplopia). After a regimen of 20 mg twice daily of intravenous thiamine, all neurological signs diminished. In light of this, postoperative RYGBP and gastric-banding patients presenting with persistent vomiting are referred for a surgical evaluation, and multivitamin/mineral supplementation is augmented when deemed necessary, with parenteral thiamine initiated when indicated by the physician.

Other vitamin and mineral deficiencies include vitamin A, noted in 10%; hypokalemia in 56%; and hypomagnesemia in 34% of RYGBP patients (11). However, these figures were not considered significant, because no patient experienced night blindness, and low potassium and magnesium levels were easily corrected with oral supplementation. The fat-soluble vitamins (A, D, E, K) are also at risk for deficiency in patients who undergo malabsorptive procedures. These vitamins are absorbed predominantly in the distal ileum, which is bypassed by these operations (18,25). Patients undergoing these procedures must take vitamin supplements containing the recommended daily allowance for these vitamins. In addition, serum levels must be monitored yearly and deficiencies treated.

WEIGHT LOSS FAILURE

Weight loss failure occurs in approximately 20%–25% of patients after RYGBP (49). Few failures can be traced to technical errors. In most cases, dietary noncompliance or behavioral changes are to blame. In these cases, patients chronically overeat and/or abuse calorie-dense foods, candies, or sweets. Patients may present with chronic vomiting, increasing appetite, increasing meal capacity, and gradual weight gain. Most will also have abandoned exercise. The treatment for someone who fails a bariatric procedure is controversial. Revision is an option but carries a higher morbidity than the original procedure. Many surgeons would opt to revise the prior procedure and to convert to a more radical operation. However, there are no publications to support that shrinking a dilated pouch or revising a dilated anastomosis will lead to renewed weight loss. Limb lengthening is also poorly studied. Although dramatically decreasing the common channel, thus enhancing the malabsorptive component of the operation will likely succeed in achieving weight loss, it may do so at increased nutritional risks. Restapling after gastrogastric fistula would also be likely to succeed in renewed weight loss. However, because most failures are due to dietary noncompliance and/or behavioral changes, no procedure guarantees success; the decision to revise should be carefully analyzed and individualized for each patient.

APPROPRIATELY FEEDING THE CRITICALLY ILL/SEVERELY OBESE

Standard nutritional support practices can be harmful for the obese patient. A nutritional formulation that restricts calories and, in particular, calories from glucose may be more beneficial. This approach, often referred to as *hypocaloric* feeding, is based on the theory that an energy deficit caused by restricting calorie administration below actual requirements can be safely compensated for by the mobilization of endogenous fat. In addition, by providing adequate protein, nitrogen homeostasis would be maintained.

Hypocaloric Nutritional Support

A protein-sparing, hypocaloric approach to nutritional support may have several potential short-term benefits for use in the critically ill obese (50–52) (see Table 6–4).

Although dextrose is the sole source for nonprotein calories, elevated blood sugars are rarely seen. Because the likelihood of hyperglycemia is reduced, many of the dextrose-associated complications are avoided. Therefore, one would anticipate less wound infections, enhanced immune function, the promotion of diuresis instead of fluid retention, and decreased carbon dioxide production. The reduction in carbon dioxide production may decrease respiratory work, potentially decreasing the need for mechanical ventilatory support. In addition, despite the deliberate restriction in energy provision, protein anabolism and successful wound healing have been reported in critically ill obese patients placed on this feeding regimen (51,52). Another beneficial attribute of the hypocaloric feeding approach is that while insulin secretion is decreased, the need for exogenous insulin administration is markedly diminished or even avoided altogether (even in diabetic patients).

Table 6–4 Theoretical Advantages of Hypocaloric Feeding

Avoidance of glucose-related complications
Avoidance of hyperglycemia
Decrease in endogenous insulin secretion
Marked decrease of, or the avoidance of, the need for exogenous insulin, even in diabetic patients
Improved ventilatory mechanics
Improved diuresis
Decreased CO_2 production
Enhanced protein anabolism
Promotion of positive nitrogen balance
Enhanced wound healing
Improved immune function

Although a hypocaloric feeding regimen may have several theoretical benefits for the severely obese patient, its success is based predominantly on the premise that the critically ill obese patient can oxidize stored fat to compensate for the calorie deficit and spare protein stores. This concept has to date not been conclusively validated. In the nonstressed patient, decreased insulin secretion and insufficient calorie administration would favor fat oxidation. However, critical illness may alter normal metabolic pathways. Currently, only two studies have considered this issue. Jeevanandam and colleagues demonstrated poor fat oxidation in a population of fasted obese critically ill patients (53). In contrast, using indirect calorimetry to analyze substrate utilization, Dickerson et al. estimated fat oxidation at 68% of nonprotein energy expenditure in a similar population of stressed postoperative obese patients who were receiving hypocaloric PN (51).

No reports in the literature to date have found any adverse effects with hypocaloric feeding. Despite the limited use (or absolute avoidance) of lipid, an essential fatty acid deficiency is unlikely to develop. Linoleic acid, the most important essential fatty acid, comprises approximately 10% of the stored lipid. Mobilization of fat releases more than the 2–3.5 gm of linoleic acid required daily (54). Even if lipolysis and fat oxidation are less efficient in the stressed obese patient, most patients would only require this form of nutritional support for a relatively limited period of time. If a patient requires longer support, an intralipid infusion can be given once weekly to prevent an essential fatty acid deficiency.

ESTIMATING ENERGY REQUIREMENTS

The estimation of energy expenditure can be difficult in this population of patients. Most equations for calculating energy expenditure have not been derived for the extremely obese. Firstly, body composition is quite different. As compared to the nonobese, the majority of overweight patients have both an increased fat mass and increased lean body mass (55,56). However, the proportion of lean body mass to fat mass can vary greatly.

Other obesity-associated factors may also affect body composition. Obesity in adults is often associated with hypertension, edema, and congestive heart failure, all of which may be secondary to overexpansion of the extracellular fluid (ECF). It has been shown that total body water, ECF, intracellular fluid (ICF) and the ratio of ECF/ICF are significantly increased in obese women compared to normal weight subjects (57). Therefore, these derangements in body composition—and the great variability from patient to patient—make using ideal body weight in standard energy expenditure equations inaccurate. Given the larger lean body mass, using ideal body weight will generally underestimate caloric requirements. However, using actual body weight may massively overestimate energy expenditure because fat is less metabolically active than fat-free tissue and body fluid is inactive. Using an adjusted body weight may better estimate lean body mass in the obese; however, this approach has not been validated (58).

Numerous formulas are available to estimate energy requirements for patients, but all suffer from inaccuracies that have been described elsewhere (59–61). Most rely on weight as a gross estimate of lean body mass. Some differentiate men from women and the young from the old. Most have been criticized for lack of accuracy for the critically ill. Few even consider obesity as an independent variable (62,63). Das et al. found that predicted energy expenditure deviated from measured expenditure for both equations thought to be useful for the obese (64). Unfortunately, her study was performed in noncritically ill obese patients. Indirect calorimetry may also be considered; however, there are no published studies to validate its accuracy in critically ill/morbidly obese patients.

ENTERAL HYPOCALORIC FEEDING

Although the hypocaloric protein-sparing approach was originally conceived for PN support, there is no reason that it cannot be applied to enteral feeding. However, because most enteral formulations are provided ready made from the manufacturer, this approach can be challenging. To produce a hypocaloric, protein-sparing enteral formula, one must construct an enteral formulation entirely out of modular protein and dextrose components or modify a commercially prepared product. There are several high-protein, low-fat formulas that can be used as a basis for the latter. More standard products may also be used and are usually more cost effective.

Daily administration of a standard formulation may be based on the provision of 60% of the calculated energy requirements. Additional protein can be added to meet 100% of the protein needs. Although these formulas tend to provide approximately 30% of the total calories as lipid, with a hypocaloric regimen, the lipid contribution will be minimized and of no significance.

Most standard commercially available enteral products contain the sufficient vitamins and minerals to meet the FDA guidelines when 2000 kcal are administered daily. Because hypocaloric feeding generally will provide less than 2000 kcal/day, additional micronutrient supplementation may be required.

THE APPLICATION OF HYPOCALORIC FEEDING

Although the concept of a specialized approach for nourishing the severely ill obese patient has been considered for a number of years, few studies in the literature evaluate this technique, and even fewer prospective randomized trials compare it to standard feeding regimens.

In a nonrandomized trial, Dickerson et al. placed 13 obese patients requiring PN for postoperative complications on a hypocaloric regimen (51). The researchers reported net protein anabolism, complete tissue healing, and lack of major complications. Burge and colleagues, in a randomized, prospective trial of noncritically ill obese patients, compared a hypocaloric parenteral formulation with a standard approach (52). In both groups, positive nitrogen balance was achieved. However, the researchers did not report the incidence of complications or the effect on outcome. In a second prospective, randomized trial by the same group of investigators, Choban and colleagues studied hypocaloric feeding in both critically ill and noncritically ill obese patients (65). Positive nitrogen balance was again achieved in both groups. Glucose control was better in the hypocaloric-fed group, but did not reach statistical significance. This may have been due to the small study size. Complication rates were equivalent and there were no untoward effects noted in the group given the lower energy formulations. Importantly, they were able to obtain these results without the need for indirect calorimetry. Unfortunately, effects on outcome were not reported.

ACCESS ISSUES

Although little is written describing the possible difficulties of establishing feeding access in the severely obese, most clinicians are very familiar with them. Obese patients are probably more prone to access-related complications due to their body habitus and concomitant medical conditions. Central venous access is complicated by the lack of reliable anatomical landmarks and the respiratory risk of placing one of these patients in the Trendelenburg position (angling the bed with the legs up and the head down) commonly used for catheter placement.

Obtaining enteral access can also be challenging (66). Gastric feeding may be undesirable secondary to the increased risk of aspiration because many severely obese patients suffer from aspiration risk factors such as gastroesophageal reflux disease, gastroparesis, increased intraabdominal pressure, and the like. Postpyloric tube placement may also be challenging in this patient population. Blind nasalenteric placement is made more difficult by the increased adiposity of the soft tissues of the palate and pharynx. Fluoroscopic tube placement may be impossible for patients weighing over 400 pounds, because many fluoroscopy tables are not designed for patients who weigh more than 350 pounds. Surgical tube placement carries all of the potential problems associated with surgery. These include complications associated with medical diseases (cardiac, pulmonary, thromboembolic, etc.) and those associated with the surgery. The operative incision is more prone to infection and healing complications. Although laparoscopic surgery minimizes problems associated with an incision, it is not immune to other complications. Patients still require general anesthesia for laparoscopy. The carbon dioxide gas used to create the pneumoperitoneum may lead to carbon dioxide retention in patients with pulmonary insufficiency. Standard trocars and laparoscopic instruments may be too short to be used for patients with massive abdominal walls. The increased intraabdominal pressure created by the pneumoperitoneum (necessary to elevate the anterior abdominal wall to create a work space), and the heavy abdominal wall can cause derangements in venous blood return to the heart.

CONCLUSION

Surgical therapy is the most effective modality for treatment of severe obesity. Improvements in patient safety and the incorporation of laparoscopic techniques have dramatically increased surgical access for the estimated 20 million Americans who could benefit greatly from successfully losing weight. The current group of bariatric procedures achieves a high likelihood of weight-loss success at a relatively low perioperative risk. However, the reduction in dietary intake, changes in eating habits, possible dysfunctional eating, vomiting, and/or nutrient malabsorption can lead to both macro- and micronutrient deficiencies. These deficiencies may present years after the surgery and be initially insidious, but could result in severe consequences. Additionally, these procedures are unique and have their own specific complications that may develop and require prompt recognition and treatment. Such operations will require a lifetime commitment between patients and their health care professionals. When the severely obese become critically ill, providing safe nutritional support has its own set of problems. It is safe to state that all clinicians will be asked to care for the morbidly obese. Therefore, all must be familiar with the potential nutritional consequences of the procedures currently being performed and be prepared to treat them appropriately.

REFERENCES

1. Allison DB, Fontaine KR, Manson JE, Stevens J, Vanltallie TB. Annual deaths attributable to obesity in the United States. *JAMA.* 1999;282:1530–1538.
2. Mokdad AH, Marks JS, Stroup DF, Gerberding JL. Actual causes of death in the United States, 2000. *JAMA.* 2004;291:1238–1245.
3. Buchwald H, Avidor Y, Braunwald E, et al. Bariatric surgery: A systematic review and meta-analysis. *JAMA.* 2004;292:1724–1737.
4. Das SK, Roberts SB, McCrory MA, et al. Long-term changes in energy expenditure and body composition after massive weight loss induced by gastric bypass surgery. *Am J Clin Nutr.* 2003;78:22–30.

5. Bothe A, Bistrian BR, Greenberg I. Energy regulation in morbid obesity by multidisciplinary therapy. *Surg Clin North Am.* 1979;59:1017–1031.

6. Scopinaro N, Gianetta E, Adami GF, et al. Biliopancreatic diversion for obesity at eighteen years. *Surgery.* 1996;119:261–268.

7. Tacchino RM, Mancini A, Perrelli M, et al. Body composition and energy expenditure: Relationship and changes in obese subjects before and after biliopancreatic diversion. *Metabolism.* 2003;52:552–558.

8. Hess DS, Hess DW. Biliopancreatic diversion with a duodenal switch. *Obesity Surgery.* 1998;8:267–282.

9. Pories WJ, Swanson MS, MacDonald KG, et al. Who would have thought it? An operation proves to be the most effective therapy for adult-onset diabetes mellitus. *Ann Surg.* 1995;222: 339–352.

10. Avinoah E, Ovnat A, Charuzi I. Nutritional status seven years after Roux-en-Y gastric bypass surgery. *Surgery.* 1992;111:137–142.

11. Halverson JD. Micronutrient deficiencies after gastric bypass for morbid obesity. *Am Surg.* 1986;52:594–598.

12. Amaral JF, Thompson WR, Caldwell MD, Martin HF, Randall HT. Prospective hematologic evaluation of gastric exclusion surgery for morbid obesity. *Ann Surg.* 1985;201:186–192.

13. Rhode BM, Arseneau P, Cooper BA, Katz M, Gilfix BM, MacLean LD. Vitamin B-12 deficiency after gastric bypass surgery for obesity. *Am J Clin Nutr.* 1996;63:103–109.

14. Printen KJ, Halverson JD. Hemic micronutrients following vertical banded gastroplasty. *Am Surg.* 1988;54:267–268.

15. Smith CD, Herkes SB, Behrns KE, Fairbanks VF, Kelly KA, Sarr MG. Gastric acid secretion and vitamin B_{12} absorption after vertical Roux-en-Y gastric bypass for morbid obesity. *Ann Surg.* 1993;218:91–96.

16. Sugerman HJ. Bariatric surgery for severe obesity. *J Assoc Acad Minor Phys.* 2001;12:129–136.

17. Elliot K. Nutritional considerations after bariatric surgery. *Crit Care Nurs Q.* 2003;26:133–138.

18. Slater GH, Ren CJ, Siegel N, et al. Serum fat-soluble vitamin deficiency and abnormal calcium metabolism after malabsorptive bariatric surgery. *J Gastrointest Surg.* 2004;8:48–55.

19. Brolin RE, La Marca LB, Kenler HA, Cody RP. Malabsorptive gastric bypass in patients with superobesity. *J Gastrointest Surg.* 2002;6:195–203.

20. Skroubis G, Sakellaropoulos G, Pouggouras K, Mead N, Nikiforidis G, Kalfarentzos F. Comparison of nutritional deficiencies after Roux-en-Y gastric bypass and after biliopancreatic diversion with Roux-en-Y gastric bypass. *Obes Surg.* 2002;12:551–558.

21. Goldner WS, O'Dorisio TM, Dillon JS, Mason EE. Severe metabolic bone disease as a long-term complication of obesity surgery. *Obes Surg.* 2002;12:685–692.

22. Kushner R. Managing the obese patient after bariatric surgery: A case report of severe malnutrition and review of the literature. *JPEN.* 2000;24:126–132.

23. Marceau P, Biron S, Lebel S, et al. Does bone change after biliopancreatic diversion? *J Gastrointest Surg.* 2002;6:690–698.

24. Brolin RE, Leung M. Survey of vitamin and mineral supplementation after gastric bypass and biliopancreatic diversion for morbid obesity. *Obes Surg.* 1999;9:150–154.

25. Hatizifotis M, Dolan K, Newbury L, Fielding G. Symptomatic vitamin A deficiency following biliopancreatic diversion. *Obes Surg.* 2003;13:655–657.

26. Newbury L, Dolan K, Hatzifotis M, Low N, Fielding G. Calcium and vitamin D depletion and elevated parathyroid hormone following biliopancreatic diversion. *Obes Surg.* 2003;13:893–895.

27. Papini-Berto SJ, Burini RC. Causes of malnutrition in post-gastrectomy patient. *Arq Gastroenterol.* 2001;38:272–275.

28. Rhode BM, Shustik C, Christou NV, MacLean LD. Iron absorption and therapy after gastric bypass. *Obes Surg*. 1999;9:17–21.

29. Schilling RF, Gohdes PN, Hardie GH. Vitamin B_{12} deficiency after gastric bypass for obesity. *Ann Int Med*. 1984;101:501–512.

30. Hoffman R, Benz E, Shattil S, Furie B, Cohen H, Silberstein L, et al. Disorders of iron metabolism: Iron deficiency and overload. In: *Hematology: Basic Principles and Practice*. 3rd ed. New York, N.Y.: Churchill Livingstone, Harcourt Brace & Co.; 2000.

31. Simon SR, Zemel R, Betancourt S, et al. Hematologic complications of gastric bypass for morbid obesity. *South Med J*. 1989;82:1108–1110.

32. Centers for Disease Control and Prevention. CDC Recommendations to prevent and control iron deficiency in the United States. *MMWR Recomm Rep*. 1998;47:1–29.

33. Brolin RE, Gorman JH, Gorman RC, et al. Are vitamin B_{12} and folate deficiency clinically important after Roux-en-Y gastric bypass? *J Gastrointest Surg*. 1998;2:436–442.

34. Mahmud K, Ripley D, Dolscherholmen A. Vitamin B_{12} absorption tests: Their unreliability in postgastrectomy states. *JAMA*. 1971;216:1167–1171.

35. Crowley LV, Olson RW. Megaloblastic anemia after gastric bypass for obesity. *Am J Gastroenterol*. 1984;79:850–860.

36. Marcuard SP, Sinar DR, Swanson MS, Silverman JF, Levine JS. Absence of luminal intrinsic factor after gastric bypass surgery for morbid obesity. *Dig Dis Sci*. 1989;34:1238–1242.

37. Halverson JD. Metabolic risk of obesity surgery and long-term follow-up. *Am J Clin Nutr*. 1992;55(2 suppl):602S–605S.

38. Alverez-Leite JL. Nutrient deficiencies secondary to bariatric surgery. *Curr Opin Clin Nutr Metab Care*. 2004;7569–7575.

39. Goode LR, Brolin RE, Chowdhury HA, et al. Bone and gastric bypass surgery: Effects of dietary calcium and vitamin D. *Obes Res*. 2004;12:40–47.

40. Coates PS, Fernstrom JD, Fernstrom MH, et al. Gastric bypass surgery for morbid obesity leads to increase in bone turnover and a decrease in bone mass. *J Clin Endo Metab*. 2004;89:1061–1065.

41. Shaker JL, Norton AJ, Woods MF, et al. Secondary hyperparathyroidism and osteopenia in women following gastric exclusion surgery for obesity. *Osteopor Int*. 1991:77–81.

42. Bell NH. Bone loss and gastric bypass surgery for morbid obesity. *J Clini Endocrinol Metab*. 2004;89:1059–1060.

43. Pugnale N, Giusti V, Suter M, et al. Bone metabolism and risk of secondary hyperparathyroidism 12 months after gastric banding in obese pre-menopausal women. *Int J Obes Relat Metab Disord*. 2003;27:110–116.

44. Loh Y, Watson WE, Verma A, et al. Acute Wernicke's encephalopathy following bariatric surgery: Clinical course and MRI correlation. *Obes Surg*. 2004;14:129–132.

45. Sola E, Morillas C, Garzon S, Ferrer JM, Martin J, Hernandez-Mijares A. Rapid onset of Wernicke's encephalopathy following gastric restrictive surgery. *Obes Surg*. 2003;13:661–662.

46. Salas-Salvado J, Garcia-Lorda P, Cuatrecasas G, et al. Wernicke's syndrome after bariatric surgery. *Clin Nutr*. 2000;19:371–373.

47. Chaves LC, Faintuch J, Kahwage S, Alencar Fde A. A cluster of polyneuropathy and Wernicke-Korsakoff syndrome in a bariatric unit. *Obes Surg*. 2002;12:328–334.

48. Bozbora A, Coskin H, Ozamagan S, et al. A rare complication of adjustable gastric banding: Wernicke's encephalopathy. *Obes Surg*. 2000;10:274–285.

49. Maclean LD, Rhode BM, Sampalis J, Forse RA. Results of the surgical treatment of obesity. *Am J Surg*. 1993;165:155–162.

50. Baxter JK, Bistrian BR. Moderate hypocaloric parenteral nutrition in the critically ill, obese patient. *Nutr Clin Pract*. 1989;4:133–135.

51. Dickerson RN, Rosato EF, Mullen JL. Net protein anabolism with hypocaloric parenteral nutrition in obese stressed patients. *Am J Clin Nutr.* 1986;44:747–755.

52. Burge JC, Goon A, Choban PS, et al. Efficacy of hypocaloric total parenteral nutrition in hospitalized obese patients: A prospective, double-blind randomized trial. *JPEN.* 1994;18:203–207.

53. Jeevanandam M, Young DH, Schiller WR. Obesity and the metabolic response to severe multiple trauma in man. *J Clin Invest.* 1991;87:262–269.

54. Mascioli EA, Smith MF, Trerice MS, et al. Effect of total parenteral nutrition with cycling on essential fatty acid deficiency. *JPEN.* 1979;3:171–173.

55. Benedetti G, Mingrone G, Marcoccia S, et al. Body composition and energy expenditure after weight loss following bariatric surgery. *J Am Coll Nutr.* 2000;19:270–274.

56. Das SK, Roberts SB, Kehayias JJ, et al. Body composition assessment in extreme obesity and after massive weight loss induced by gastric bypass surgery. *Am J Physiol.* 2003;284:E1080–E1088.

57. Heymsfield SB, Lichtman S, Baumgartner RN, et al. Assessment of body composition: An overview. In: Bjorntorp P, Brodoff BN, eds. *Obesity.* Philadelphia, Pa.: J.B. Lippincott Co.; 1992:37–54.

58. Wilkens, K. Adjustment for obesity. *ADA Renal Practice Group Newsletter.* Winter 1984.

59. Osborne BJ, Saba AK, Wood SJ, et al. Clinical comparison of three methods to determine resting energy expenditure. *Nutr Clin Pract.* 1994;9:241–246.

60. Daly JM, Heymsfield SB, Head CA, et al. Human energy expenditure: Overestimation by widely used prediction equations. *Am J Clin Nutr.* 1985;42:1170–1174.

61. Cortes B, Nelson LD. Errors in estimating energy expenditure in critically ill surgical patients. *Arch Surg.* 1989;124:287–290.

62. Ireton-Jones CS. Evaluation of energy expenditure in obese patients. *Nutr Clin Pract.* 1989;4:127–129.

63. Bernstein RS, Thornton JC, Yang MU, et al. Prediction of the resting metabolic rate in obese patients. *Am J Clin Nutr.* 1983;37:595–602.

64. Das SK, Saltzman E, McCrory MA, et al. Energy expenditure is very high in extremely obese women. *J Nutr.* 2004;134:1412–1416.

65. Choban PS, Burge JC, Scales D, et al. Hypoenergetic nutrition support in hospitalized obese patients. A simplified method for clinical application. *Am J Clin Nutr.* 1997;66:546–550.

66. Shikora SA. Enteral feeding tube placement in obese patients: Considerations for nutrition support. *Nutr Clin Pract.* 1997;12:S9–S13.

CHAPTER 7

Nutritional Management for Neurosurgical Patients

Dema Halasa-Esper, MS, RD, CNSD

INTRODUCTION

Injury to the central nervous system (CNS), either from trauma, neoplasm, autoimmune disease, or ischemia can profoundly affect neurologic function. Acute neurologic injury, can trigger systemic pathophysiologic processes that can affect organ function, metabolism, nutritional status, and immune function, contributing to sepsis and multiple organ failure (1). Furthermore, intracranial processes seen in acute neurologic injury include elevated intracranial pressure, reduced cerebral blood flow, decreased tissue oxygen supply, and decreased total systemic blood volume (2). These abnormalities are prevalent primarily in severely ill patients, increasing their risk for morbidity and mortality.

Specialized nutrition support is often required, utilizing either enteral or parenteral nutrition, because altered mental status, dysphagia, and mechanical ventilation are commonly seen with acute neurologic injury, and all inhibit oral nutrition intake. Enteral nutrition (EN) is preferred; however, parenteral nutrition (PN) may be required when gastrointestinal intolerance occurs. Prior to the 1980s, a paucity of studies was available regarding the role of nutrition support in neurologic injury. The standard of care in patients with severe neurologic injury was to delay nutrition support until normal gastrointestinal function returned, because nutritional support was thought to play an equivocal role in this subgroup of critically ill patients who were at high risk for in-hospital morbidity and mortality.

In the past decades, the role of nutrition support in neurologic injury has evolved due to advances in research and increased knowledge of the pathophysiology following injury. Although most of the attention has focused on the medical and nutritional management of patients with traumatic brain injury (TBI), acute ischemic and hemorrhagic brain injury and other critical neurologic illnesses also present with similar metabolic and nutritional challenges (3). The purpose of this chapter is to review the metabolic, physiologic, and nutritional management during the acute neurologic injury phase in TBI, spinal cord injury, and ischemic and hemorrhagic brain injuries.

OVERVIEW OF THE CENTRAL NERVOUS SYSTEM

The nervous system is subdivided into CNS and the peripheral nervous system (PNS), and is unique in that its structural features and pathways are symmetrical. The CNS includes the brain and the spinal cord, whereas the PNS consists of the nerves that connect the CNS with muscles and other organ systems.

The brain is encapsulated within the skull and divided into the cerebrum, brain-stem, and cerebellum (see Figure 7–1). The cerebrum houses the largest portion of the brain, the cerebral hemispheres. Inferior to the hemispheres is the diencephalon, which contains the thalamus, hypothalamus, and the pineal gland. The brainstem consists of the midbrain, pons, and medulla. The lower portion of the brainstem is

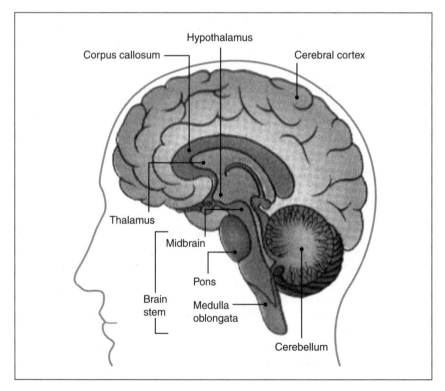

Figure 7–1 Neuroanatomy. Human Brain and Its Three Main Parts: The Cerebrum, Cerebellum, and the Brain Stem.

Source: http://www.sirinet.net/~jgjohnso/brain.html

called the bulb or bulbar region. The cerebellum is located dorsal to the pons. Extending from the medulla is the spinal cord, which is a slender cylindrical tube of nervous tissue at the center of the vertebral column that extends from the skull to the lumbar vertebral area. The spinal cord transmits neural messages to and from the brain, connecting it to the environment (see Figure 7–2) (4).

The PNS is composed of the nerves emerging from the brain (cranial nerves) and the spinal cord (spinal nerves) and is responsible for conveying neural messages from sensory receptors to the CNS and from the CNS outward to muscles and glands in the body.

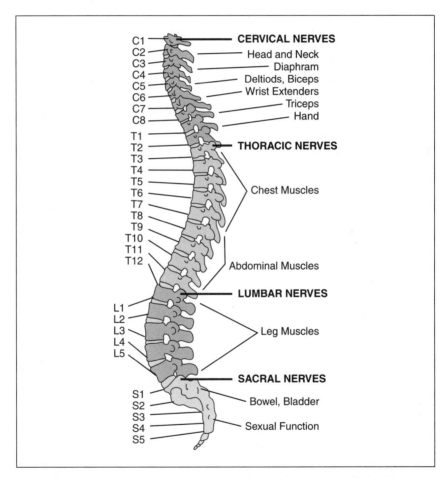

Figure 7–2 Neuroanatomy. Spinal Cord Divided into Its Specific Neurological Segments. The Spinal Cord Provides the Link between the Brain and the Rest of the Body.

Source: http://www.spinalinjury.net/html/_anatomy_of_the_spinal_cord_co.html

The autonomic nervous system (ANS) and the somatic nervous system (SNS) are additional components of the nervous system that are involved in conveying and processing sensory information. The SNS is involved in processing conscious and unconscious sensory information, such as vision, pain, and touch from the head, body, and extremities to the CNS. It also is responsible for motor control of voluntary muscles (5). The ANS, divided into the sympathetic and the parasympathetic systems, controls sensory activities from visceral organs, including the digestive system, cardiovascular system, smooth muscles, and glands. The sympathetic system prepares the body for crisis situations, known as the "fight-or-flight response." When stimulated, the sympathetic nervous system causes an increase in heart rate and blood pressure, shunting of blood flow from internal organs to the muscles, and inhibition of the digestive system (6). The parasympathetic system maintains the day-to-day activities of the body and causes an opposite effect when stimulated: heart rate slows, blood pressure decreases, and activities of the gastrointestinal system increase. Injury and dysfunction of the CNS can deleteriously affect these two systems, which can worsen symptomatology (i.e., autonomic dysfunction) in patients with neurological impairment (4).

METABOLIC RESPONSE TO NEUROLOGIC INJURY

Following acute neurologic injury, physiologic changes occur in substrate metabolism, hormone secretion, and immune function similar to that seen in sepsis and trauma (1,7,8). The primary goal following acute neurologic injury is to maintain oxygen delivery to vital organs and attain hemodynamic stability. Once these vital tasks are achieved, other acute management needs such as medical nutrition therapy can be addressed (9). The initial metabolic response following injury, often referred to as the *shock* or *ebb phase*, includes a decrease in body temperature and cardiac output, and a reduction of energy expenditure. Following this phase, an increase in metabolism and subsequent catabolism occurs. This process is mediated by the release of counterregulatory hormones such as cortisol, epinephrine, and norepinephrine. This phase can last for several days to a few weeks, depending on the severity of the injury. The metabolic shift from anabolism to catabolism occurs after injury and stress, and the body mobilizes glucose, protein, and fat for energy. Furthermore, circulating levels of insulin increase following metabolic stress, but the response to insulin is blunted in tissues. This predominantly occurs in skeletal muscle. Insulin resistance and glucose intolerance is believed to be caused by the effects of counterregulatory hormones (9). As a result, hyperglycemia is commonly seen in metabolically stressed patients. The primary nutritional goal during this time is to provide an adequate amount of energy and protein to attenuate the increased metabolic demand seen with neurologic injury, as well as controlling elevated blood glucose levels with insulin. Hyperglycemia is associated with adverse outcomes in critically ill patients, as well as effects of neurologic recovery in neurotrauma patients (10,11). Using insulin therapy in adult critically ill patients may decrease mortality, and the main determinant for this is related to targeting euglycemia (12).

NUTRITION ASSESSMENT

Nutrition assessment in neurologic injury is imperative in identifying the presence of or risk for malnutrition. Trauma patients, such as those with TBI, often are healthy prior to the unforeseen injury; however, screening a patient's past medical, surgical, and social history is important in identifying conditions and diseases that may possibly influence nutrition status (e.g., liver disease, diabetes, renal dysfunction, prior GI surgery, and alcohol abuse, to name a few). See Chapter 1 for a more in-depth discussion (9).

Dysphagia is characteristically seen in severe brain injury, stroke patients, and in many degenerative neurologic diseases, including Parkinson's disease, multiple sclerosis, and amyotrophic lateral sclerosis. Proper screening and management of dysphagia can expedite the recovery process. Misdiagnosis not only impedes nutritional status, but is also associated other complications such as aspiration and pneumonia. For instance, Odderson et al. (13) reported that early screening for dysphagia in patients with acute stroke provided not only a salutary effect for patients, but a cost-effective benefit as well, with a reduction in length of hospital stay and reduced incidence of aspiration pneumonia.

Attaining accurate anthropometric measurements in the critical care setting remains a challenge for clinicians. For instance, assessment of anthropometric measurements in the critical care setting is not a reliable predictor of lean body mass, but rather reflects changes in fluid balance (14). Hence, fluctuations in measured body weight should be interpreted with caution during acute illness and injury. Obtaining an estimate of usual body weight is helpful when comparing changes in weight status and determining energy needs. However, it is essential to identify weight changes in the later stages of neurologic disease because immobilization causes muscle wasting and changes in body stature, particularly in spinal cord injuries (15). During a physical exam, it is important to assess overall fat and muscle stores, muscle tone, and evidence of edema. Each of these variables provides evidence of declining nutrition status; in particular, poor muscle stores and tone along with evidence of muscle wasting indicate the presence of malnutrition.

The use of surrogate markers, such as albumin, prealbumin, and transferrin are often used to assess and define malnutrition in hospitalized patients; however, the validity of their use is questionable (16). Once the patient is hemodynamically stable and nutrition support has been initiated, serum protein levels can be monitored (9). Selection of serum protein levels with a shorter half-life (e.g., prealbumin) is more applicable in the acute care setting. Plasma concentration of visceral proteins can increase or decrease in response to systemic changes. For instance, during trauma and illness, hepatic reprioritization occurs in which the synthesis of acute phase proteins (i.e., C-reactive protein, serum amyloid A, and ferritin) increase, while the synthesis of certain plasma proteins (i.e., albumin, transferrin, and transthyretin) decrease (17). Cytokines are intercellular signaling polypeptides produced during the inflammatory process and are mediators in stimulating the production of acute-phase proteins. The cytokines involved in the inflammatory response include IL-6, IL-1, tumor necrosis factor, and interferon-y (17). Hence, changes in visceral protein levels seen during the physiologic changes associated with disease and trauma should be interpreted with caution; low serum levels indicate that a patient is very ill and requires close nutrition monitoring and intervention (18). Increasing serum visceral protein values can be interpreted as an improvement in metabolic profile from catabolism to anabolism, particularly when the acute phase response has subsided in such events as trauma, sepsis, and/or injury.

ENERGY EXPENDITURE

Metabolic rate reflects the activity of body cell mass and is the central indicator of metabolic activity (19). Fat-free mass correlates with body weight, although factors such as age, sex, and height can influence variations in fat-free mass (20). Metabolic rate and activity is affected by changes in body cell mass. Specifically, metabolic rate increases with illness and injury due to changes in substrate metabolism. This, in turn, causes an increase in energy expenditure (21). Hypermetabolism is characterized by an increase in energy expenditure, oxygen consumption (VO_2), and carbon dioxide production, which, in turn, leads to an increase in caloric energy requirements (22).

Energy expenditure following acute neurologic injuries and neurotrauma can vary depending on the severity and site of injury. Furthermore, other factors such as medications, presence of sepsis, nutrition support, and body temperature are other variables that can affect energy expenditure (23–25). Generally, critically ill patients in the neurosurgery/neurocritical care unit (NCCU) are hypermetabolic and hypercatabolic within the initial weeks after injury. The following will discuss the energy expenditure changes in TBI, spinal cord injury, and ischemic and hemorrhagic stroke during the acute phase of neurologic injury.

Traumatic Brain Injury

In the 1980s, investigators used indirect calorimetry (IC) studies to examine the metabolic alterations following severe head injury. These studies found that neurological impairment profoundly affects energy expenditure in a form similar to that seen in trauma and burn patients (10). Nonsedated patients with TBI may experience an increase in energy expenditure of 140% to 200% above resting energy expenditure (REE) (8). The degree of hypermetabolism is inversely correlated with the Glasgow Coma Score (GCS), a scoring system used to quantify level of consciousness following severe head injury (see Table 7–1) (26).

Furthermore, elevated intracranial pressure (ICP) is associated with increased oxygen consumption, protein catabolism, and systemic hypermetabolism in the

Table 7–1 Common Scales used in Neurosurgery/ Neurocritical Illness

Glasgow Coma Score (GCS)	Accumulative scores from eye opening, verbal, and motor function. Common scale used in head/ trauma patients.	Normal: 15 Mild head injury: 13 to 15 Moderate head injury: 9 to 12 Severe head injury: 3 to 8
Intracranial pressure (ICP)	Measured by lumbar puncture or an ICP monitor in head injury and patients with SAH/ICH.	Normal range: 0 to 15 mm Hg Elevated range: greater than 20 mm Hg
Fischer grading system of CT scan	Grading of blood on the CT in stroke patients with SAH.	Grade 1: No clot seen Grade 2: Diffuse thin layer of blood <1 mm thick Grade 3: Localized clot or diffusely distributed hemorrhage ≥1 mm in thickness Grade 4: Intracerebral or intraventricular hemorrhage Grade 5: Greatest risk of subsequent vasospasm
Hunt Hess grading system	System used to measure severity of and prognosis in patients with SAH.	Grade 0: asymptomatic, unruptured aneurysm. Grade 1: mildly symptomatic with headache Grade 2: Severe headache, nuchal rigidity and possibly a cranial nerve deficit Grade 3: Lethargy, confusion; mild focal deficit Grade 4: Stupor, moderate to severe hemiparesis Grade 5: Comatose, decerebrate rigidity or flaccidity

SAH: subarachnoid hemorrhage; ICH: intracerebral hemorrhage

early posttrauma phase of severe head trauma (27). Elevated ICP is a complication of neurologic injury and occurs when measured ICP is above 15 mm Hg in adults. Increased ICP is mostly seen in traumatic brain injury; however, ICP monitoring is also warranted in patients with stroke, intracerebral hemorrhage, hydrocephalus, and subarachnoid hemorrhage (28).

Intracranial pressure affects cerebral perfusion pressure (CPP). CPP is the difference between mean arterial pressure (MAP) and ICP. This is represented by the equation:

$$CPP = MAP - ICP$$

Any rise in ICP is detrimental to brain blood flow and can cause ischemia and hypoxia to the brain because of a corresponding drop in CPP. This must be treated rapidly and urgently to prevent permanent anoxic injury. In order to increase CPP, medications are administered with the purpose of either raising MAP or lowering ICP. Medications used to raise MAP include vasoconstricting agents such as neosynephrine or norepinephrine; however, the mainstay of treatment is to administer osmotic solutions to decrease intracerebral edema. Such agents include mannitol and hypertonic saline. These agents help to decrease cerebral edema, which, in turn, lowers ICP. Occasionally, when these measures do not attain the desired effect, barbiturates and benzodiazepines can be administered intravenously to decrease cerebral metabolic demand. This response in turn lowers the ICP. However, these pharmacologic agents can decrease energy expenditure by 20% to 30% and should thus be considered when determining energy needs (10). Medications that may decrease energy expenditure are available in Table 7–2 (29).

Acute Spinal Cord Injury

The initial management in acute spinal cord injury (ASCI) is to protect the patient from further spinal cord damage, treat spinal cord edema with high-dose methyprednisolone, monitor fluid and electrolytes, and prevent respiratory compromise (4,30). The nutritional management of ASCI patients is complex and based on several factors. First, energy expenditure can vary from patient to patient depending on the severity and site of the spinal cord injury. In particular, energy expenditure in ASCI is affected by the extent of neuronal connectivity and neurogenic stimuli (muscle tone) to the musculoskeletal system that remains after injury (31). Patients with complete spinal cord injury experience no function below the level of injury as well as any sensation and ability for voluntary movement, such as seen in tetraplegia. As

Table 7–2 Medications that May Decrease Energy Expenditure (29)

Barbiturates (e.g., phenobarbital)
Neuromuscular blocking agents (e.g., vecuronium, pancuronium)
Opioids (e.g., morphine)
Sedation agents (e.g., midazolam, fentanyl)

Source: Dickerson RN, Roth-Yousey L. Medication effects on metabolic rate: A systematic review (part 1). *J Am Diet Assoc.* 2005;105:835–843.

for incomplete or lower spinal cord injury (i.e., paraplegia), patients experience some function below the primary area of injury, with an ability to move one limb more than another as well as having sensation in parts of the body that cannot move. Patients with incomplete injuries experience an increase in energy requirements postinjury while the opposite occurs in patients with complete level injury due to less muscle tone (32). Flaccidity of denervated musculature below the level of injury appears to contribute to the reduction in energy needs and lower REE. However, energy expenditure appears to improve as the patient regains motor function (31).

Secondly, the initial systemic effect after spinal cord trauma is hypermetabolic and hypercatabolic response. This stress response is mediated by the neuroendocrine and sympathetic nervous systems (33). Third, in addition to the trauma and any surgical intervention needed after ASCI, patients may also experience fever, infectious complications, and sepsis, all of which may further exaggerate the catabolic response. The initial metabolic response in ASCI follows an acute traumatic insult; however, these patients lapse into a chronic phase (greater than 3 weeks), which is characterized by marked reduction in substrate use and metabolic activity, prolonged nitrogen excretion, calcium wasting, and weight loss (15,34,35). Energy expenditure changes in the later phase of spinal cord injury, and thus energy requirements should be adjusted accordingly in order to prevent metabolic complications of overfeeding.

Ischemic and Hemorrhagic Stroke

Patients with hemorrhagic stroke are managed differently than those with ischemic stroke. Hemorrhagic stroke patients are managed in a similar fashion as patients with actual or potentially increased ICP; ischemic stroke is treated with thrombolytic therapy in the face of symptomatology of 3 hours or less (4). The metabolic response following nontraumatic intracranial hemorrhage (IH) and other forms of stroke resembles that of mild to moderate head injury (36,37). Preestablished criteria for calculating energy needs in this patient population are scarce, and clinicians rely on experience and the use of predicted equations in order to determine energy requirements.

Kasuya and coworkers (37) reported that subarachnoid hemorrhage (SAH) patients treated with early craniotomy for aneurysm clipping experienced a profound increase in metabolic rate, particularly among the severely ill. Of the three study periods (day 4, day 10, and discharged), patients with mild and severe SAH experienced the highest increase in basal energy expenditure on day 10, at $146 \pm 24\%$ and $198 \pm 78\%$, respectively. Also, there was a significant difference of the change in nitrogen balance in patients at days 4 and 10 among the two groups. The group of patients with severe SAH experienced greatest nitrogen loss ($P = 0.0037$). However, patients with surgical complications and those on ventilators were excluded, and thus the study findings cannot be generalized to patients dependent on mechanical ventilation. Hence, patients who are intubated usually present with poorer grades and an increase in systematic and metabolic stress; energy expenditure may rise with increasing Hunt and Hess grade (38). Further randomized clinical control trials are needed in this patient population to confirm these findings.

Based on a recent study, however, investigators compared measured energy expenditure based on IC in nontraumatic IH patients to patients with TBI. The authors reported a similar increase in metabolic rate between these two cohorts within the first week following the injury (39). The study's findings are preliminary, because a larger study is needed to understand if the energy needs of critically ill stroke patients are at high risk of being underestimated, with subsequent inadequate nutrition as their metabolic rate is estimated under conventional nutrition practice. Further clinical studies are needed to verify the metabolic response in critically ill patients with hemorrhagic and ischemic strokes.

In conclusion, energy expenditure is quantified by either measuring energy expenditure as determined by IC or by calculating resting energy expenditure through the use of predictive equations. Routine use of IC in the NCCU is warranted due to the high variability of metabolic response seen with neurologic injury. For example, spinal cord injury may elicit reduced resting energy expenditure unlike that seen in TBI (40). Hence, serial IC studies are suggested in order to capture the fluctuating metabolic rate and energy requirements seen within this population. IC itself presents with limitations, however. Exclusion criteria for IC study include medical or surgical instability, fraction of inspired oxygen (FiO_2) $\geq 60\%$, positive end-expiratory pressure ≥ 5 mm Hg, failure to cooperate, agitation, seizure activity, and spasticity (41). Adherence to guidelines and protocols for the performance of IC, as well as having an experienced technician to perform the IC study, are some of the requirements needed for valid IC measurements.

PROTEIN CATABOLISM

Skeletal muscle is the largest amino acid compartment in the body. Changes in muscle protein metabolism are characteristically seen in sepsis and injury, which subsequently impacts whole-body protein balance (42). Muscle breakdown during injury is mediated by cytokines and hormones, as well as increased expression of intracellular protein degradation in skeletal muscle. Among hormones, gluococorticoids have been shown to play a key role in muscle protein breakdown (43). In particular, elevated cortisol levels are seen in sepsis and trauma and are common in acute stroke patients (36).

Neurologic injury can profoundly affect the whole-body protein balance. For instance, TBI is associated with nitrogen losses ranging between 10 and 40 grams per day. Nitrogen excretion peaks approximately 7 to 10 days postinjury in nonspinal injured patients, with an improvement in nitrogen retention by the second to third week postinjury (8). However, in ASCI patients, negative nitrogen balance remains longer and can last up to 7 weeks postinjury, ostensibly due to the denervation of lean muscle mass (15). Furthermore, Chalela and associates (36) studied 27 critically ill stroke patients and reported that 44% of these patients experienced a negative nitrogen balance within 5 days of insult (2–11 days). Nitrogen balance studies were completed 24 hours after EN reached goal rate. Traditionally, stroke patients are not viewed as being hypercatabolic; however, this study may suggest that critically ill stroke patients may experience proteolysis during the acute phase of injury and may require higher protein requirements. None of the patients enrolled had any underlying catabolic illnesses, and none of the following variables was associated with negative nitrogen balance: gender, glucose 6.6 mmol/L or more, age 80 years or older, National Institutes of Health Stroke Scale (NIHSS) 20 or higher, mechanical ventilation, and diabetes mellitus. Limitations to this study include a small sample size and lack of serial nitrogen balance measurements beyond the median 5 days (2–11) from onset of stroke to nitrogen balance measurement.

NUTRIENT REQUIREMENTS

Energy Requirements

Energy requirements for hemorrhagic and ischemic strokes and other neurologic injuries have not adequately been studied with randomized clinical controlled trials. Of the investigations available, TBI has been the primary focus of these studies, and guidelines for energy requirements are readily available (10). Other factors, including site of injury, medication, and surgical procedures such as elective craniotomy, can all affect REE in neurologic injury (44). Patients with neurologic injury have been reported to be hypermetabolic as well as hypometabolic. For instance, during epileptic seizures or *decerebrate posturing* (involuntary extension of extremities that indicates brain stem damage) REE can increase to 300% of basal metabolic rate during the episode (average of 191%); while in between the seizure event, REE may be only be 140% of basal energy needs (44). Also, the neurologically injured patient may experience pharmacologically induced paralysis or hypothermia, which can reduce energy need to basal metabolic rate or lower.

Various studies have compared energy expenditure with IC to predicted equations, such as the Harris-Benedict equation (HBEE) in ASCI. Table 7–3 provides a summary of these trials. All of these studies have different results and there is no consensus on energy requirements in ASCI. These trials are limited by the small number of patients enrolled, as well as the lack of homogeneity in the populations studied, study design, and application of activity and injury factors with HBEE (31). Larger prospective, randomized, controlled clinical trials are needed for better understanding of the energy requirements in the ASCI population. Until the results of such trials are available, measurement of resting metabolic rate (RMR) may provide the best approach in determining energy needs in ASCI patients.

With the potential for such variance in energy requirements, IC measurements are recommended in acute neurologic injury to determine accurate energy needs. If IC is not available, then predicted equations can be used. The HBEE with a stress factor has been mostly used to determine energy needs in neurotrauma. Researchers recommend HBEE × 1.4–1.6 for neurotrauma patients who are not pharmacologically paralyzed and HBEE × 1.0 for patients who are medically paralyzed (10).

Table 7–3 Studies That Evaluated Energy Expenditure in ASCI (26, 34, 45–48)

Investigators	N	Study Aims	Study Results
Barco et al., 2002	11	Compared MTEE with HBE in pts with isolated ASCIs	HBE strongly correlated with MTEE
Rodriguez et al., 1997	12	Compared MREE with HBE in pts with varying ASCIs	HBE significantly overestimated energy requirements
Peruzzi et al., 1994	7	Compared HBE and MREE in pts with complete ASCIs	HBE and MREE correlated in the first 3 days postinjury; but significantly different on days 4 and 5
Kearns et al., 1992	10	Compared MREE with HBE in pts with isolated ASCIs	MREE was 10% below HBE, but increased over time as muscle function regained
Kolpek et al., 1989	6	Compared MREE with HBE; included pts with tetraplegia and paraplegia	HBE correlated with MREE
Young et al., 1987	4	Compared MREE with HBE in pts with quadriplegia	Indirect calorimetry is more accurate in determining energy requirements

ASCI: acute spinal cord injury; HBE: Harris-Benedict equation; MTEE: measured total energy expenditure; Pts: patients

Source: Adapted with permission: Marian M. Acute spinal cord injuries: Nutrition management. *Support Line.* 2004;26(2):3–8.

However, HBEE with stress factor may underestimate or overestimate RMR, depending on the stress factor used and patient condition. There are other predicted illness-modified equations used for critically ill patients that predict RMR (e.g., Ireton-Jones and Penn State equations) but these equations have not been studied in neurotrauma patients. Further research is needed to understand the use of these equations in this patient population.

Furthermore, energy requirements can be calculated by using weight-based estimates of 25–35 calories/kg/day based on preinjury weight status (44). Recalculation of energy needs is suggested during the course of treatment as changes occur in medical care (including the use of medications that affect REE) and clinical status. Energy requirements for different neurologic injuries are described in Table 7–4.

Table 7–4 Energy Need of Patients with Neurologic Injuries (4,10,35,39)

	Percentage above BEE
Traumatic head injury	
Mild–moderate head injury	130%–150%
Severe head injury	150%–200%
Decerebrate posturing	200%
Neuromuscular blockade	100%
Spinal cord injury (later phase)	94%
Quadriplegia	23 kcal/kg/d
Paraplegia	28 kcal/kg/d
Stroke, hemorrhagic and ischemic	130%–150%

BEE: Basal energy expenditure

Protein Requirements

Following neurotrauma, protein requirements increase due to a hypermetabolic and hypercatabolic state (49). Patients with neurologic injury require 15%–25% of total calories as protein, which is equal to 1.5 to 2.0 g/kg based on preinjury weight (protein needs should be based on an adjusted body weight when percent of ideal body weight is greater than 130%) (10). Although the goal for patients with neurological injuries is to provide adequate protein for repletion, a positive nitrogen balance may not be achieved for several weeks during the acute injury phase. The provision of high amounts of protein does not abolish the hypermetabolic response or the obligatory losses seen in traumatic brain and spinal cord injuries (3). For instance, patients with ASCI may experience a negative nitrogen balance for as long as 7 weeks after the acute event due to the loss of muscle innervation and immobilization (15). Furthermore, patients with spinal cord injury may lose as much as 10% to 20% of their body weight within 4 weeks postinjury, with 85% of this reflecting a loss of lean body mass (34,50). Hence, a higher protein requirement, in the range of 2.0–2.3 gm/kg/day, may be needed (15).

In addition, the use of steroid therapy can further exacerbate nitrogen losses, depending on the dose and duration of therapy. The current standard of care does not encourage the use of steroid treatment in TBI but high-dose steroid therapy may be used to treat spinal cord edema in ASCI (4,40). A high-protein enteral formula may be recommended during the acute injury phase to attenuate the negative nitrogen balance seen in acute neurologic injury and trauma. Adjustments should be made accordingly based on nitrogen balance studies. Protein can be adjusted upward to achieve nitrogen equilibrium as long as renal and liver function can handle the higher nitrogen load.

Fat Requirements

It is recommended that 10%–30% of total energy needs during critical illness come from fat calories, with a minimum of 2% as EFAs to prevent deficiency (9). When calculating fat calorie needs, it important to assess if the sedative agent propofol is being used. It is commonly used for short-term sedation and mechanical ventilator management, as well as allowing for frequent neurologic examinations in neurosurgical/neurocritical care patients. It is a lipid-in-water–based emulsion that provides 1.1 calories/mL and should be calculated into daily energy needs to prevent overfeeding. Recommendations for the use of nutrition support along with propofol include limiting total lipid calories in parenteral solutions to 1.0 g/kg/d; enterally fed patients may require a low-fat, high-protein formula when propofol or other lipid-based sedatives are prescribed (4,51).

FLUID MANAGEMENT

The management of fluid therapy in patients with neurologic injury has evolved from fluid restriction to advocating euvolemia. Optimal fluid balance is essential to the maintenance of CPP and ICP, which, in turn, is vital to neurological outcome. This change in practice has allowed nutrition support to be initiated earlier, rather than it being secondary to maintaining serum osmolality and ICP (22). Fluid resuscitation is important in the initial management of TBI, and the type of fluid and rate of delivery is debatable. Traditionally, hypersomolar therapy (e.g., mannitol) has been used to reduce elevated ICP; however, there is a growing interest in using hypertonic saline for both resuscitation and maintenance in head-injured patients (52). It is imperative to discuss fluid status with the medical team along with the role of nutrition therapy in the fluid management of patients with neurologic injury.

Hyponatremia is a common clinical and metabolic complication seen in the NCCU and is defined as a serum sodium concentration that is less than 135 mg/dl. Hyponatremia typically relates to either inappropriate water retention or excess sodium excretion. There are primarily two noniatrogenic causes of hyponatremia in intracranial disease: the syndrome of inappropriate secretion of antidiuretic hormone (SIADH) and cerebral salt wasting (CSW). A clinical distinction exists between these two disorders, and accurate assessment of fluid status is imperative in distinguishing these differences. Incorrect diagnosis and inappropriate management and treatment can lead to irreparable clinical outcomes (e.g., exacerbation of cerebral edema and ischemia and death) (53). For instance, SIADH presents as a euvolemic or hypervolemic state, and thus the primary treatment is fluid restriction; whereas CSW presents in a patient with a volume-depleted status, requiring fluid replacement and maintenance of positive salt balance. Further review of the differences in SIADH and CSW is available in a review by Rabinstein and Wijdicks (53). See Table 7–5.

Table 7–5 Differential Diagnosis between CSW and SIADH

Variables	CSW	SIADH
Body weight	⇊	⇈ or no change
Fluid balance	Negative	Normal or ⇈
Appearance of dehydration	Present	Absent
Sodium balance	Negative	Balance
Serum osmolality	⇈ or normal	Decreased
Urine volume	Normal or ⇈	Normal or ⇊
Extracellular fluid volume	⇊	⇈
Fluid restriction	Not indicated	Indicated

CSW, cerebral salt wasting syndrome; SIADH, syndrome of inappropriate antidiuretic hormone. ⇊—decrease, ⇈—increase

NUTRITIONAL CONSIDERATIONS

Early and adequate nutrition support is thought to improve neurologic outcome and decrease morbidity and mortality (10,54). Studies recommend ideally initiating nutrition support within 48 hours of injury (55). The benefit of early nutrition support includes improved survival, lower infection risk, reduced rate of disability, and possibly reducing length of stay (56,57). Furthermore, investigators have shown that early EN support improves nutrient delivery in head-injured patients fed either via the nasogastric or nasointestinal route (56). However, a pilot study failed to detect similar results in ASCI (58). The use of immune-enhancing formulations and the role of specific nutrients in reducing oxidative stress have scarcely been studied in this population, and may be beneficial in improving clinical and nutritional outcomes.

Various obstacles preclude the provision of adequate nutrition support. For instance, delayed gastric emptying has been reported in neurologic injury, and the causes are thought to be multifactorial. Injury or damage to the higher centers of the CNS impacts gut function and motility, because gastrointestinal activity is regulated by the ANS. Furthermore, ASCI patients may experience paralytic ileus for 72 hours and up to 1 week due to autonomic disruption and the complications related to acute spinal cord trauma (33). Delayed gastric emptying is further exacerbated by increased ICP, as well as certain medications that are used to control elevated ICP (e.g., opioids, paralytic agents, and barbiturates). Once ICPs are within normal range, gastric function normalizes, but the exact mechanism remains unclear. Delayed gastric emptying and feeding intolerance is also associated with the severity of head injury. Patients with GCS less than 8 are more likely to experience feeding intolerance due to the severity of the brain injury. Lastly, cytokines, particularly increased levels of IL-1, significantly affect gastric emptying (59).

Several studies over the past decade have compared the use of small bowel feeding with gastric feeding in neurologic injury in order to provide more timely and adequate delivery of nutrition support (40). The former has been shown to be safe and effective in preventing aspiration and improving outcome (55). Ensuring and maintaining postpyloric feeding placement remains a clinical challenge, and investigators have reported that gastric feedings can successfully be used in this population (60–62). Taylor and associates compared the gradual increase in EN when gastric residual volumes were less than 50 ml on two consecutive measurements compared to an enhanced EN route in which EN feeding rate was started at full nutritional requirements by day 1 postinjury (56). The enhanced EN group experienced a higher percentage of nutrient delivery within the first week after injury, had fewer infectious complications, and better neurologic outcome at 3 months than the control patients. The investigators allowed for a higher gastric residual in the enhanced group (EN was stopped with gastric residuals >200 ml), which may have assisted with higher nutrient delivery and tolerance.

Earlier nutrition support studies reported PN to be more effective in providing necessary calories, protein, and fluid following neurologic injury (59). However, although EN has been shown to be more beneficial than PN in preserving gut integrity, improving immune competence, and attenuating the metabolic response to stress during critical illness, successful use of EN may be a challenge in patients with neurological injuries because these patients are at risk for delayed gastric emptying (62,63). However, transpyloric tube placement has been found to circumvent this problem. Small bowel feeding tube placement may be needed in patients who require supine positioning, heavy sedation, and those with large gastric residual volume and at risk for aspiration pneumonia (64). For instance, in one study, 23 of 30 neurosurgical patients in a pentobarbital-induced coma for intractable intracranial hypertension received at least 75% of their calorie needs through postpyloric enteral feedings (65). Physiologic changes associated with primary injury to the brain, combined with the pharmacodynamic influences of barbiturate therapy, contribute to the difficulties of initiating aggressive nutrition support (66).

In patients with gastrointestinal injury, prolonged ileus, and those who cannot tolerate EN, PN can be added as a supplemental or complete source of nutrition support. Hyperglycemia is a common PN-induced complication as well as an increased risk for infection (64). Hyperglycemia adversely affects neurological function; thus, aggressively controlling elevated blood sugar with insulin is warranted (67). However, if managed appropriately, hyperglycemia can be avoided when using PN.

There have been no studies that have assessed the efficacy of the route and timing of feeding in spinal cord injury and stroke patients; however, the previously listed recommendations should also hold true to all patients with neurological injury.

CONCLUSION

Critically ill patients in a NICU present with a multitude of metabolic, physiologic, and nutritional challenges. The use of nutrition support is clearly needed in this population. Early enteral nutrition, given at less than 72 hours after injury, is recommended to obtain the numerous benefits associated with the use of early EN (see Chapter 3 for a more in-depth discussion). Although guidelines for TBI are available, further studies in assessing energy expenditure and route of nutrient delivery are needed in ASCI, intracranial hemorrhage, and ischemic brain injury. Furthermore, inadequate nutritional support can negatively affect clinical outcomes in critically ill patients; hence, the use of IC monitoring is suggested in this subgroup of patients until further studies can define the actual nutritional requirements needed in this subset of the neurologically injured population.

REFERENCES

1. Sunderland PM, Heilbrun MP. Estimating energy expenditure in traumatic brain injury: Comparison of indirect calorimetry with predictive formulas. *Neurosurgery.* 1992;31:246–252; discussion 252–253.

2. Daverat P, Castel JP, Dartigues JF, Orgogozo JM. Death and functional outcome after spontaneous intracerebral hemorrhage. A prospective study of 166 cases using multivariate analysis. *Stroke.* 1991;22:1–6.

3. Twyman D. Nutritional management of the critically ill neurologic patient. *Crit Care Clin.* 1997;13:39–49.

4. Varella L, Jastremski CA. Neurological impairement. In: *The Science and Practice of Nutrition Support: A Case-Based Core Curriculum.* Dubuque, Iowa: Kendell/Hunt Publishing Company; 2001.

5. Noback CR SN, Demarest RJ, Ruggiero DA. *The Human Nervous System.* 6th ed. Totowa, N.J.: Human Press; 2005.

6. Schunn CD, Daly JM. Small bowel necrosis associated with postoperative jejunal tube feeding. *J Am Coll Surg.* 1995;180:410–416.

7. Frayn KN. Hormonal control of metabolism in trauma and sepsis. *Clin Endocrinol.* 1986;24: 577–599.

8. Clifton GL, Robertson CS, Grossman RG, Hodge S, Foltz R, Garza C. The metabolic response to severe head injury. *J Neurosurg.* 1984;60:687–696.

9. Cresci GA, Martindale RG. Nutrition support in trauma. In Gottschlich M, ed. *The Science and Practice of Nutrition Support: A Case-Based Core Curriculum.* Dubuque, Iowa: Kendall/Hunt Publishing Company; 2001.

10. Bullock R CR, Clifton G, et al. *Guidelines for the Management of Severe Head Injury.* New York, N.Y.: Brain Trauma Foundation and American Association of Neurological Surgeons; 1995.

11. Lam AM, Winn HR, Cullen BF, Sundling N. Hyperglycemia and neurological outcome in patients with head injury. *J Neurosurg.* 1991;75:545–551.

12. Pittas AG, Siegel RD, Lau J. Insulin therapy and in-hospital mortality in critically ill patients: Systematic review and meta-analysis of randomized controlled trials. *JPEN.* 2006;30:164–172.

13. Odderson R KJ, McKenna BS. Swallowing management in patients on an acute stroke pathway: Quality is cost effective. *Arch Phys Med Rehabil.* 1995;76:1130–1133.

14. Bistrian BR, Blackburn GL, Vitale J, Cochran D, Naylor J. Prevalence of malnutrition in general medical patients. *JAMA.* 1976;235:1567–1570.

15. Rodriguez DJ, Benzel EC, Clevenger FW. The metabolic response to spinal cord injury. *Spinal Cord.* 1997;35:599–604.

16. Seres DS. Surrogate nutrition markers, malnutrition, and adequacy of nutrition support. *Nutr Clin Pract.* 2005;20:308–313.

17. Gabay C, Kushner I. Acute-phase proteins and other systemic responses to inflammation. *N Engl J Med.* 1999;340:448–454.

18. Fuhrman MP, Charney P, Mueller CM. Hepatic proteins and nutrition assessment. *J Am Diet Assoc.* 2004;104:1258–1264.

19. Moore F. Energy and the maintenance of the body cell mass. *JPEN.* 1980;4:228–260.

20. Frankenfield D, Rowe WA, Cooney RN, Smith JS, Becker D. Limits of body mass index to detect obesity and predict body composition. *Nutrition.* 2001;17:26–30.

21. Frankenfield D. Energy requirements in the critically ill. *Support Line.* 2005;27:3–7.

22. Donaldson J, Borzatta MA, Matossian D. Nutrition strategies in neurotrauma. *Crit Care Nurs Clin North Am.* 2000;12:465–475.

23. Long CL, Nelson KM, Akin JM Jr., Geiger JW, Merrick HW, Blakemore WS. A physiologic basis for the provision of fuel mixtures in normal and stressed patients. *J Trauma.* 1990;30:1077–1085; discussion 1085–106.

24. Long CL, Schaffel N, Geiger JW, Schiller WR, Blakemore WS. Metabolic response to injury and illness: Estimation of energy and protein needs from indirect calorimetry and nitrogen balance. *JPEN.* 1979;3:452–456.

25. Rouby JJ, Eurin B, Glaser P, et al. Hemodynamic and metabolic effects of morphine in the critically ill. *Circulation.* 1981;64:53–59.

26. Robertson CS, Clifton GL, Grossman RG. Oxygen utilization and cardiovascular function in head-injured patients. *Neurosurgery.* 1984;15:307–314.

27. Bucci MN, Dechert RE, Arnoldi DK, Campbell J, McGillicuddy JE, Bartlett RH. Elevated intracranial pressure associated with hypermetabolism in isolated head trauma. *Acta Neurochir (Wein).* 1988;93:133–136.

28. Smith ER, Amin-Hanjani S. Evaluation and management of elecated intracranial pressure in adults. Available at: www.uptodate.com. Accessed November 17, 2005.

29. Dickerson RN, Roth-Yousey L. Medication effects on metabolic rate: A systematic review (part 1). *J Am Diet Assoc.* 2005;105:835–843.

30. Bracken MB, Shepard MJ, Collins WF, et al. A randomized, controlled trial of methylprednisolone or naloxone in the treatment of acute spinal-cord injury. Results of the Second National Acute Spinal Cord Injury Study. *N Engl J Med.* 1990;322:1405–1411.

31. Marian M. Acute spinal cord injuries: Nutrition management. *Support Line.* 2004;2:3–8.

32. Hadley MN, Walters BC, Grabb PA, et al. Guidelines for the management of acute cervical spine and spinal cord injuries. *Clin Neurosurg.* 2002;49:407–498.

33. Blissitt PA. Nutrition in acute spinal cord injury. *Crit Care Nurs Clin North Am.* 1990;2:375–384.

34. Kearns PJ, Thompson JD, Werner PC, Pipp TL, Wilmot CB. Nutritional and metabolic response to acute spinal-cord injury. *JPEN.* 1992;16:11–15.

35. Cox SA, Weiss SM, Posuniak EA, Worthington P, Prioleau M, Heffley G. Energy expenditure after spinal cord injury: An evaluation of stable rehabilitating patients. *J Trauma.* 1985;25:419–423.

36. Chalela J, Haymore J, Schellinger P, Kang D, Warach S. Acute stroke patients are being underfed. A nitrogen balance study. *Neurocritical Care.* 2004;1:331–334.

37. Kasuya H, Kawashima A, Namiki K, Shimizu T, Takakura K. Metabolic profiles of patients with subarachnoid hemorrhage treated by early surgery. *Neurosurgery.* 1998;42:1268–1274; discussion 1274–1275.

38. Leira R, Davalos A, Silva Y, et al. Early neurologic deterioration in intracerebral hemorrhage: Predictors and associated factors. *Neurology.* 2004;63:461–467.

39. Esper DH, Coplin WM, Carhuapoma JR. Energy expenditure in patients with nontraumatic intracranial hemorrhage. *JPEN.* 2006;30:71–75.

40. ASPEN Board of Directors and the Clinical Guideline Task Force. Guidelines for the use of parenteral and enteral nutrition in adult and pediatric patients. *JPEN.* 2002;26:1SA–128SA.

41. McClave SA, McClain CJ, Snider HL. Should indirect calorimetry be used as part of nutritional assessment? *J Clin Gastroenterol.* 2001;33:14–19.

42. Wray CJ, Mammen JM, Hasselgren PO. Catabolic response to stress and potential benefits of nutrition support. *Nutrition.* 2002;18:971–977.

43. Hasselgren P. Glucocorticoids and muscle catabolism. *Curr Opin Clin Nutr Metab Care.* 1999;2: 201.

44. Militsa B. Nutrition in neurologic and neurological critical care. *Neurology India.* 2001;49: S75–S79.

45. Barco KT, Smith RA, Peerless JR, Plaisier BR, Chima CS. Energy expenditure assessment and validation after acute spinal cord injury. *Nutr Clin Pract.* 2002;17:309–313.

46. Peruzzi WT, Shapiro B, Cane R. Resting energy expenditure in the acute phase of spinal cord injury (abstract). *Crit Care Clin.* 1994;22:A208.

47. Kolpek JH, Ott LG, Record KE, et al. Comparison of urinary urea nitrogen excretion and measured energy expenditure in spinal cord injury and nonsteroid-treated severe head trauma patients. *JPEN.* 1989;13:277–280.

48. Young B, Ott L, Rapp R, Norton J. The patient with critical neurological disease. *Crit Care Clin.* 1987;3:217–233.

49. Ott L, Young B, Phillips R, McClain C. Brain injury and nutrition. *Nutr Clin Pract.* 1990;5:68–73.

50. Laven GT, Huang CT, DeVivo MJ, Stover SL, Kuhlemeier KV, Fine PR. Nutritional status during the acute stage of spinal cord injury. *Arch Phys Med Rehabil.* 1989;70:277–282.

51. Mirenda J, Broyles G. Propofol as used for sedation in the ICU. *Chest.* 1995;108:539–548.

52. Doyle JA, Davis DP, Hoyt DB. The use of hypertonic saline in the treatment of traumatic brain injury. *J Trauma.* 2001;50:367–383.

53. Rabinstein AA, Wijdicks EF. Hyponatremia in critically ill neurological patients. *Neurologist.* 2003;9:290–300.

54. Rapp RP, Young B, Twyman D, et al. The favorable effect of early parenteral feeding on survival in head-injured patients. *J Neurosurg.* 1987;58:906–911.

55. Yanagawa T, Bunn F, Roberts I, Wentz R, Pierro A. Nutritional support for head-injured patients (Cochrane Review). In: The Cochrane Library, Update software, Oxford. 2005:1–20.

56. Taylor SJ, Fettes SB, Jewkes C, Nelson RJ. Prospective, randomized, controlled trial to determine the effect of early enhanced enteral nutrition on clinical outcome in mechanically ventilated patients suffering head injury. *Crit Care Med.* 1999;27:2525–2531.

57. Nyswonger GD, Helmchen RH. Early enteral nutrition and length of stay in stroke patients. *J Neurosci Nurs.* 1992;24:220–223.

58. Dvorak MF, Noonan VK, Belanger L, et al. Early versus late enteral feeding in patients with acute cervical spinal cord injury: A pilot study. *Spine.* 2004;29:E175–E180.

59. Ott L, Young B, Phillips R, et al. Altered gastric emptying in the head-injured patient: Relationship to feeding intolerance. *J Neurosurg.* 1991;74:738–742.

60. Spain DA, DeWeese RC, Reynolds MA, Richardson JD. Transpyloric passage of feeding tubes in patients with head injuries does not decrease complications. *J Trauma.* 1995;39:1100–1102.

61. Rhoney DH, Parker Jr D, Formea CM, Yap C, Coplin WM. Tolerability of bolus versus continuous gastric feeding in brain-injured patients. *Neurol Res.* 2002;24:613–620.

62. Klodell CT, Carroll M, Carrillo EH, Spain DA. Routine intragastric feeding following traumatic brain injury is safe and well tolerated. *Am J Surg.* 2000;179:168–171.

63. Maynard ND, Bihari DJ. Postoperative feeding. *BMJ.* 1991;303:1007–1008.

64. Heyland DK, Dhaliwal R, Drover JW, Gramlich L, Dodek P. Canadian clinical practice guidelines for nutrition support in mechanically ventilated, critically ill adult patients. *JPEN.* 2003;27: 355–373.

65. Magnuson B, Hatton J, Williams S, Loan T. Tolerance and efficacy of enteral nutrition for neurosurgical patients in pentobarbital coma. *Nutr Clin Pract.* 1999;14:131–134.

66. Magnuson B, Hatton J, Zweng TN, Young B. Pentobarbital coma in neurosurgical patients: Nutrition considerations. *Nutr Clin Pract.* 1994;9:146–150.

67. Boulanger BR, Nayman R, McLean RF, Phillips E, Rizoli SB. What are the clinical determinants of early energy expenditure in critically injured adults? *J Trauma.* 1994;37:969–974.

CHAPTER 8

Surgical Oncology

Mary Marian, MS, RD; and Mary Russell, MS, RD, CNSD

INTRODUCTION

The incidence of new cancers in the United States is approximately 1.4 million cases per year with cancer the cause of death in 25% of deaths from all causes (1). When deaths are aggregated by age, cancer has surpassed heart disease as the leading cause of death for individuals under the age of 85 (2). Prostate cancer is the most commonly diagnosed cancer in men followed by lung and bronchus, colon, and rectum (2). For women, breast, lung, and bronchus, followed by colon and rectal cancers are the most common (2). In 2006 approximately 564,830 Americans died from cancer, or about 1,550 per day. Cancers of the lung and bronchus, prostate, and colon and rectum in men, and cancers of the lung and bronchus, breast, and colon and rectum in women continue to be the most common fatal cancers. These four cancers account for one half of the total cancer deaths among men and women (1).

The continuum of cancer survival includes treatment and recovery, life after recovery, and living with advanced cancer. Each stage is associated with different challenges because the presence of cancer and the oncological therapies often utilized for the treatment of cancer can have a profound effect on nutritional status. Therefore, for patients newly diagnosed with cancer, undergoing treatment, or recovering from therapy as well as in remission, nutrition is an important component of medical care. Nutrition intervention goals include the following:

- prevention or reversal of nutritional deficiencies
- prevention or improvement in treatment-related symptoms
- enhanced response to therapy
- decreased morbidity related to disease/treatment
- prevention or improvement in functional ability
- prevention or improvement in quality of life

Surgery, chemotherapy, radiation, and immunotherapy are commonly utilized antineoplastic therapies, and their side effects are significant contributors to alterations in nutritional status. It is well documented that nutritional issues and

169

malnutrition afflict many cancer patients with malnutrition often the ultimate cause of mortality (3,4). Reportedly, 40% to 80% of oncology patients develop detectable malnutrition during their illness (5,6). Additionally, it is common practice in medicine to evaluate patients for the presence of a malignancy when significant weight loss is unintentional. Malnutrition can result due to the disease process, oncologic treatment, or both.

CANCER ANOREXIA-CACHEXIA SYNDROME

Malnutrition can develop due to a wasting syndrome known as *cancer anorexia-cachexia syndrome* (*CACS*), which is derived from the Greek words *kakos*, meaning "bad," and *hexis*, meaning "condition" (7). Cachexia is often manifested by not only weight loss but also anorexia, early satiety, dysgeusia, nausea, constipation, fatigue, anemia, and edema. Cachexia is also commonly associated with other inflammatory conditions such as cardiac failure, rheumatoid arthritis, and chronic obstructive pulmonary disease. Warren reported as early as 1932 that upon autopsy, severe malnutrition was the immediate cause of death in 22% of patients with cancer and up to two thirds of the remaining patients exhibiting some degree of cachexia (3). In a retrospective analysis of more than 3000 patients treated by nine different oncologic protocols, the Eastern Cooperative Oncology Group (ECOG) reported that weight loss (as little as 6%) predicted response to therapy, decreased overall survival, and correlated with performance status, productivity, and quality of life, all of which declined concurrently with weight (8). Furthermore, approximately 80% of the study patients presented with weight loss before being diagnosed with cancer.

Tumor type and stage of disease have been shown to impact nutritional status because patients with gastric, esophageal, and pancreatic cancer reportedly are more malnourished than patients with breast cancer and hematologic malignancies. About 48%–61% of patients with colon, prostate, lung cancer, and unfavorable non-Hodgkin's lymphoma experience some weight loss while patients with advanced cancer experience malnutrition the most frequently (8,9). Patients with similar types of cancer and disease stage may vary significantly in the development of cachexia, illustrating that tumor phenotype and host response also contribute to this complex condition.

Treatment for CACS generally includes treatment of the underlying malignancy as well as amelioration of the other factors influencing the ability to consume adequate nutrition. Individual cancers appear to have different mechanisms for CACS, including cytokines, akinetic effects of the gastrointestinal system, and factors that cause nausea by targeting the feeding centers located in the hypothalamus. Pharmacologic management (e.g., megestrol acetate, corticosteroids) of cancer-associated symptoms can also be successfully employed to aid in the control of CACS.

Mechanisms

Although the syndrome is not well understood, a variety of mechanisms that likely contribute to nutritional deterioration and ultimately cancer cachexia have been implicated. Cachexia can be exhibited by patients with localized as well as metastatic disease. The progressive wasting of skeletal muscle exhibited by patients with cancer cachexia is clearly very different from that of patients with simple starvation. Decreased hepatic protein synthesis, reduced hepatic mass, and preferential utilization of fat stores over lean body mass characterize simple starvation. Although inanition in itself explains the body composition changes seen in simple starvation, reduced nutritional intake alone does not explain why malnutrition occurs in so many cancer patients because cachexia may still occur in patients consuming what appear to be adequate calories.

A number of cytokines mediators have been implicated in orchestrating the complex scenario of events that potentially facilitates the development of malnutrition in cancer patients (10). Cytokines are protein mediators secreted by a wide variety of cell types, including macrophages, monocytes, lymphocytes, and endothelial and epithelial cells in response to malignancy, trauma, or sepsis. The proinflammatory cytokines including TNF α, IL-1, IL-6, and interferon gamma (IFN γ) have been linked with the onset of cancer cachexia (7). In animals, administration of these cytokines subsequently results in anorexia, weight loss, proteolysis, and lipolysis, accompanied by increases in cortisol and glucagon levels, and increases in energy expenditure. These cytokines are thought to work in concert rather than individually in their promotion of malnutrition. Other mediators that may play a role in the development of cancer cachexia include PIF, a 24-kd glycoprotein protelysis-inducing factor that has been isolated from the urine of weight-losing cancer patients but not in those losing weight from other causes (11).

Several neurotransmitter systems within the hypothalamus have also been implicated in cancer cachexia, primarily anorexia (7). Seratonin and melanocortin, in particular, have been identified as possible contributors although their precise role has yet to be identified.

It is important to classify cachexia as primary or secondary and differentiate between the two types. The etiology of primary cachexia is not well understood and therefore difficult to treat. Alterations in metabolic pathways, abnormal substrate metabolism, and altered energy expenditure have been postulated as potential causes. On the other hand, the causes of secondary cachexia (a functional inability to consume adequate oral intake) may be more treatable, because malnutrition may develop due to mechanical factors (e.g., obstruction, mucositis) or treatment modalities.

Antineoplastic Treatments

Antineoplastic therapies, including surgery, chemotherapy, and radiation, are known contributors to malnutrition (see Table 8–1).

Table 8–1 Antineoplastic Therapies That May Impact Nutritional Status

Treatment	Potential Nutritional Impact
Surgery	Increased nutrient needs for recovery and wound healing, malabsorption, early satiety, dehydration, abdominal cramping, diarrhea bloating/gas, fluid/electrolyte imbalance, lactose intolerance, hyperglycemia
Chemotherapy	
Cytotoxic	Nausea, vomiting, anorexia, diarrhea, immunosuppression, fatigue, mucositis, peripheral neuropathy, dysgeusia, heightened sensitivity to tastes, metallic taste
Hormonal (glucocorticoids, anti-androgens/estrogens, gonadotropin-releasing hormone analog)	Hyperglycemia, edema, osteoporosis, nausea, vomiting, bone pain, hot flashes, hypercalcemia
Immunotherapy (interleukins, Interferon alfa, monoclonal antibodies)	Anorexia, nausea, vomiting, diarrhea, fatigue, immunosuppression
Radiation	Thorax area: anorexia, dysphagia, esophagitis, heartburn, early satiety, fatigue Abdomin/pelvic area: nausea, vomiting, diarrhea, abdominal cramping/bloating/gas, lactose intolerance, malabsorption, chronic colitis and enteritis

Surgically induced malnutrition is generally related to reduced gastrointestinal absorptive capacity for nutrients or increased metabolic demands for tissue repair postoperatively in the face of inadequate nutrition intake. Chemotherapy can result in a number of symptom-related side effects related to treatment as described in Table 8–1. Radiation therapy (see Table 8–1) also actively promotes nutritional deterioration when the organs associated with the mechanics of eating or nutrient absorption are affected by the radiotherapy field. Because of the prevalence of malnutrition associated with these oncologic therapies, symptom-related side effects should be aggressively treated. Table 8–2 provides strategies for combating these challenges.

Table 8–2 Nutritional Strategies for Management of Treatment-Related Symptoms

Symptom	Etiology	Recommendations
Anorexia	Radiation, chemotherapy Cytokines, oncological therapies, pain, depression	Small, frequent nutrient-dense meals, avoid drinking fluids with meals, avoid low-calorie filler foods, increase physical activity, appetite stimulants
Constipation & Diarrhea	Antineoplastic therapies	Low-fat, lactose-free, increase soluble fiber intake, avoid spicy foods, avoid caffeine, drink plenty of liquids, probiotics
Dysphagia	Tumor burden, antineoplastic therapies	Thickened, moist, soft or ground/pureed foods
Early satiety	Antineoplastic therapies	Small, frequent nutrient-dense meals, avoid drinking fluids with meals
Fatigue	Tumor burden, antineoplastic therapies, anemia, dehydration, chronic pain, medications, stress depression, poor nutrition	Small, frequent nutrient-dense meals, physical activity, meal planning/ assistance with shopping/meal preparation, manage stress and depression
Nausea/vomiting	Antineoplastic therapies	Small, frequent, low-fat, low-fiber meals, avoid spicy foods and caffeine, try not eating 1 to 2 hours before treatment, antiemetics; hypnosis, acupuncture, music therapy also effective
Stomatitis, mucositis	Antineoplastic therapies	Soft, nonirritating foods, nutrient-dense liquids/ nutritional supplements, miracle mouth/viscous lidocaine swishes, lemon/glycerine swabs

(*continues*)

Table 8–2 Continued

Symptom	Etiology	Recommendations
Weight loss	Tumor burden, cytokines, antineoplastic therapies	Small, frequent nutrient-dense meals, try liquid/powder nutritional supplements, consume high-calorie/protein foods
Weight gain	Antineoplastic therapies, edema	Low-fat diet with lean meats, low-fat dairy products, whole grains, fruits and veggies
Xerostomia	Tumor burden, antineoplastic therapies	Drink/swallow small amounts of food at one time, sip water/fluid after each bite, try sweet or tart foods, soft/pureed foods, suck on hard candies, artificial saliva

NUTRITION SCREENING AND ASSESSMENT

Malnutrition can be insidious in onset; therefore, early detection and intervention are essential to correct existing nutritional deficiencies or to promote maintenance of optimal nutritional status. The Joint Commission on the Accreditation of Healthcare Organizations (JCAHO) mandates that all hospitalized patients be screened for nutritional risk. However, the majority of patients with cancer are likely to receive therapy in an outpatient setting, where nutrition screening and intervention protocols are less likely to be established. Therefore, the first step in nutrition intervention is to determine, in all settings, which patients may benefit from nutrition intervention.

Ideally, patients should be screened for nutritional risk (see following criteria) *before* antineoplastic therapies are initiated—especially since the results of the ECOG study revealed that the presence of a 5% or more weight loss from usual body weight prior to initiation of therapy had a negative impact on outcome in terms of quality of life and survival (8). Although anorexia has been reported as the most common problem affecting the ability of patients with cancer to consume adequate oral nutrition, newly diagnosed patients with advanced cancer also complained of abdominal fullness (60%), constipation (58%), taste changes (46%), mouth dryness (40%), nausea (39%), and vomiting (27%) prior to initiation of oncologic treatment (12).

Severe malnutrition has been defined in the literature in two ways: functional (increased risk of morbidity and/or mortality) and by degree of weight loss (greater than 2% per week, 5% per month, 7.5% per 3 months, and 10% per 6 months) (13,14). The National Cancer Institute Grading System for weight loss is as follows: grade 0 = less than 5.0% loss, grade 1 = 5.0%–9.9%, grade 2 = 10.0%–19.9%, grade 3 = greater than 20.0% (15). Unfortunately, this grading system does not take into account the baseline deficit or the length of time that has elapsed. Attention to weight loss at an earlier time point is required to successfully prevent deterioration of weight, body composition, and performance status.

The patient-generated subjective global assessment (PG-SGA) is an assessment tool that provides a comprehensive evaluation of nutritional status specific for oncology patients. Based on the data obtained, patients can then be triaged into the appropriate nutrition intervention categories. Serial assessments are necessary to monitor any changes in nutritional status, because there is a high risk for nutritional deterioration in this population over time. CACS should be considered when the patient presents with an involuntary weight loss of 5% over 6 months, especially when muscle wasting is manifested (16).

NUTRITION INTERVENTION

Adequate intake of calories, protein, and micronutrients can improve nutritional status for most patients with cancer (17). The nutritional principles outlined by the American Cancer Society's guidelines on diet, nutrition, and cancer prevention should be used for the basis of a healthy diet for all patients with cancer, including those who are well nourished, during as well as after treatment (1). However, patients with cancer may experience challenges consuming adequate oral intake or other short-term and long-term issues (e.g., diarrhea, xerostomia, mucositis, etc.) that impact on nutritional status and are not addressed by these guidelines. A discussion regarding these particular issues will be forthcoming later in this chapter.

Patients identified at moderate- and high-nutritional risk should receive a comprehensive nutritional assessment that includes evaluation of anthropometric measurements (including weight for height, weight history, BMI, waist-to-hip ratio), nutrition history, physical examination for signs of nutritional deficiencies and laboratory data (e.g., electrolytes, renal function, glucose, serum albumin, and prealbumin, and hemoglobin/hematocrit together with MCV, MCHC). Assessment of performance status and quality of life should also be considered part of a comprehensive nutritional assessment. An *individualized* plan for nutrition intervention should be developed for patients identified with malnutrition that includes goals for clinical outcomes as well as plans for intervention. This plan should coincide with not only the medical team desires but also with the patient's and/or caregiver's wishes. Furthermore, the nutrition care plan should be based on the risks and burdens associated the provision of nutrition and expected outcomes to be accrued. Patients should be reassessed on a regular basis to allow for evaluation of the intervention's success and to determine if the nutrition care plan should be revised based on the patient's clinical status, treatment plan, and such. Possible goals of intervention include:

- Maintenance/improvement in nutritional status
- Maintenance/improvement in body weight; specifically lean body mass
- Adequate intake of macro- and micronutrients
- Prevention/improvement in symptoms related to treatment(s)
- Maintenance/improved functional status and quality of life

Several investigators have assessed the impact of both preoperative and perioperative nutrition and effect on clinical outcomes (18–20), specifically the utilization of specialized enteral formulations containing immunonutrients (arginine, omega-3 fatty acids, and nucleotides) compared with standard formulations (21–24). Braga et al. evaluated the impact of using commercially prepared immune-enhancing diets (IEDs) both preoperatively and postoperatively in patients with gastrointestinal cancers (20). Patients were randomized to three groups. The first group, the preoperative nutrition group, consumed 1 L/day of an oral IED for 5 days prior to surgery. These patients also received an intravenous solution of 5% glucose and electrolytes until they began eating again postoperatively. The second group (the perioperative group) received the same preoperative regimen, but starting 12 hours postoperatively, were fed via a jejunostomy feeding tube with the same preoperative IED. The third group (traditional therapy) received no pre- or perioperative IED, but postoperatively received an intravenous solution of 5% glucose and electrolytes until oral nutrition was started. The three groups were comparable in all nutrition and surgical variables. A significant reduction in postoperative infections was found in both the preoperative and perioperative groups when compared with the group receiving standard care. Additionally, the number of patients with noninfectious or any complications was lower (although not statistically significant) in both the pre- and perioperative groups when compared with the group receiving standard care. The rates of all types of complications were similar between the pre- and perioperative groups. The mean length of hospitalization was also significantly shorter for patients receiving both the pre- and perioperative IED. Braga and colleagues also investigated whether using IEDs pre- and perioperatively when compared with conventional therapy or nonimmune-enhancing diets for patients with colorectal cancer would be of benefit (25). Patients receiving the IEDs had fewer postoperative infectious complications when compared with the conventional and non-IED study groups and increased gut perfusion. In another study utilizing IEDs perioperatively, patients receiving IEDs had fewer infectious complications including pneumonia and wound infections (18). Inflammatory markers such as C-reactive protein and IL-6 were also reduced in the IED group. Lastly, perioperative consumption of IEDs reportedly reduced infectious complications in well-nourished patients (22).

Based on the results of these studies, the European Society for Parenteral and Enteral Nutrition (ESPEN) clinical guidelines for EN support recommends the initiation of preoperative EN for 5–7 days, using IEDs containing arginine, omega-3 fatty acids, and nucleotides, for patients scheduled to undergo surgery for upper-gastrointestinal cancer regardless of nutritional status (26). Others caution that before the use of IEDs can be recommended on a more global basis that further study is warranted. Overall, the results of clinical studies using IEDs have been mixed. This is likely due to study design, differing patient populations, study size, and the delivery of nutrients in various amounts. Oncology patients, in particular, differ by type of disease and tumor, stage of disease, and type of treatment. Moreover, it appears that to gain the greatest benefits related to using IEDs, in terms of modulating the inflammatory response, that the particular nutrients must have been consumed before the time of injury or insult (such as surgery).

NUTRITIONAL SUPPLEMENTS

Oral nutrition is the preferred method for the provision of adequate nutrition. Because nutritional status may affect the progression of the disease, tolerance to treatment, ability to complete treatment, and increased overall morbidity and mortality, the ability to consume adequate oral nutrition should be reassessed often. The strategies for maintaining adequate oral intake depend on the challenges experienced by the individual. Table 8–1 provides recommendations that have been found to successfully maintain oral intake when treatment-related symptoms are problematic (27). Aggressive management of symptoms related to treatment has also been shown to not only improve/maintain nutritional status but also improve quality of life and social interactions (28,29).

The use of commercially prepared nutritional supplements has resulted in better weight gain and reduced incidence of postoperative complications in patients undergoing surgery for gastrointestinal cancers (30). Omega-3 (specifically eicosapentaenoic acid [EPA]) enriched nutritional supplements have been found to reverse weight loss, increase lean body mass, and improve quality of life and survival in some clinical studies (31–33). EPA has been associated with an anti-inflammatory response, including down-regulation of both proinflammatory cytokine synthesis and the acute phase response in both healthy individuals and patients with cancer. Conversely, other studies have found no improvements (33–35). However, in the Fearon et al. study, patients with gastrointestinal cancers who received EPA experienced a significant increase in body weight compared to placebo (33). This data also suggests that consumption of 2 gms daily of EPA is necessary to obtain any benefit from supplementation. Higher doses do not appear to confer additional benefits. However, before EPA supplementation is commonly recommended, further studies are needed to better elucidate the benefits of omega-3 fatty acid supplementation including optimum dosage, specific formulations, route of administration, impact on body composition, quality of life, survival, and the specific patient populations likely to benefit.

NUTRITION SUPPORT

When oral nutritional intake is insufficient to maintain nutritional status or is contraindicated, nutrition support should be considered. The time at which nutrition support should be instituted for patients with cancer is controversial. This may be due in part to the fact that many use the term "supportive nutrition" interchangeably with parenteral nutrition (PN), because it was previously thought that cancer-associated malnutrition could be prevented and that survival and nutritional status could be improved with the use of PN. In their review of more than 40 randomized prospective trials of patients undergoing surgical, chemotherapy, or radiation treatment for cancer, Klein and Koretz concluded that few studies found any statistically significant difference in clinical endpoints (postoperative complications or mortality rates) between patients receiving nutrition support (PN or enteral tube feeding) and those who did not (36). While these results may suggest that the therapeutic benefits of nutrition support are limited in cancer patients, one must remember that the quality of these trials is affected by many factors, including small sample size, heterogeneous populations (differences in tumor type and disease stage), and variation in initiation and duration of nutrition support, thereby obscuring any nutritional benefits. A multitude of options is currently available for providing nutrition-support interventions for oncology patients at risk for as well as those presenting with malnutrition. The most appropriate intervention(s) should be chosen after a comprehensive assessment of factors including nutritional status, oncologic treatment planned, patient wishes, and degree of aggressive intervention warranted (see Chapter 3 for further details regarding the indications/contraindications for nutrition support). If aggressive antineoplastic therapies are planned, then nutritional intervention should be actively pursued.

ENTERAL NUTRITION

EN support is clearly preferred over PN when specialized nutrition support is warranted (see Chapter 3 for further discussion). In the meta-analysis of 27 prospective, randomized controlled studies investigating the use of early EN in hospitalized patients with a variety of medical conditions, including surgical oncology patients, Marik et al. noted a significant reduction in hospital length of stay and infectious complications with early EN (37). In addition to a reduction in infectious complications and LOS, EN is associated with positive clinical measures such as earlier reduction in inflammatory markers such as C-reactive protein levels, improved APACHE II scores, and shorter duration of nutrition support (38–40). The current evidence available suggests that EN should be initiated within 24–48 hours following injury or hospital admission in order to gain such benefits. The exact percentage of goal calories to achieve these clinical outcomes is currently not clear. Although previously thought to be beneficial, a number of recent studies have shown that "trickle feedings" or "trophic feeds" (e.g., 10–30 mL/hour) are neither sufficient to maintain gut integrity nor to achieve positive clinical outcomes (41,42).

A review of the current literature reflects that the delivery of approximately 14–18 kcal/kg/d or 60%–70% of enteral feeding goal is recommended to achieve favorable outcomes (42–44).

The American Society for Parenteral and Enteral Nutrition (ASPEN) clinical guidelines recommend that specialized nutrition support should be initiated for patients with an inadequate oral intake for 7 to 14 days or in patients in whom inadequate oral intake is expected for a 7- to 14-day period (45). EN should be considered for patients unable to consume adequate oral nutrition when the gastrointestinal tract can be safely used.

PARENTERAL NUTRITION

PN for patients receiving chemotherapy with or without radiation can result in increased weight and body fat mass, correction of vitamin and mineral deficiencies, and improved hydration (46). However, data from 26 randomized controlled trials of PN in cancer patients suggested that the therapy was associated with net harm, leading the American College of Physicians to recommend that "routine use of PN for patients undergoing chemotherapy should be discouraged" (47). In its technical review, the American Gastroenterological Society concluded that PN was associated with decreased tumor response and increased complications and infections and had no effect on survival of patients receiving chemotherapy or radiation (48). Zaloga describes several studies in cancer patients in which EN, compared with PN, resulted in fewer infections, lower cost, and/or fewer complications (49). In contrast, a report by Fan et al. notes lower mortality, reduced preoperative morbidity, and fewer infections in hepatocellular carcinoma patients who received PN, compared with those who received EN (50).

The VA Cooperative Study, which included many patients with lung or gastrointestinal cancer, demonstrated that major infections were significantly greater in patients who received PN and were not severely malnourished, and that patients who were moderately to severely malnourished and received PN for at least 7 days had significantly fewer complications than did patients who received an oral diet (51). The National Institutes of Health, ASPEN, and the American Society for Clinical Nutrition, in a consensus statement (52), noted that:

- A course of 7–10 days of preoperative PN in a malnourished patient with GI cancer results in a reduction in postoperative complications
- Routine use of postoperative PN in malnourished surgical patients who did not receive preoperative PN results in an increase in complications
- PN is indicated if, by postoperative day 5–10, the patient is unable to tolerate oral feeding or EN

The group noted that the amount and type of preoperative PN provided in many of the studies was suboptimal and that in some cases excess energy was provided.

In summary, PN should not be routinely administered to cancer patients undergoing chemotherapy, radiation, or surgery. It should be considered only in patients who are moderately to severely malnourished and unable to tolerate EN or oral diet for at least 1 week. Preoperative PN is indicated for moderately to severely malnourished patients in whom surgery may safely be delayed 7–14 days (45).

HOME NUTRITION SUPPORT

Nutrition support, especially EN, is widely used in long-term care, hospice, and other alternative care sites (53). Advances in technology and improvement in reimbursement by third-party payers, as well as patient preference, have led to significant expansion in the use of nutrition support in the home setting. ASPEN guidelines for the provision of home nutrition support stress the importance of in-depth nutrition assessment; assessment of the patient's home environment and his or her medical suitability for EN or PN, education level, and rehabilitative potential; and close evaluation of reimbursement sources prior to making a decision about home nutrition support (54). PN or EN should be terminated when the patient no longer benefits from the therapy or the burden exceeds the benefit (53–55). Howard, in 1993, reviewed the use of home nutrition support in cancer patients (56). Mean survival time with nutrition support (EN or PN) was 6 months; 25% lived more than 1 year and 20% returned to an oral diet as the sole method of nourishment (56). Children and adults with leukemia, lymphoma, or small bowel or liver neoplasms had a relatively better outcome than did other cancer patients. Patients with active cancer who received PN or EN at home had no more therapy-related readmissions than did other groups of patients, but their overall rehospitalization rate was greater.

Most literature examining the experience of home EN patients reflects the European experience. Loeser et al. studied quality of life and nutritional status in 155 patients, slightly more than half with malignant disease, who required gastrostomy tube (GT) feeding for more than 6 weeks (57). At the conclusion of the study (during which almost half of the patients either died or dropped from the study), the patients demonstrated improved quality of life and physical function, less fatigue, and stable or slightly improved nutritional status. Beer et al. (58) followed patients who had received early GT placement for 208–344 days and noted a significant reduction in treatment interruptions and malnutrition prevalence in the patients who received a GT before or within 2 weeks of initiation of radiation therapy, compared with patients who did not have the tube placed until 2 weeks to 3 months after radiation therapy began.

Schattner et al. also studied head and neck cancer survivors, who required EN for 32±39.6 months (59). Oral intake during this period was minimal to none. At the start of feeding, 51% of patients had a normal body mass index (BMI) and were assigned to weight maintenance; of these patients, 84% maintained a normal BMI and 16% were assigned to the weight gain group. Thirty-one percent of the patients had an elevated BMI and were assigned to a weight loss regimen; average BMI loss was 4 kg/m^2. On average, each patient required three feeding tubes (range 1–13); tolerance to feeding was excellent.

GT placement for decompression has been noted to be technically feasible and safe in patients with malignant bowel obstruction due to ovarian cancer and has facilitated end-of-life care at home or in an inpatient hospice for most patients (60).

Home PN offers limited benefit for most patients with widely metastatic disease and a poor prognosis (46). A study of terminally ill cancer patients in a long-term care facility suggested that most patients experienced neither hunger nor thirst (61). Buchman suggested that provision of no nutrition support and voluntary fasting may be reasonable for these patients because of the reduction in glucose oxidation and skeletal muscle catabolism from ketosis (62–64). Home PN may be indicated when there is a short-term loss of GI function associated with a cancer diagnosis or its treatment or a failure of EN (45,65). Bozzetti suggested development of specific criteria for establishing the utility of home PN for cancer patients. His suggestion was presence of a "valid medical indication" and a projected survival of at least 3 months (66). Hoda et al. noted median survival time of 5 months from initiation of PN until death in 52 patients with incurable cancer (67); 16 patients survived >1 year, and complications of PN in these patient were deemed "acceptable." Echoing others (68–70), these authors suggested that home PN could be life sustaining and indeed beneficial in a subset of patients with advanced, incurable cancer.

HEAD AND NECK CANCER

Malnutrition plays a key role in the morbidity of head and neck cancer patients receiving surgery, chemotherapy, radiotherapy, or combined modality therapy. Typically, oropharyngeal cancers are associated with weight loss prior to diagnosis of head and neck cancer (71). Following diagnosis, an additional 10% of pretherapy body weight may be lost during radiotherapy or combined-modality treatment (72). It is difficult to discern whether poor nutrition results in poor outcome because patients who receive more aggressive treatment experience greater toxicity to therapy, resulting in poor nutrition and weight loss. It has been established, however, that a reduction of greater than 20% of total body weight results in an increase in toxicity and mortality (4).

Therapeutic interventions including surgery, radiotherapy, and chemotherapy, in addition to poor intake, are the primary causes of weight loss. The paraneoplastic effect, as previously discussed, of the cancer itself is an additional factor. Severe toxicity can result in prolonged treatment times because of poor nutritional status, and prolonged treatment time has been implicated in poor clinical outcome. Swallowing function is also commonly adversely affected by treatment. Severe mucositis and neutropenia are also common sequelae of chemoradiation. In order to maintain or improve nutrition and hydration status, gastrostomy (G-tubes) or percutaneous endoscopic gastrostomy (PEG) tubes are frequently used as an avenue for the provision of nutrition in this patient population with typically 46% of patients with stage III cancer, and over 50% with stage IV head and neck cancers requiring G-tubes

(73). The dependence on EN support 6–12 months following surgical, radiotherapy, and/or chemotherapy interventions reportedly varies from 6% to 64% (74,75). Shiley et al. report the short-term (3 to 4 months) rate of G-tube dependence was 67% after chemoradiation and 50% after surgical management (76). At long-term (≥1 year) follow-up after chemoradiation, while patients without recurrence typically had at least some oral intake, one third still required supplemental enteral support due to chronic dysphagia.

Therefore, early intervention with nutritional supplementation can reduce the chance of inferior outcome in patients at high risk of weight loss, such as those with poor nutritional status prior to the initiation of therapy, those with a large tumor burden, those undergoing concurrent radiation therapy/chemotherapy, or those managed with radiotherapy fields that encompass large volumes of oropharyngeal mucosa.

Individualized nutritional counseling has been shown to effectively increase dietary intake and maintain or improve nutritional and functional status and quality of life in patients undergoing radiotherapy with a variety of head and neck cancers (77). Isenring et al. found that intense nutritional counseling beginning within 4 days of the start of radiotherapy, and continuing weekly for about 6 weeks, resulted in less weight loss and less deterioration in nutritional status and quality of life compared with patients receiving minimal nutrition intervention (78). Counseling is typically aimed at providing nutrition recommendations to meet nutritional needs in the face of symptomatic problems related to treatment (such as nausea, vomiting, early satiety, etc.), personal food preferences, and typical intake.

ESOPHAGEAL AND GASTRIC CANCERS

Patients with esophageal and gastric cancers also often present with malnutrition. Esophageal obstruction, dysphagia, anorexia, and the side effects (such as severe mucositis, vomiting, etc.) of treatment modalities including chemotherapy, radiation, and surgery individually or in combination, are commonly cited factors influencing nutrition status in this patient population (79).

Nutrition pathways, which identify whether patients with esophageal cancer are at low, moderate, or severe nutrition risk and provides patients with the appropriate nutrition intervention ranging from preventative advice for low-risk to enteral feedings for high-risk patients, are associated with less weight loss, greater radiotherapy completion rates, fewer hospital admissions, and shorter length of stay when admitted (79). Esophageal cancer frequently results in severe dysphagia or marked luminal obstruction, thereby necessitating the need for enteral support. Bozzetti and colleagues found that the administration of EN support resulted in stabilization of body weight and serum proteins, while patients receiving standard oral diets continued to experience deteriorations in both weight and serum proteins (80).

Gastric cancer is one of the most common cancers worldwide, with malnutrition commonly associated with its presence. Anorexia reportedly is experienced by approximately two thirds of patients with gastric cancer (81). Abdominal pain, anemia, and nausea and vomiting have been reported in 66%, 42%, and 32% of such patients, respectively (81).

Gastric resection is associated with an increased risk for morbidity, depending on the disease state and type of resection needed (82). The presence and type of disease dictates whether a small portion of the stomach must be removed versus a total gastrectomy. Whether a Billroth I (anastomosis of the esophagus or the remaining stomach to the duodenum) or a Billroth II (anastomosis of the esophagus or remaining stomach to the jejunum) is performed often impacts on the patient's ability to consume adequate oral nutrition postoperatively. Complications such as leaking or necrosis of the duodenal stump can also negatively impact on patient outcomes.

Dumping syndrome is a common consequence of gastric surgery, especially when the pylorus is either removed or bypassed. Dumping syndrome occurs when the food passes through the gastrointestinal tract quickly before significant absorption can occur, resulting in symptoms such as abdominal cramping, diarrhea, sweating, nausea, dizziness, and tachycardia (83), although these symptoms tend to lessen postoperatively. Symptoms usually appear within 30–60 minutes of eating and 2–3 hours after eating. Dietary modifications to help combat these symptoms include:

- eating small, frequent, bland, and low-fat meals
- avoiding spicy foods, alcohol, and sugar and sweets
- avoiding very hot or cold foods
- limiting fluids to 4 ounces during meals; drink liquids 30–45 minutes before and after eating

Depending on the type and extent of gastric surgery performed, some nutrients, vitamins, and minerals may be poorly absorbed with subsequent deficiencies in iron, calcium, folate, and B_{12}. Consuming a liquid or chewable multivitamin/mineral supplement and B_{12} shots may become necessary to avoid/correct deficiencies.

SMALL BOWEL CANCERS

EN can be critical to the prevention and treatment of the malnutrition associated with cancer, in particular in those patients with obstructions or defects of the oropharynx, esophagus, stomach, or duodenum (46). It should be considered when oral intake is insufficient to meet nutrition requirements for patients undergoing active anticancer treatment (27,83,84). If EN is not tolerated or is contraindicated, PN may be considered.

PANCREATIC CANCER

Pancreatic cancer is the fourth leading cause of cancer death in the United States, Canada, and western Europe (85). Tumor resection with curative intent is possible in only 10%–15% of subjects, with many patients facing limited therapeutic options and a poor prognosis (85). Recently, Hines and Reber (86) suggested that at some surgical centers, where a large number of pancreatic cancer surgeries are performed, survival rates may be higher.

Wignore and colleagues (87) noted that patients with pancreatic cancer had lost 15% of preillness weight by the time of diagnosis and had a median loss of 25% of preillness weight by time of death. Reduced intake is caused by a number of factors including depression, nausea, pain, anxiety, depression, and gastric outlet obstruction (85). Malabsorption and altered glucose tolerance further complicate nutritional status.

Nutritional interventions are not likely to extend the survival of a patient with advanced, progressive pancreatic cancer, but may have a role in palliative care and improvement in quality of life (85).

Brennan et al. randomized patients undergoing resection for pancreatic cancer to a postoperative regimen of PN versus IV fluid. They found no benefit to the routine use of postoperative PN, and noted that patients who received it had a significant increase in postoperative infectious complications (88). Kirby and Teran suggested that PN may have a role in blunting the progression of cachexia and weight loss and in allowing patients who may be cured the ability to better tolerate aggressive therapy (89). Bruno and colleagues demonstrated that a combination of nutrition support, pancreatic enzyme therapy, and biliary drainage prevented weight loss in patients with unresectable cancer of the pancreatic head (90).

At present, there is no strong evidence to support the use of early EN over PN or even, in some cases, IV hydration alone, for patients with pancreatic cancer. Rigorously designed clinical trials are needed to define the appropriate method of nutrition support (91–93).

LARGE BOWEL CANCERS

Early resumption of an oral diet following colorectal surgery is often possible and has been shown to be safe (94,95). EN or PN may be indicated for certain colon cancer patients with severe malnutrition and, in the latter case, inability to use the GI tract for nutrition support. Routine use of PN in patients with colon cancer has not been shown to be beneficial and is not recommended (96,97).

OSTOMIES

Ostomies are surgically created openings from the bowel to the skin that allows stool to pass through a newly created site in order to relieve the bowel of stool. Indications for ostomies are described in Table 8–3. Ostomies, such as jejunostomy, ileostomy, and colostomy, are classified based on their location in the bowel. Over 750,000 people in the United States have some type of ostomy (98). Ostomies may be temporary or permanent.

Table 8–3 Indications for Adult Ostomy Placement

Fecal Diversion

Jejunostomy
Trauma

Ileostomy
Cancer
Inflammatory bowel disease (Crohn's disease/ulcerative colitis)
Familial adenomatous polyposis (FAP)
Trauma

Cecostomy
Large bowel obstruction

Colostomy
Colon or rectal cancer
Trauma
Acute diverticulitis
Bowel rest needed

Urinary Diversion

Bladder extrophy
Cancer of the bladder
Spinal bifida
Spinal trauma

The nutritional management generally depends on the type of ostomy. The length of hospitalization following surgery for an ostomy is 7 to 10 days with diet initiation and advancement within 2 to 4 days (83).

ENTEROCUTANEOUS FISTULAS

Enterocutaneous fistulas (EFs) of the small bowel and colon may be complications of oncologic surgery. More than 75% of EFs are a result of bowel injury, inadvertent enterotomy, and/or anastomotic leakage (98). Fistula formation is more commonly associated with surgery in the presence of malignancy or inflammatory bowel disease (98). Death related to enterocutaneous fistulas remains disproportionately high compared with that associated with other surgical conditions (99). In more than published reports, sepsis was the leading cause of death, with high fistula output and presence of comorbidities in the patient important factors influencing the risk of death.

That malnutrition is associated with EF formation has been recognized for decades. Edmunds et al., in 1960, noted the relationship between malnutrition and mortality, with overall mortality of 54% in patients with small bowel fistulas compared with 16% for fistulas of the colon (100).

Once PN became widely available, it was widely adopted as the modality of choice for nutrition support of patients with EF (99). However, evidence that PN promotes healing of EF (beyond its role in providing nutrients) is not available. Gastrointestinal secretion is reduced 30%–50% in patients who receive PN (101). However, there are no published data to support the concept that PN results in earlier fistula closure (99). In one series of 1168 patients, Li et al. reported that 13.6% received PN, yet overall closure rates were high and mortality was low (102). Some authors have noted that an elemental enteral formula may reduce fistula output as much as PN (103). Levy et al. reported that 85% of 335 patients with EF in their study were converted to EN after a short period of PN (104). Among 234 patients managed conservatively, spontaneous fistula closure was seen in 38%, with a mortality rate of 19% (104). Limited data from animal models suggests that EN rather than PN increases anastomotic strength, possibly via trophic effects on the intestinal mucosa (105).

Initially, treatment of EF should concentrate on drainage of fluid collections, treatment of sepsis, management of fistula output, and correction of electrolyte and fluid imbalances (99). There is no evidence that bowel rest and restriction of enteral intake increase rates of EF closure, and in fact these practices may increase the risk of complications. High-output small bowel fistulas may require PN for optimal management, but EN should be used if at all possible. Operative repair should be delayed at least 3 months if spontaneous closure does not occur (99).

MALIGNANT BOWEL OBSTRUCTION

Malignant bowel obstruction (MBO) is common in patients with gynecological, colorectal, and advanced cancer. Although the precise etiology is unclear, MBO can be caused by a number of factors as illustrated in Table 8–4 (106). Nausea, vomiting, abdominal distention and pain, intermittent diarrhea, and constipation are symptoms typically manifested. Symptoms are rarely acute, instead developing slowly or intermittently in patients due to partial obstructions.

The diagnosis of MBO is established based on clinical presentation and confirmed with an abdominal radiograph. Treatment is individualized based on the patient presentation and past medical history, stage of disease, prognosis, treatment plans, and the patient's wishes. Surgery is generally the primary treatment; however, some patients are not surgical candidates and thus require alternative approaches for control of symptoms.

The medical management of MBO includes fluid administration to maintain hydration status and pharmacologic interventions such as analgesics, antisecretory drugs, antiemetics, and corticosteroids (106). Nasogastric suction or a venting gas-

Table 8–4 Potential Causes of Malignant Bowel Obstruction

Adhesions
Inflammatory edema
Inflammatory bowel disease
Intestinal muscle paralysis
Carcinomatosis with concurrent tumor filtration of the GI musculature and nerves
Fecal impaction
Constipating medications
Postradiation bowel damage
Hernia

trostomy may also be instituted to provide relief from nausea and vomiting when other medical avenues instituted prove ineffective.

Specialized nutrition support is also often initiated as part of the supportive care; however, this area also remains controversial within the palliative medicine arena (106). PN is typically instituted because the general diagnosis of MBO alone tends to preclude the possibility of using EN. A percutaneous endoscopic gastrostomy (PEG) tube is commonly placed to provide EN, when only the upper GI tract is occluded.

The use of PN for patients with MBO remains controversial. There is currently insufficient data to recommend the routine use of PN for all patients with MBO. Guidelines for initiation of PN for MBO are described in Table 8–5 (107). Outcomes measures and quality of life should be considered before initiation of SNS.

CONCLUSION

Medical nutrition therapy plays an important role in maintaining or improving the nutritional status of individuals with cancer. Nutrition screening plays a critical role in identifying patients who are at high risk for nutritional deterioration. Many

Table 8–5 Indications for PN in MBO (107)

Starvation likely to be the cause of death
Aggressive antineoplastic therapy planned
Survival is expected to be ≥ 3 months
Intravenous fluid required to maintain hydration status and nutrition equilibrium
Patient desires aggressive nutrition intervention
No other alternative

Source: Ripamonti C, Bruera E. Palliative management of malignant bowel obstruction. *Int J Gynecol Cancer.* 2002;12:135–143.

of the antineoplastic therapies, including surgery, are associated with a number of symptomatic side effects that can have a profound impact on nutritional status. Treatment-related symptoms should be aggressively addressed in order to maintain or improve nutritional status as well as quality of life.

REFERENCES

1. American Cancer Society. Available at: www.cancer.org. Accessed February 7, 2007.
2. Jemal A, Murray T, Ward E, et al. Cancer statistics, 2005. *CA Cancer J Clin.* 2005;55:10–30.
3. Warren S. The immediate cause of death in cancer. *Am J Med Sci.* 1932;185:610.
4. Copeland EM. Nutrition as an adjunct to cancer treatment in the adult. *Cancer Res.* 1977; 37:2451–2456.
5. Chute CG, Greenberg ER, Baron J, et al. Presenting condition of 1,539 population-based cancer patients in New Hampshire and Vermont. *Cancer.* 1985;56:2107–2111.
6. Shils ME. Principles of nutritional therapy. *Cancer.* 1979;43(suppl 5):2093–2102.
7. Barber MD. The pathophysiology and treatment of cancer cachexia. *Nutr Clin Pract.* 2002; 17:203–209.
8. DeWys WD, Begg C, Llavin PT, et al. Prognostic effect of weight loss prior to chemotherapy in cancer patients. *Am J Med.* 1980;69:491–497.
9. Meguid MM, Meguid V. Preoperative identification of the surgical cancer patient in need of postoperative supportive total parenteral nutrition. *Cancer.* 1985;55(suppl 1):258–262.
10. Tchekmedyian NW, Heber D. Clinical approaches to nutritional support in cancer. *Curr Opin Oncol.* 1993;5:633–638.
11. Todorov P, Cariuk P, McDevitt T, et al. Characterization of a cancer cachectic factor. *Nature.* 1996;379:739–742.
12. Grosvenor M, Bulcavage L, Chlebowski R. Symptoms potentially influencing weight loss in a cancer population. Correlations with primary site, nutritional status, and chemotherapy administration. *Cancer.* 1989;63:330–334.
13. Blackburn GL, Bistrian BR, Maini BS, et al. Nutritional and metabolic assessment of the hospitalized patient. *JPEN.* 1997;1:11–22
14. Ottery FD. Rethinking nutritional support of the cancer patient: The new field of nutritional oncology. *Semin Oncol.* 1994;21:770-778.
15. National Institutes of Health. National Cancer Institute, Cancer Therapy Evaluation Program. Common Toxicity criteria. Version 2.0. June 1, 1999.
16. Inui A. Cancer anorexia-cachexia syndrome: Are neuropeptides the key? *Cancer Research.* 1999;59:4493–4501.
17. Brown J, Byers T, Thompson K, et al. Nutrition during and after cancer treatment: A guide for informed choices by cancer survivors. *CA Cancer J Clin.* 2001;51:153–181.
18. Braga M, Gianotti L, Radaelli G, et al. Perioperative immunonutrition in patients undergoing cancer surgery: Results of a randomized double-blind phase 3 trial. *Arch Surg.* 1999;134:428–433.
19. Senkal M, Zumtobel V, Bauer K-H, et al. Outcome and cost-effectiveness of perioperative enteral immunonutrition in patients undergoing elective upper gastrointestinal tract surgery. *Arch Surg.* 1999;134:1309–1316.
20. Braga M, Gianotti L, Nespoli L, et al. Nutritional approach in malnourished surgical patients: A prospective randomized study. *Arch Surg.* 2002;137:174–180.

21. Gianotti L, Braga M, Nespoli L, et al. Effect of route of delivery and formulation of postoperative nutritional support in patients undergoing major operations for malignant neoplasms. *Arch Surg.* 1997;132:1222–1229.

22. Braga M, Gianotti L. Preoperative immunonutrition: Cost benefit analysis. *JPEN.* 2005;29: S57–S61.

23. Chen DW, Wei Fei Z, Zhang YC, et al. Role of enteral immunonutrition in patients with gastric carcinoma undergoing major surgery. *Asian J Surg.* 2005;28:121–124.

24. Farreras N, Artigas V, Cardona D, et al. Effect of early postoperative enteral immunonutrition on wound healing in patients undergoing surgery for gastric cancer. *Clin Nutr.* 2005;24:55–65.

25. Braga M, Gianotti L, Vignali A, Carlo VD. Preoperative oral arginine and omega-3 fatty acid supplementation improves the immunometabolic host response and outcome after colorectal resection for cancer. *Surgery.* 2002;132:805–814.

26. Weimann A, Braga M, Harsanya L, et al. ESPEN guidelines on enteral nutrition: Surgery including organ transplantation. *Clin Nutr.* 2006;25:224–244.

27. Nitenberg G, Raynard B. Nutritional support of the cancer patient: Issues and dilemmas. *Crit Rev Oncl Hematol.* 2000;34:137–168.

28. Clifford C, Kramer B. Diet as risk and therapy for cancer. *Med Clin N Am.* 1993;77:725–744.

29. Grindel CG, Whitmer K, Barsevick A. Quality of life and nutritional support in patients with cancer. *Cancer Pract.* 1996;4:81–87.

30. Keele AM, Bray MJ, Emery PW, et al. Two phase-randomized controlled clinical trial of postoperative oral dietary supplements in surgical patients. *Gut.* 1997;40:393–399.

31. Gogos CA, Ginopoulos P, Salsa B, et al. Dietary omega-3 polyunsaturated fatty acids plus vitamin E restore immunodeficiency and prolong survival for severely ill patients with generalized malignancy. A randomized controlled trial. *Cancer.* 1998;82:395–402.

32. Barber MD, Ross JA, Preston T, et al. Fish oil-enriched nutritional supplement attenuates progression of the acute phase response in weight-losing patients with advanced pancreatic cancer. *J Nutr.* 1999;129:1120–1125.

33. Fearon KC, Barber MD, Moses AG, et al. Double-blind, placebo-controlled, randomized study of eicosapentaenoic acid diester in patients with cancer cachexia. *J Clin Oncol.* 2006;24:3401–3407.

34. Jatoi A, Rowland K, Loprinzi CL, et al. An eicosapentaenoic acid supplement versus megestrol acetate versus both for patients with cancer-associated wasting: A North Central Cancer Treatment Group and National Cancer Institute of Canada collaborative effort. *J Clin Oncol.* 2004;22: 2469–2476.

35. Burns CP, Halabi S, Clamon G, et al. Phase II study of high-dose fish oil capsules for patients with cancer related cachexia. *Cancer.* 2004;101:370–378.

36. Klein S, Koretz RL. Nutrition support in patients with cancer: What do the data really show? *Nutr Clin Pract.* 1994;9:91–100.

37. Marik PE, Zaloga GP. Early EN in acutely ill patients: A systematic review. *Crit Care Med.* 2001;29:2264–2270.

38. Wu GH, Zhang YW, Wu ZH. Modulation of postoperative immune and inflammatory response by immune-enhancing enteral diet in gastrointestinal cancer patients. *World J Gastroenterol.* 2001;7:357–362.

39. Magnotti LJ, Deitch EA. Burns, bacterial translocation, gut barrier function, and failure. *J Burn Care Rehabil.* 2005;26:383–391.

40. Abou-Assi S, Craig K, O'Keefe SJ. Hypocaloric jejunal feeding is better than total parenteral nutrition in acute pancreatitis. *Am J Gastroenterol.* 2002;97:2255–2262.

41. McClave SA. Optmizing what is delivered: Dosing, formula, additives. ASPEN Clinical Nutrition Week. Orlando, Florida, 2005.

42. Taylor S, Fettes S, Jewkes C, et al. Prospective, randomized, controlled trial to determine the effect of early enhanced enteral nutrition on clinical outcome in mechanically ventilated patients suffering head injury. *Crit Care Med.* 1999;27:2525–2531.

43. Ziegler TR, Smith RJ, O'Dwyer ST, et al. Increased intestinal permeability associated with infection in burn patients. *Arch Surg.* 1992;127:26–30.

44. McClave SA, Sexton LK, Spain DA, et al. Enteral tube feeding in the intensive care unit: Factors impeding adequate delivery. *Crit Care Med.* 1999;27:1252–1256.

45. ASPEN Board of Directors and the Clinical Guidelines Task Force. Guidelines for the use of parenteral and enteral nutrition in adult and pediatric patients. *JPEN.* 2002;26:1SA–138SA.

46. Schattner M, Shike M. Nutrition support of the patient with cancer. In: Shils ME, Shike M, Ross AC, Caballero B, Cousins RT, eds. *Modern Nutrition in Health and Disease.* 10th ed. Baltimore, Md.: Lippincott Williams and Wilkins; 2005:1290–1313.

47. American College of Physicians. Parenteral nutrition in patients receiving cancer chemotherapy. *Ann Intern Med.* 1989;110:734–736.

48. American Gastroenterological Association Clinical Practice and Practice Economics Committee. AGA technical review on parenteral nutrition. *Gastroenterology.* 2001;121:970–1001.

49. Zaloga G. Parenteral nutrition in adults with functioning gastrointestinal tracts: Assessment of outcomes. *Lancet.* 2006;367:1101–1111.

50. Fan ST, Lo CM, Lai ECS, Chu KM, Liu CL, Wong J. Perioperative nutritional support in patients undergoing hepatectomy for hepatocellular carcinoma. *N Engl J Med.* 1994;331:1547–1552.

51. The Veterans Affairs Total Parenteral Nutrition Cooperative Study Group. Peroperative total parenteral nutrition in surgical patients. *N Engl J Med.* 1991;325:525–532.

52. Klein S, Kinney J, Jeejeebhoy MB, et al. Nutrition support in clinical practice: Review of published data and recommendations for future research directions. *JPEN.* 1997;21:133–150.

53. Ireton-Jones C. Home care. In: Matarese LE, Gottschlich MM, eds. *Contemporary Nutrition Support Practice: A Clinical Guide.* 2nd ed. Philadelphia, Pa.: Saunders; 2003:301–314.

54. American Society for Parenteral and Enteral Nutrition Board of Directors and the Standards for Specialized Nutrition Support Task Force. Standards for home nutrition support: Home care patients. *Nutr Clin Prac.* 2005;20:579–590.

55. American Dietetic Association Board of Directors. Position of the American Dietetic Association: Ethical and legal issues in nutrition, hydration, and feeding. *J Am Diet Assoc.* 2002;102:716–726.

56. Howard L. Home parenteral and enteral nutrition in cancer patients. *Cancer.* 1993;72:3531–3541.

57. Loeser C, von Hetrz U, Küchler T, Rzehak P, Müller M. Quality of life and nutritional state in patients on home enteral tube feeding. *Nutrition.* 2003;19:605–611.

58. Beer K, Krause K, Zuercher T, Stanga Z. Early percutaneous endoscopic gastrostomy insertion maintains nutritional state in patients with aerodigestive tract cancer. *Nutr Cancer.* 2005;52:29–34.

59. Schattner M, Willis H, Raykher A, et al. Long-term enteral nutrition facilitates optimization of body weight. *JPEN.* 2005;29:198–203.

60. Pothur B, Montemarano M, Gerardi M, et al. Percutaneous endoscopic gastrostomy tube placement in patients with malignant bowel obstruction due to ovarian carcinoma. *Gynecol Obstet.* 2005;96:330–334.

61. McCann RM, Hall WJ, Groth-Junker A. Comfort care for terminally ill patients. The appropriate use of nutrition and hydration. *JAMA.* 1994;272:1263–1266.

62. Buchman AL. Must every cancer patient die with a central venous catheter? *Clin Nutr.* 2002;21:269–271.

63. Owen OE, Caprio S, Reichard Jr GA, Mozzoli MA, Boden G, Owen RS. Ketosis of starvation: A revisit and new perspectives. *Clin Endocrinol Metabol.* 1983;12:357–379.

64. Heber D, Byerley LO, Chi J, et al. Pathophysiology of malnutrition in the adult cancer patient. *Cancer.* 1986;58:1867–1873.

65. Howard L, Ament M, Fleming R, Shike M, Steiger E. Current use and clinical outcome of home parenteral and enteral nutrition therapies in the United States. *Gastroenterology.* 1995;109: 355–365.

66. Bozzetti F, Cozzaglio E, Biganzoli E, et al. Quality of life and length of survival in advanced cancer patients on home parenteral nutrition. *Clin Nutr.* 2002;21:281–288.

67. Hoda D, Jatoi A, Lopinzi C, Kelly D. Should patients with advanced, incurable cancers ever be sent home with total parenteral nutrition? A single institution's 20-year experience. *Cancer.* 2005;103:863–868.

68. August DA, Thorn D, Fischer RL, Welchek CM. Home parenteral nutrition for patients with inoperable malignant bowel obstruction. *JPEN.* 1991;15:323–327.

69. Ripamonti C, Twycross R, Baines M, et al. Clinical practice recommendations for the management of bowel obstruction in patients with end stage cancer. *Support Care Cancer.* 2001;9: 223–233.

70. Whitworth MK, Whitfield A, Holm S, Shaffer J, Makin W, Jayson GC. Doctor, does this mean I'm going to starve to death? *J Clin Oncol.* 2004;22:199–201.

71. Nguyen TV, Yueh B. Weight loss predicts mortality after recurrent oral cavity and oropharyngeal carcinomas. *Cancer.* 2002;95(3):553–562.

72. Yueh B, Feinstein AR, Weaver EM, Sasaki CT, Concato J. Prognostic staging system for recurrent, persistent, and second primary cancers of the oral cavity and oropharynx. *Arch Otolaryngol Head Neck Surg.* 1998;124:975–981.

73. Ahmed KA, Samant S, Vieira F. Gastrostomy tubes in patients with advanced head and neck cancer. *Laryngoscope.* 2005;115:44–47.

74. Seikaly H, Rieger J, Wolfaardt J, et al. Functional outcomes after primary oropharyngeal cancer resection and reconstruction with the radial forearm free flap. *Laryngoscope.* 2003;113: 897–904.

75. Tsue TT, Desyatnikova SS, Deleyiannis FW, et al. Comparison of cost and function in reconstruction of the posterior oral cavity and oropharynx. Free vs. pedicled soft tissue transfer. *Arch Otolaryngol Head Neck Surg.* 1997;123:731–737.

76. Shiley SG, Hargunani CA, Skoner JM. Swallowing function after chemoradiation for advanced stage oropharyngeal cancer. *Otolaryngol Head Neck Surg.* 2006;134:455–459.

77. Ravasco P, Monteiro-Grillo I, Marques V, et al. Impact of nutrition on outcome: A prospective randomized controlled trial in patients with head and neck cancer undergoing radiotherapy. *Head Neck.* 2005;27:659–668.

78. Isenring E, Capra S, Bauer J. Patient satisfaction is rated higher by radiation oncology outpatients receiving nutrition intervention compared with usual care. *J Hum Nutr Det.* 2004;17: 145–152.

79. Odelli C, Burgess D, Bateman L, et al. Nutrition support improves patient outcomes, treatment tolerance and admission characteristics in oesophageal cancer. *Clin Oncol* (R Coll Radiol). 2005;17:639–645.

80. Bozzetti F, Cozzaglio L, Gavazzi C, et al. Nutritional support in patients with cancer of the esophagus: Impact on nutritional status, patient compliance to therapy, and survival. *Tumori.* 1998;84:681–686.

81. Symreng T, Larsson J, Schildt B, Wetterfors J. Nutritional assessment reflects muscle energy metabolism in gastric carcinoma. *Ann Surg.*1983;198:146–150.

82. Sax HC. Immunonutrition and upper gastrointestinal surgery: What really matters. *Nutr Clin Pract.* 2005;20:540–543.

83. Jackson/Siegelbaum Gastroenterology. Anti-dumping post-gastrectomy diet. Available at: www.gicare.com. Accessed August 31, 2006.

84. Scolapio JS. A review of the trends in the use of enteral and parenteral nutrition support. *J Clin Gastroenterol.* 2004;38:403–407.

85. Chandu A, Smith ACH, Douglas M. Percutaneous endoscopic gastrostomy in patients undergoing resection for oral tumors: A retrospective review of complications and outcomes. *J Oral Maxillofac Surg.* 2003;61:1279–1284.

86. Ellisom NM, Chevlen E, Still C, Dubagunta S. Supportive care for patients with pancreatic adenocarcinoma: Symptom control and nutrition. *Hematol Oncol Clin N Am.* 2002;16:105–121.

87. Hines OJ, Reber HA. Pancreatic surgery. *Curr Opin Gastro.* 2006;22:520–526.

88. Wigmore S, Plester C, Richardson R, Fearon K. Changes in nutritional status associated with unresectable pancreatic cancer. *Br J Cancer.* 1997;75:106–109.

89. Brennan MF, Pfisters PWT, Posner M, Quesada O, Shike M. A prospective randomized trial of total parenteral nutrition after major pancreatic resection for malignancy. *Ann Surg.* 1994;220: 436–441.

90. Kirby D, Teran J. Enteral feeding in critical care, gastrointestinal diseases and cancer. *Gastrointes Endosc Clin N Am.* 1998;3:623–643.

91. Bruno M, Heverkort E, Tijssen G, Tytgat G, van Leeuwen D. Placebo controlled trial of enteric coated pancreatin microsphere in patients with unresectable cancer of the pancreatic head region. *Gut.* 1998;42:92–96.

92. Lipman TO. Grains or veins: Is enteral nutrition really better than parenteral nutrition? *JPEN.* 1998;22:167–182.

93. Jeejeebhoy KN. Total parenteral potion or poison? *Am J Clin Nutr.* 2001;74:1650–1653.

94. Arnoletti JP, Aiko S. Esophageal/gastric/pancreatic cancer. In: Rolandelli R, Bankhead R, Boulatta J, Compher C, eds. *Clinical Nutrition: Enteral and Tube Feeding.* 4th ed. Philadelphia, Pa.: Elesevier Saunders; 2005:526–520.

95. Bufo A, Feldman S, Daniels G, Lieberman R. Early postoperative feeding. *Dis Colon Rectum.* 1994;37:1260–1265.

96. Reissman P, Teoh T, Cohen S, Weiss E, Nogueras J, Wexner S. Is early oral feeding safe after elective colorectal surgery? A prospective randomized trial. *Ann Surg.* 1995;222:73–77.

97. Fasth S, Hulten L, Magnusson O, Nordgren S, Warnold I. Postoperative complications in colorectal surgery in relation to preoperative clinical and nutritional state and postoperative nutritional treatment. *Int J Colorec Dis.* 1987;2:87–92.

98. Vitello J. Nutritional assessment and the role of preoperative parenteral nutrition in the colon cancer patient. *Sem Surg Oncol.* 1994;10:183–194.

99. Berry S, Fischer J. Classification and pathophysiology of enterocutaneous fistulas. *Surg Clin North Am.* 1996;76:1009–1018.

100. Lloyd D, Gabe S, Windsor ACJ. Nutrition and management of enterocutaneous fistulas. *Br J Surg.* 2006;93:1045–1055.

101. Edmunds Jr LH, Williams G, Welch C. External fistulas arising from the gastro-intestinal tract. *Ann Surg.* 1960;152:445–471.

102. Gonzalez-Pinto I, Gonzalez E. Optimising the treatment of upper gastrointestinal fistulae. *Gut.* 2001;49(suppl 4):iv22–iv31.

103. Li J, Ren J, Zhu W, Yin L, Han J. Management of enterocutaneous fistulas: 30-year clinical experience. *Chin Med J.* (Engl) 2003;116:171–175.

104. Deitel M. Elemental diet and enterocutaneous fistula. *World J Surg.* 1983;7:451–454.

105. Levy E, Frileux P, Cugnenc P, Honiger J, Ollivier J, Parc R. High-output external fistulae of the small bowel: Management with continuous enteral nutrition. *Br J Surg.* 1989;76:676–679.

106. Kiyama T, Efron D, Tantry U, Barbul A. Effect of nutritional route on colonic anastomotic healing in the rat. *J Gastrointest Surg.* 1999;3:441–446.

107. McKinlay AW. Nutritional support in patients with advanced cancer: Permission to fall out? *Proc Nutr Soc.* 2004;63:431–435.

CHAPTER 9

Trauma

Jennifer Lefton, MS, RD, LD/N, CNSD

INTRODUCTION

Trauma is an injury caused by physical force and is the leading cause of death among Americans between the ages of 1 and 44 years (1). Traumatic injuries may be categorized as blunt (e.g., a motor vehicle crash) or penetrating (e.g., gun shot wound or knife stab wound); blunt trauma is more common. Optimal trauma care relies on the expeditious and timely coordinated efforts of a multidisciplinary medical team to promote the greatest potential for survival and other clinical outcomes such as morbidity and rehabilitation. The availability of this coordinated care can mean the difference between life and death.

The basics of trauma management include prevention of hypoxemia and prevention/treatment of shock. As a result of blood loss and shifting of fluid from the intravascular to the interstitial space, hemodynamic stability is a primary concern. Control of bleeding, administration of blood products if necessary, and fluid resuscitation are part of the initial therapy provided to trauma victims. Cardiac function and urine output are closely monitored during this therapy (2). Impaired gas exchange may also result from the reduced circulating volume but can also occur as a result of direct injury to the lungs (2). Once adequate oxygenation is achieved and the patient is adequately resuscitated and hemodynamically stable, nutrition support should be initiated.

METABOLIC RESPONSE

Metabolic changes that occur after a traumatic injury are categorized into three phases: shock or resuscitation, acute catabolic, and anabolic (see Figure 9–1).

The shock phase, previously referred to as the ebb phase, occurs during the first 24–48 hours postinjury. It is characterized by hypometabolism, with energy expenditure less than normal and low insulin levels. Loss of plasma volume and low cardiac output may result in hypotension, poor tissue perfusion, and eventually shock.

Figure 9–1 Characteristics of the Metabolic Response to Trauma

Shock/resuscitative phase
- Decreased energy expenditure
- Decreased oxygen consumption
- Decreased cardiac output
- Decreased circulating blood volume
- Hypotension
- Poor tissue perfusion
- Shock

Acute catabolic phase
- Increased counterregulatory hormones
- Increased energy expenditure
- Increased oxygen consumption
- Increased gluconeogenesis
- Increased proteolysis
- Increased ureagenesis
- Catabolism
- Hyperglycemia

Anabolic phase
- Normal energy expenditure
- Decreased counterregulatory hormones
- Anabolism

Sources: Adapted from various sources (4,5,7).

At 24–48 hours posttrauma, a rise in counterregulatory hormones (glucagon, cortisol, epinephrine, norepinephrine) leads the transition to the acute catabolic phase. Production of proinflammatory cytokines such as tumor necrosis factor (TNF), and the interleukins (IL) 1, 2, and 6 are also increased. These factors mediate many of the metabolic changes that occur in this phase (3). A rise in glucagon stimulates hepatic glucose production through glycogenolysis and gluconeogenesis, but glycogen stores may have been depleted by this time (4). Protein is broken down to amino acids, which are transferred to the liver where they may be used as a source of energy via the gluconeogenesis pathway; for protein synthesis it may be converted to urea and excreted through the urine. The increase in protein degradation cannot keep pace with protein synthesis, resulting in net protein losses, and these losses are generally not corrected by provision of nutrition support (5). The liver reprioritizes protein synthesis to produce more positive acute-phase proteins (e.g., C-reactive protein) and fewer negative-acute phase proteins (e.g., albumin, prealbumin) (6). There is an increase in ureagenesis and nitrogen excretion in trauma patients. It is not unusual for trauma patients to lose more than 15–20 g

Figure 9–2 Manifestations of Systemic Inflammatory Response Syndrome (SIRS)

At least two of the following are present:

- Febrile (>38° C) or hypothermic (<36° C)
- Tachycardia (heart rate >90 beats per minute)
- Tachypnea (respiratory rate >20 breaths per minute) or $PaCO_2$ <32 mm Hg
- Abnormal WBC (WBC >12,000 cells/mm^3 or <4,000 cells/mm^3), or >10% immature band forms

Source: American College of Chest Physicians/Society of Critical Care Medicine Consensus Conference Committee (1992).

---

nitrogen/day (7). An increase in lipolysis results in an increase of circulating free fatty acids, which are not a preferred source of energy during this phase (7). The overall picture during this phase is hypermetabolism, increased energy expenditure, and significant protein loss. The length of this phase varies greatly; additional insults (infection, sepsis, and surgery) may reinitiate the cascade of hormonal changes that mediate the hypermetabolic response and/or cause shock.

This metabolic response is an important component of the systemic inflammatory response syndrome (SIRS) (see Figure 9–2) (8). SIRS affects more than 50% of intensive care unit patients; trauma patients are at particularly high risk for developing SIRS (9).

The anabolic phase occurs when catabolic hormones return to normal levels. Energy expenditure decreases; however, patients are capable of using extra energy to support lean body mass recovery in conjunction with rehabilitative therapies. The overall picture during this phase is convalescence and anabolism.

NUTRITIONAL REQUIREMENTS

Energy

Determining the energy needs of trauma patients can be challenging (10). Generally, energy expenditure and, hence, requirements are increased. Underfeeding may result in impairments in wound healing and organ (including respiratory muscle strength leading to failure to wean from mechanical ventilation) and immune function (7). Overfeeding can be just as detrimental, resulting in hyperglycemia (11), azotemia (12), electrolyte abnormalities, pulmonary compromise (13,14) and failure to wean from mechanical ventilation (15), and hepatic steatosis (16).

Indirect calorimetry remains the ideal method for determining energy needs, but not all health care facilities have access to this equipment. Additionally, many trauma patients have chest tubes or require high ventilator settings (FiO_2 >60%), both of which result in inaccurate indirect calorimetry measurements. Therefore, many clinicians must rely on predictive equations (see Table 9–1) to determine energy needs (10).

Although developed over 90 years ago, the Harris Benedict energy equation (HBEE) (17) is still used in some situations to predict energy requirements. The HBEE is typically multiplied by a factor to account for the increased energy needs as a result of the inflammatory response. Mean resting energy expenditure (REE)

Table 9–1 Selected Predictive Equations Used to Determine Energy Needs of Trauma Patients

Formulas	Equations
Harris Benedict	EE male = 13.75 (W) + 5 (H) − 6.76 (A) + 66.47 EE female = 9.56 (W) + 1.85 (H) − 4.68 (A) + 655.1 Injury factors range from 1.2 to 1.5
Ireton-Jones, 1992	Spontaneously breathing patients IJEE(s) = 629 − 11 (A) + 25 (W) − 609 (O) Ventilator-dependent patients IJEE(v) = 192 − 10 (A) + 5 (W) + 281 (S) + 292 (T) + 851 (B)
Ireton-Jones, 2002	Spontaneously breathing patients IJEE(s) = 629 − 11 (A) + 25 (W) − 609 (O) Ventilator-dependent patients IJEE(v) = 1784 − 11 (A) + 5 (W) + 244 (S) + 239 (T) + 804 (B)
Penn State	EE = HBEE (0.85) + V_E (33) + T_{max} (175) − 6433
Frankenfield	EE = HBEE (1.1) + V_E (32) + T_{max} (140) − 5340
Swinamer	EE = 945 (BSA) − 6.4(A) + 108 (Temp) + 24.2 (f) + 817 (VT) − 4349
Kcals/kg	25–30 kcals/kg

W = weight (kg)

H = height (cm)

A = age (years)

O = obesity (1 = present; 0 = not present)

S = sex (1 = male; 0 = female)

T = trauma (1 = present; 0 = not present)

B = burn (1 = present; 0 = not present)

HBEE = Harris Benedict energy equation

V_E = minute ventilation (L/min)

T_{max} = maximum temperature over previous 24 hours (degrees centigrade)

BSA = body surface area (m²)

Temp = current temperature (degrees centigrade)

f = respiratory rate (breath/minute)

VT = tidal volume (L/min)

Source: Adapted from various sources (17–23).

has been reported to be 120%–155% above predicted normal levels for 25 days posttrauma (18).

Another option is to use the Ireton Jones energy equation (IJEE) that provides options for spontaneously breathing or ventilated patients (see Table 9–1). This formula adds factors for trauma or burn injury (19) and a revised version has been developed (20). Additional formulas suggested for critically ill patients (although not exclusively trauma patients) have been proposed. The Swinamer equation (21) and Penn State equation (22) rely on continuous dependent variables that relate to the degree of inflammation. A recent study validated that the Penn State equation was most accurate when compared to the Ireton Jones and Frankenfield equations (22). The Penn State equation relies on minute ventilation and maximum temperature and includes the HBEE. The HBEE is calculated using the patient's actual weight whether the patient is obese or not (22).

Other guidelines have suggested 25–30 kcal/kg body weight/day or 120%–140% of HBEE posttrauma (23).

Protein

Proteins play a critical role in tissue, cell, and organelle structure and as enzymes and hormones (24). Provision of inadequate protein can lead to greater nitrogen losses and impaired wound healing; conversely, excessive protein intake may lead to azotemia and dehydration (11).

Protein needs of trauma patients are elevated as a result of catabolism and the need for acute-phase protein substrate, wound healing, and immune function. Protein requirements have been suggested to be as high as 1.5–2.0 g protein/kg body weight/day for patients posttrauma. However, research has shown that providing protein in amounts of 1.25 g protein/kg/day should be sufficient in early posttrauma (25). Others have found 1.0–1.2 g protein/kg/day to be a fair approximation of optimal protein needs (26). Although most patients can tolerate more protein, older adults are more likely to become azotemic when excessive amounts of protein are provided (27,28). Patients with significant wound healing needs (e.g., burns, pressure ulcers, etc.) may require up to 2 g protein/kg/day. Provision of high-protein regimens may reduce protein losses but protein sparing is not further improved by providing protein in amounts greater than 1.5 g protein/kg/d (25,29,30). Loss of skeletal muscle tissue is not avoidable in critically ill trauma patients (31) and the goal of nutritional support is to minimize these losses (32,33).

Carbohydrates

Carbohydrates are the primary source of energy (glucose) in the body serving as an oxidative fuel for the brain, erythrocytes, and leukocytes (24). Glycogen stores are depleted in 12–24 hours posttrauma. Trauma and starvation both result in the endogenous production of glucose from gluconeogenic pathways. However, during stress states after trauma, the provision of an exogenous source of glucose does not suppress the body's endogenous production of glucose, making hyperglycemia a common complication. Oxidized glucose from lipid and amino acid substrates can provide as much as 2 mg/kg/minute of glucose (7). Providing insufficient amounts of carbohydrate can lead to impaired wound healing and immune response. Over-feeding of carbohydrate can result in hyperglycemia (11), hypercapnia (13–15), and fatty infiltrates in the liver (16). Minimum carbohydrate needs are 100–150 grams daily and normal metabolism to maximize protein sparing. The provision of dextrose greater than 4 mg/kg/minute should be avoided in trauma patients receiving parenteral nutrition (PN) (or 50%–60% of total daily calories) (34) in order to avoid the deleterious complications associated with the provision of excess glucose. Recent trauma guidelines similarly suggested no more than 5 mg/kg/minute for burn patients and less amounts in the nonburn population (23). When evaluating carbohydrate intake, it is important to consider additional sources such as intravenous (IV) fluids and medications containing dextrose.

Fat

Fat is a concentrated source of energy and provides essential fatty acids (EFA). Providing too little fat can lead to an essential fatty acid deficiency (EFAD). Signs of EFAD include dermatitis, alopecia, thrombocytopenia, anemia, and poor wound healing. At a minimum, 2%–4% of total calories should be given as essential fatty acids to prevent EFAD (30). Fat can be used to meet energy needs to help avoid using too much carbohydrate. Fat also spares protein as well as carbohydrate from being used as an energy source. Excessive fat administration can lead to hyper-triglyceridemia or fat overload, which manifests as respiratory distress and abnormal liver function tests, although abnormal liver function tests are more often the result of excessive carbohydrate administration (35). The effects of overfeeding fat are seen with PN and not necessarily with EN. Although the total amount of lipid given may not lead to these complications, a high infusion rate of any amount of intravenous fat emulsions (IVFE) can be problematic. IVFE should not be infused at <0.11 grams/kg/hour (36).

The calories provided from fat should not exceed more than 10%–30% of total calories provided. Enteral formulas used in trauma patients should not exceed 30% of total calories as fat. Quantities of IVFE can be manipulated to avoid providing more than 30% of total calories as fat, especially in patients receiving lipid-based medications (e.g., propofol). Propofol is a sedative that is given in a 10% fat emulsion providing 1.1 kcal/mL. IVFE are contraindicated in patients with egg allergy and should be used cautiously in patients with hypertriglyceridemia. The general guidelines for IVFE administration recommend maintaining serum triglyceride levels less than 400 mg/dl (34). IVFE in the United States contain only long-chain triglycerides from soy and safflower oils, which are thought to be immunosuppressive and proinflammatory because they are metabolized to prostaglandins of the 2 series and leukotrienes of the 4 series (37).

Micronutrients

Little is known regarding the micronutrient requirement of trauma patients. As with many other patient populations, trauma patients should receive at a minimum the recommended dietary allowance (RDA) for vitamins and minerals. Some patients may require further supplementation beyond the RDA for certain micronutrients to make up for greater losses through wounds or surgical drains. For example, additional zinc may be needed for patients with high gastrointestinal losses after abdominal surgery.

Interest has grown in the possible role that antioxidants may play in critically ill trauma patients. A small study of trauma patients found that supplemental vitamin C, vitamin E, selenium, and N-acetylcysteine resulted in fewer infectious complications and less organ dysfunction (38). A larger study that provided enteral alpha-tocopherol and parenteral ascorbic acid also reduced the incidence of organ failure and shortened ICU length of stay (LOS) (39). Crimi et al. showed that trauma patients receiving enteral feedings supplemented with 500 mg/d vitamin C and 400 IU/d vitamin E for just 10 days had a significantly lower 28-day mortality rate compared to control subjects (40).

Selenium has been of particular interest in patients with SIRS. Patients with lower selenium levels early in their hospital stay were three times more likely to develop ventilator-associated pneumonia, organ dysfunction, or die (41). Selenium supplementation, in patients with renal insufficiency and SIRS, reduced the need for dialysis (42); however, no randomized controlled trials have been completed that have included trauma patients.

Most enteral formulations provide the RDA amounts of vitamins and minerals within 1000–1500 mL of formula. Some formulations may contain supplemental amounts of certain micronutrients and clinicians should be aware of the overall micronutrient content of enteral feeding formulations used at their institutions. In the rare instance that a formula may not meet the vitamin and mineral RDAs, a multivitamin with minerals supplement should be provided. Patients on PN should have vitamin and trace element solutions added daily (43).

Fluid and Electrolytes

Fluid and electrolyte needs vary greatly among individuals posttrauma because there is an enormous variation in fluid requirements depending on the individual's clinical status. Fluid needs may be very high initially during resuscitation. Additional fluids may be needed to replace losses through surgical drains, gastric output, or other gastrointestinal losses. In some circumstances, patients may require a fluid restriction. Generally, fluids and electrolytes are given to maintain adequate urine output and normal serum electrolyte levels. Fluid needs can be estimated at approximately 30–40 mL/kg body weight depending on age, size, and organ function in stable patients. Knowledge of the electrolyte composition of body fluids and intravenous fluids can help to guide replacement therapy (see Tables 9–2 and 9–3) (44).

Table 9–2 Composition of Gastrointestinal Secretions

	Volume (mL/24 hours)	Sodium (mmol/L)	Potassium (mmol/L)	Chloride (mmol/L)	Bicarbonate (mmol/L)
Saliva	1500 (500–2000)	10	20	10	20
Stomach	1500 (100–4000)	60	10	130	0
Duodenum	100–2000	140	5	104	0
Ileum	3000 (100–9000)	140 (80–150)	5 (2–8)	104 (43–137)	30
Colon		60	30	40	
Pancreas	(100–800)	140 (113–185)	5 (3–7)	75 (54–95)	115
Bile	(50–800)	145 (131–164)	5 (3–12)	100 (89–180)	35

Source: Reprinted with permission from Shires III GT, Barber A, Shires GT. Fluid and electrolyte management of the surgical patient. In: Schwartz SI, ed. *Principles of Surgery.* 7th ed. New York, NY: McGraw-Hill; 1999:55–56.

NUTRITION SUPPORT

Route of Nutrition Support

One of the first studies evaluating EN (within 12 hours postop) versus PN (day 6) found that patients receiving EN had a better nitrogen balance, higher lymphocyte count, and fewer major infections (45). The same group later compared early EN versus early PN, finding no difference in nitrogen balance but significantly fewer infections in the enterally fed group (46). Others have affirmed these findings that not only are there fewer major septic complications in patients receiving enteral feedings but also significantly more catheter-related sepsis in patient populations receiving PN (47). A meta-analysis conducted that same year concluded that one or more infectious complications developed in twice as many patients given PN compared to EN (48). Therefore, patients with blunt and penetrating abdominal injuries should be fed enterally when feasible because of the lower incidence of septic complications compared to parenterally fed patients (23). PN should be reserved for patients in whom enteral feeding has not been (or is anticipated to not be) successful for 7 days (23).

Enteral Access

Practically any type of enteral access may be used dependent on the surgical intervention required to treat the injury. Patients undergoing laparotomy often have

Table 9–3 Composition of Intravenous Fluids

	Glucose (g/dL)	Sodium (mEq/L)	Potassium (mEq/L)	Calcium (mEq/L)	Chloride (mEq/L)	Lactate (mEq/L)	Osmolarity (mOsm/L)
Lactated ringers	—	130	4	3	109	28	273
0.9% NaCl (normal saline)	—	154	—	—	154	—	308
0.45% NaCl (half normal saline)	—	77	—	—	77	—	154
5% dextrose in water	5	—	—	—	—	—	253
5% dextrose in 0.45% NaCl	5	77	—	—	77	—	407
5% dextrose in 0.9% NaCl	5	154	—	—	154	—	560
3% sodium chloride	—	513	—	—	513	—	1026

Source: Reprinted with permission from Shires III GT, Barber A, Shires GT. Fluid and electrolyte management of the surgical patient. In: Schwartz SI, ed. *Principles of Surgery.* 7th ed. New York, NY: McGraw-Hill; 1999:55–56.

203

small bowel feeding tubes placed during the operative procedure; whereas, nasogastric or nasointestinal feeding tubes can be inserted in patients who do not require laparotomy.

Studies evaluating outcomes of patients receiving nasogastric versus nasointestinal feedings have not demonstrated improved outcomes by either method. One
study found that it took longer to reach and tolerate a goal enteral volume in gastric fed patients (49). Another reported a greater percentage of calorie and nitrogen
intake in the nasointestinal fed group (50). However, small bowel feeding access
could not be achieved, and many patients in the nasointestinal group were actually
fed in the stomach. No studies comparing gastric and small bowel feedings in the
trauma population have found any difference in length of stay, pneumonia, ventilator days, or mortality (49–52).

Current recommendations are to initiate enteral feedings even if postpyloric access cannot be achieved (23). Small bowel feeding access should be attempted in patients with persistently high gastric residual volumes (greater than 250 mL on two
consecutive measurements), documented reflux, or when the risk of aspiration is elevated (52). Patients requiring supine position or receiving high amounts of sedatives and paralytic agents may also be candidates for small bowel feedings (5,12).
Patients should be adequately resuscitated and hemodynamically stable prior to
starting small bowel feedings due to the risk of developing bowel ischemia.

Initiating Nutrition Support

Finding the optimal time to initiate enteral feedings can be challenging. Although
some studies have reported a benefit of starting enteral feedings as early as 12–18
hours postlaparotomy (53), recent guidelines report that there is insufficient evidence to suggest starting feedings within 24 hours of the injury results in better
outcomes compared to starting feedings within 72 hours after the injury (23).

Generally, once a trauma patient has been adequately resuscitated and is hemodynamically stable, enteral feedings may be started. The following markers of
adequate resuscitation have been suggested: base excess <2.5 mEq/L, lactate <2.5
mmol/L, heart rate <120 beats per minute, no vasopressors, inotropic agents at a
rate <5 mcg/kg/minute (54). Many facilities have adopted protocols to guide the
initiation of enteral feedings and achieve early tolerance (55). A suggested algorithm
is shown in Figure 9–3 (23).

When tolerance of at least 50% of the enteral feeding goal cannot be achieved
by postinjury day 7, PN should be initiated (23). When initiating PN, goal amounts
of protein and lipid can be provided initially without causing harm, whereas dextrose is generally started at about one half the amount needed to meet energy needs.
The amount of dextrose is gradually increased over a few days while maintaining
glycemic control and normal electrolyte levels. If possible, concurrent small
amounts of EN may help support the gut's metabolic needs and may be beneficial
in patients requiring long-term PN (56). See Chapter 3 for a more in-depth discussion on specialized nutrition support.

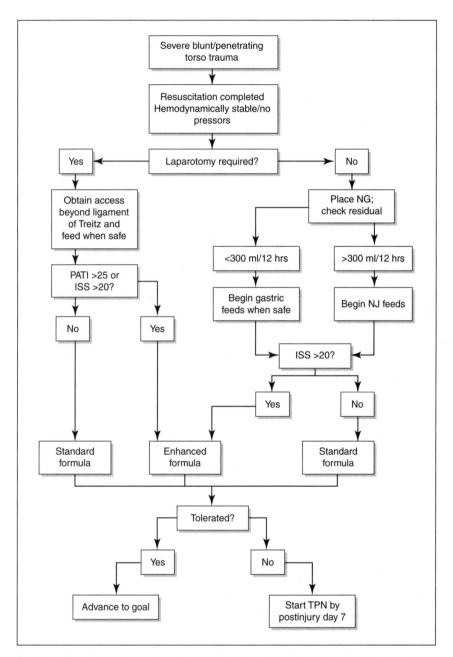

Figure 9–3 A Suggested Algorithm for Initiating Enteral Feedings in Trauma Patients

Source: Adapted with permission from Jacobs DG, Jacobs DO, Kudsk KA, et al. Practice management guidelines for nutritional support of the trauma patient. *J Trauma*. 2004;57:660–679.

Enteral Formulations

Due to elevated protein requirements posttrauma, high-nitrogen formulations are typically recommended to optimally meet nutrition requirements. Most patients can tolerate a standard polymeric high-nitrogen formulation with or without fiber; patients receiving fiber-supplemented formulas should be monitored closely. Cases of small bowel obstruction have been reported in patients given fiber-containing formulas (57,58).

Although considerable controversy remains, some patients may benefit from immune-enhancing formulations. Immune-enhancing formulations tend to have two or more of the following in greater amounts when compared to standard formulas: arginine, glutamine, omega-3 fatty acids, and nucleic acids. Several studies including trauma patients have compared immune-enhancing formulations to a control formulation. Brown et al. (59) compared a feeding formula with supplemental arginine, alpha-linolenic acid, and beta-carotene to a standard formula in 37 trauma patients. The study formula resulted in fewer infections and significantly greater change in nitrogen balance compared to the control. However, patients receiving the study formula were fed significantly more calories than the control. In a larger multicenter trial, Moore et al. (60) compared an immune-enhanced diet to an elemental formula. The elemental formula provided significantly less protein per liter than the immune-enhancing formula; therefore, it is difficult to determine if the favorable outcomes (significantly fewer abdominal abscesses and less multiple organ failure) reported were due to the immune-enhancing components or the greater protein content. Kudsk et al. (61) then compared an immune-enhancing formulation to an isocaloric, isonitrogenous control. There were significantly fewer infectious complications and intraabdominal abscesses in those receiving the immune-enhancing formulation. The need for therapeutic antibiotics and the hospital length of stay (LOS) was also significantly less. Additionally, Weimann et al. found significantly fewer SIRS days with an immune-enhancing formulation compared to a control (62). One study has shown no improvement with the immune-enhancing formulation (63). Table 9–4 provides a summary of outcomes studies.

Multiple studies evaluating the use of immune-enhancing formulations led to the publication of several meta-analyses. Beale et al. (64) concluded that immune-enhancing formulations reduced infection rates, ventilator days, and hospital LOS but had no effect on mortality. Heys et al. (65) also found reduced infectious complications and overall hospital LOS. More recently, Heyland et al. (66) completed a systematic review and also found that immune-enhancing formulations were associated with fewer infectious complications, although treatment effects varied among individual studies depending on the intervention, population studied, and the quality of the methods of the study.

Studies of immune-enhancing formulations have evaluated various patient populations, used different feeding formulations, compared immune-enhancing formulations to standard products containing less protein, measured different clinical and laboratory outcomes, and were inconsistent in timing, initiation, or duration of feeding as well as the actual quantity of the feeding delivered.

Table 9–4 Studies of Immune-Enhancing Enteral Formulations in Trauma Patients

Author	Year	No.	Study Design	Outcomes
Brown RO et al.	1994	78	IEF versus standard formulation	• Fewer nosocomial infections with IEF
Moore FA et al.	1994	203	IEF versus elemental formulation	• Fewer intraabdominal abscesses, MOF with IEF
Kudsk KA et al.	1996	72	IEF versus standard formulation	• Fewer intraabdominal abscesses, antibiotic days, and LOS with IEF
Mendez C et al.	1997	102	IEF versus standard formulation	• No improvement with IEF
Weimann A et al.	1998	71	IEF versus standard formulation	• Fewer days with SIRS and less MOF with IEF

N = number of study participants

Source: Adapted from various sources (59–62).

Recent guidelines suggest that the use of enteral formulations enhanced with adequate doses of arginine and glutamine appear to reduce LOS and septic morbidity in severely injured trauma patients (injury severity score [ISS] >20, abdominal trauma index [ATI] >25), although the precise dose and length of treatment with arginine and glutamine required to obtain this effect have not yet been determined. Whether there is additional benefit from omega-3 fatty acids, nucleotides, and trace elements is unclear (23). An industry-supported summit on immune enhancing formulations suggests that trauma patients with an ISS >18 or an ATI >20 should receive enteral feedings with an immune-enhancing formulation (67).

Glutamine

Glutamine, the most abundant amino acid in skeletal muscle, is thought to become an essential amino acid during critical illness. Glutamine has several roles including regulating acid-base balance, synthesis of nucleotides and nucleic acids, and as the preferred energy source for enterocytes (68). Plasma and muscle glutamine levels are often depleted in trauma patients (68,69). Minimizing oxidant damage, reducing cytokine production and gut bacterial translocation, and improving nitrogen balance are potential mechanisms by which glutamine may enhance the recovery from critical illness.

Enteral feedings with a higher glutamine concentration have blunted the hyper-aminoacidemia and aromatic amino acid response to injury (70). Another study of multiple trauma patients found that enteral feedings with supplemental glutamine resulted in less pneumonia, bacteremia, and sepsis (71). However, the addition of glutamine to a standard feeding formulation did not have a positive effect on infectious complications, antiobiotic therapy, and 6-month mortality, although only a quarter of the patients studied were trauma patients (72). A recent larger study compared standard formula, standard formula plus glutamine, and immune-enhancing formula plus glutamine. Study results showed that neither using a formulation with the addition of glutamine nor using an immune-enhancing formula resulted in improved outcomes because there was no difference between groups with regards to ventilator days, ICU days, hospital days, infectious complications, or mortality (73).

Parenteral sources of glutamine have also been studied. Provision of dipeptide alanyl-glutamine was found to improve insulin sensitivity (74) and reduce the incidence of hyperglycemia (75). One study found a significant reduction in the incidence of pneumonia in patients receiving parenteral glutamine (75). Additional studies have reported favorable outcomes with parenteral glutamine supplementation in critically ill patients (76–78), but these studies included mixed ICU populations and very few trauma patients.

Several meta-analyses have evaluated the usefulness of supplemental glutamine in critically ill patients. Novak et al. found that the greatest benefit tended to be seen with high-dose parenteral glutamine solutions in surgical patients (79). A 2003 systematic review found a statistically significant reduction in mortality and a trend toward a significant decrease in infectious complications with glutamine in critical illness (79). The authors further recommended that critically ill trauma patients receive 15–25 g glutamine/day for greater than 5 days (80). The Canadian practice guidelines also suggest that glutamine supplementation should be considered for trauma patients (81). Despite the positive benefits associated with glutamine supplements, the data do not clearly show that supplementation improves clinical outcomes in trauma patients. Therefore, before glutamine supplementation can be recommended on a more global basis for trauma patients, further research is needed.

MONITORING NUTRITION SUPPORT

Monitoring the efficacy and outcomes of nutritional support in trauma patients can be challenging. Many of the parameters frequently used in nutritional assessment and monitoring are affected by many factors other than just nutritional intake. See Chapter 1 for a more in-depth discussion.

Adequacy of Nutrition Support

It is important to monitor the actual nutrient intake as compared to the prescribed volume. Frequent diagnostic tests and operative procedures can result in interruptions to the enteral feedings. Commonly used measures of tolerance (e.g., gastric residual volumes) also result in frequent interruptions of the feedings. The average energy intake in critically ill patients ranges from 51% to 71% of what is prescribed (82,83). One study demonstrated a decrease in infections and shorter LOS in patients receiving an immune-enhanced formulation providing only 18 kcal/kg body weight/day (61). This suggests that early provision of a lesser volume than prescribed can still result in improved outcomes.

Patients receiving PN tend to receive closer to the full amount prescribed compared to EN (83). This is most likely because PN does not require interruption to delivery for many of the tests and procedures that require holding the EN.

Tolerance to Nutrition Support

The patients' tolerance to nutritional support should be continually reassessed in order to assure the safe provision of support, to troubleshoot problems early, and to avoid potential adverse complications to support. Intake and output data (I/Os), assessment of GI function, and laboratory indices are routine parameters evaluated. Markers of GI tolerance to EN commonly assessed include gastric residual volumes, abdominal distention, presence of emesis, and I/Os. Bowel sounds do not need to be present in order to initiate or continue enteral feedings.

Gastric residual volumes (GRV) have been traditionally used as a marker for risk of regurgitation and aspiration of enteral feedings. There is insufficient data to support the routine use of GRV as a marker for the risk of aspiration (84). A single elevated gastric residual volume (GRV) does not equate to EN intolerance, nor does a low GRV mean tolerance to the EN regimen. A high GRV should prompt further evaluation of EN tolerance. Feedings should be delayed if high GRVs are accompanied by abdominal distention and discomfort or emesis. In the absence of these findings, feedings may be continued regardless of the GRV.

Diarrhea is another common complication in critically ill and tube-fed patients. The enteral formulation is rarely the sole cause of the diarrhea. The presence of toxins (e.g., clostridium difficile) should be ruled out and a careful evaluation of medications may help to reduce/avoid diarrhea. Antibiotics, elixirs, phosphorus supplements, magnesium-containing antacids, laxatives, and prokinetic agents can all lead to diarrhea. The addition of soluble fiber may help reduce diarrhea. Once the presence of toxins is ruled out, antidiarrheal medications can safely be provided. They should be given as a scheduled dose rather than as needed (85).

Monitoring laboratory indices aid in the assessment of adequacy and tolerance to specialized nutrition support. A basic metabolic profile facilitates the evaluation of the patient's clinical status including electrolyte levels, acid-base balance, hydration status, and tolerance to nutrient intake. Arterial blood gases provide further data for assessing acid-base balance. The frequency of glucose monitoring is dependent on levels, the source of exogenous insulin, the patient's clinical status, and the institution's protocol for managing hyperglycemia.

In summary, ongoing assessment of support is key to ensuring that the administration of nutrition is maintained, new complications have not developed, and that nutrition support goals are being achieved. Furthermore, the provision of support often requires adjustments in the regimen as the patient's clinical status changes.

Weight

Weight measurements are often inaccurate in trauma patients. Large volumes of resuscitative fluid given early posttrauma, daily fluid administration, lack of diuresis, and third spacing of fluids lead to fluid accumulation and weight gain. Serial weight measurements can be followed as trends and may be more helpful to monitor during the anabolic and recovery phases.

Serum Hepatic Proteins

Serum hepatic protein levels (e.g., albumin and prealbumin) have been commonly used to assess nutrition status and intake. However, these levels are too affected by many nonnutritional factors. In the early phases posttrauma, albumin and prealbumin levels are reduced secondary to the acute-phase response (6). Studies examining serum albumin and prealbumin levels in stress states found that these markers reflect the severity of injury and prognosis but neither nutritional status nor adequacy of their nutritional support (86).

Trends in serum protein levels can be monitored as surrogate indicators of morbidity and mortality. New sources of inflammation (infection, sepsis, or surgery) will reinitiate the acute-phase response potentially resulting in a reduction in serum protein levels. As patients reach a point of convalescence, trends in hepatic proteins are useful as part of a more global assessment of the overall clinical status.

Nitrogen Balance

Nitrogen balance may be used to determine the adequacy of the nutrition regimen. Nitrogen is lost through urine (urine urea nitrogen), stool, wounds, and skin. Urine urea nitrogen (UUN) is often used to predict total urea nitrogen (TUN), based on the assumption that UUN comprises 80% of TUN (87). Total nitrogen output is the UUN multiplied by 1.25. An additional 2–4 grams of nitrogen is added to the total losses to account for insensible losses.

However, the practicality of utilizing nitrogen balance studies in clinical practice is often limited due to difficulties in collecting urine and recording protein intake accurately as well as the large variations in nonurea nitrogen losses. Following trends result in a more accurate picture of nitrogen balance than will relying upon one measurement.

ANABOLIC AGENTS

Oxandralone, a testosterone analog with minimal androgenic effects, has decreased weight and nitrogen loss and improved donor site wound healing in burn patients

(88,89). Two studies have evaluated the use of oxandralone in trauma patients, neither of which showed improved outcome. A study comparing oxandralone to placebo found no nutritional or clinical benefit with oxandralone (90). A more recent study found that surgical and trauma ventilator dependent patients given 10 mg oxandralone twice daily spent a greater amount of time on the ventilator (91).

CONCLUSION

Patients sustaining acute trauma have altered nutritional requirements due to the underlying injury(ies) and often require specialized nutrition support (SNS). A wealth of evidence has accumulated that for patients with blunt and penetrating trauma, EN is preferred over PN when SNS is warranted. Additionally, EN should be initiated early, ideally within 24–48 hours, once patients are fully resuscitated and stabilized. The utilization of enhanced enteral formulations has been shown to be beneficial, in terms of decreasing infectious complications, when combined with initiation of early EN and the provision of adequate nutrients. However, PN should be considered when EN is contraindicated or enteral access is not available in order to minimize catabolism due to the hypermetabolism associated with trauma. Furthermore, PN should be initiated when patients have failed to tolerate >50% of EN by posttrauma day 7.

REFERENCES

1. Department of Health and Human Services Centers for Disease Control and Prevention. 10 Leading Causes of Death by Age Group—2003. Available at: www.cdc.gov. Accessed October 2006.

2. Huggins B. Trauma physiology. *Nurs Clin North Am.* 1990;25:1–9.

3. Hill AG. Initiators and propagators of the metabolic response to injury. *World J Surg.* 2000; 24:624–629.

4. Chiolero R, Revelly J, Tappy L. Energy metabolism in sepsis and injury. *Nutrition.* 1997;13 (suppl):45S–51S.

5. Cerra FB, Siegel JH, Coleman B, et al. Septic autocannabalism: A failure of exogenous nutritional support. *Ann Surg.* 1980;192:570–580.

6. Gabay C, Kushner I. Acute-phase proteins and other systemic responses to inflammation. *N Engl J Med.* 1999;340:448–454.

7. Cresci GA, Martindale RG. Nutrition support in trauma. In: Gottschlich M, et al., eds. *The Science and Practice of Nutrition Support: A Case-Based Core Curriculum.* Dubuque, Ia.: Kendall/ Hunt Publishing; 2000:445–460.

8. American College of Chest Physicians/Society of Critical Care Medicine Consensus Conference Committee. American College of Chest Physicians/Society of Critical Care Medicine Consensus Conference: Definitions for sepsis and organ failure and guidelines for the use of innovative therapies in sepsis. *Crit Care Med.* 1992;20:864–874.

9. Brun-Buisson C. The epidemiology of the systemic inflammatory response. *Intensive Care Med.* 2000;26:S64–S74.

10. Frankenfeld D. Energy expenditure and protein requirements after traumatic injury. *Nutr Clin Prac.* 2006;21:430–437.

11. Rosmarin DK, Wardlaw GM, Mirtallo J. Hyperglycemia associated with high, continuous infusion rates of total parenteral nutrition dextrose. *Nutr Clin Pract.* 1996;11:151–156.

12. Gault MH, Dixon ME, Doyle M, Cohen WM. Hypernatremia, azotemia, and dehydration due to high-protein tube feeding. *Ann Intern Med.* 1968;68:778–791.

13. Askanazi J, Elwyn DH, Silverberg PA, Rosenbaum SH, Kinney JM. Respiratory distress secondary to a high carbohydrate load: A case report. *Surgery.* 1980;87:596–598.

14. Covelli HD, Black JW, Olsen MS, Beekman JF. Respiratory failure precipitated by high carbohydrate loads. *Ann Intern Med.* 1982;95:579–581.

15. Dark DS, Pingleton SK, Kerby GR. Hypercapnia during weaning: A complication of nutritional support. *Chest.* 1985;88:141–143.

16. Kaminski DL, Adams A, Jellinek M. The effect of hyperalimentation on hepatic lipid content and lipogenic enzyme activity in rats and man. *Surgery.* 1980;88:93–100.

17. Harris JA, Benedict FG. Biometric studies of basal metabolism in man. Publication no. 270. Washington, D.C.: Carnegie Institution of Washington; 1919.

18. Monk D, Plank L, Franch-Arcas G, et al. Sequential changes in the metabolic response in critically injured patients during the first 25 days after blunt trauma. *Ann Surg.* 1996;223:395–405.

19. Ireton-Jones CS, Turner WW, Liepa GU, Baxter CR. Equations for the estimation of energy expenditure in patients with burns with special reference to ventilatory status. *J Burn Care Rehabil.* 1992;13:330–333.

20. Ireton-Jones C, Jones JD. Improved equations for predicting energy expenditure in patients: The Ireton-Jones equations. *Nutr Clin Pract.* 2002;17:29–31.

21. Frankenfield D, Smith JS, Cooney RN. Validation of 2 approaches to predicting resting metabolic rate in critically ill patients. *JPEN.* 2004;28:259–264.

22. Swinamer DL, Grace MG, Hamilton SM, et al. Predictive equation for assessing energy expenditure in mechanically ventilated critically ill patients. *Crit Care Med.* 1990;18:657–661.

23. Jacobs DG, Jacobs DO, Kudsk KA, et al. for the East Practice Management Guidelines Work Group. Practice management guidelines for nutritional support of the trauma patient. *J Trauma.* 2004;57:660–679.

24. Frakenfield D. Energy and macrosubstrate requirements. In: Gottschlich MM, ed. *The Science and Practice of Nutrition Support—A Case-Based Core Curriculum.* Dubuque, Ia.: Kendall/Hunt Publishing; 2001:31–52.

25. Larsson J, Lennmarken C, Martensson J, Sandstedt S, Vinnars E. Nitrogen requirements in severely injured patients. *Br J Surg.* 1990;77:413–416.

26. Ishibashi N, Plank LD, Sando K, Hill GL. Optimal protein requirements during the first 2 weeks after onset of critical illness. *Crit Care Med.* 1998;26:1529–1535.

27. Frankenfield D, Cooney RN, Smith JS, Rowe WA. Age-related differences in the metabolic response to injury. *J Trauma.* 2000;48:49–57.

28. Clevenger FW, et al. Protein and energy tolerance by stressed geriatric patients. *J Surg Research.* 1992;52:135–139.

29. Shaw JHF, Wildbore M, Wolfe RR. Whole body protein kinetics in severely septic patients: The response to glucose infusion and total parenteral nutrition. *Ann Surg.* 1987;205:288–294.

30. Hoffer LJ. Protein and energy provision in critical illness. *Am J Clin Nutr.* 2003;78:906–911.

31. Streat SJ, Beddoe AH, Hill GL. Aggressive nutritional support does not prevent protein loss despite fat gain in septic intensive care patients. *J Trauma.* 1987;27:262–266.

32. Shaw JH, Wolfe RR. An integrated analysis of glucose, fat, and protein metabolism in severely traumatized patients. Studies in the basal state and the response to total parenteral nutrition. *Ann Surg.* 1989;209:63–72.

33. Frankenfield DC, Smith JS, Cooney RN. Accelerated nitrogen loss after traumatic injury is not attenuated by achievement of energy balance. *JPEN*. 1997;21:324–329.

34. ASPEN Board of Directors and the Clinical Guidelines Task Force. Guidelines for the use of parenteral and enteral nutrition in adult and pediatric patients. *JPEN*. 2002;26:1SA–138SA.

35. Klein CJ, Stanek GS, Wiles CE. Overfeeding macronutrients to critically ill patients: Metabolic complications. *J Am Diet Assoc*. 1998;98:795–806.

36. Klein S, Miles JM. Metabolic effects of long-chain and medium chain triglycerides in humans. *JPEN*. 1994;18:396–397.

37. Lee S, Gura K, Kim S, et al. Current clinical applications of omega-6 and omega-3 fatty acids. *Nutr Clin Pract*. 2006;21:323–341.

38. Porter JM, Ivatury RR, Azimuddin K, Swami R. Antioxidant therapy in the prevention of organ dysfunction syndrome and infectious complications after trauma: Early results of a prospective randomized study. *Am Surg*. 1999;65:478–483.

39. Nathans AB, Neff MJ, Jurkovish GJ, et al. Randomized, prospective trial on antioxidant supplementation in critically ill surgical patients. *Ann Surg*. 2002;236:814–822.

40. Crimi E, Liguori A, Condorelli M, et al. The beneficial effects of antioxidant supplementation in enteral feeding in critically ill patients: A prospective, randomized, double-blind, placebo-controlled trial. *Anesth Analg*. 2004;99:857–863.

41. Forceville X, Vitoux, D, Gauzit R, et al. Selenium, systemic immune response syndrome, sepsis, and outcome in critically ill patients. *Crit Care Med*. 1998;26:1536–1544.

42. Angstwurm MWA, Schottdorf J, Schopohl J, Gaertner R. Selenium replacement in patients with severe systemic inflammatory response syndrome improves clinical outcome. *Crit Care Med*. 1999;27:1807–1813.

43. Task Force for the Revision of Safe Practices for Parenteral Nutrition. Safe practices for parenteral nutrition. *JPEN*. 2004;28:S39–S70.

44. Shires III GT, Barber A, Shires GT. Fluid and electrolyte management of the surgical patient. In: Schwartz SI, ed. *Principles of Surgery*. 7th ed. New York, NY: McGraw-Hill; 1999:55–56.

45. Moore EE, Jones TN. Benefits of immediate jejunal feeding after major abdominal trauma: A prospective randomized study. *J Trauma*. 1986;26:874–881.

46. Moore FA, Moore EE, Jones TN. TEN versus TPN following major abdominal trauma reduced septic morbidity. *J Trauma*. 1989;29:916–922.

47. Kudsk KA, Croce MA, Fabian TC, et al. Enteral versus parenteral feeding. Effects of septic morbidity after blunt and penetrating abdominal trauma. *Ann Surg*. 1992;215:503–513.

48. Moore FA, Feliciano DV, Andrassy RJ, et al. Early enteral feeding, compared with parenteral, reduces postoperative septic complications. The results of a meta-analysis. *Ann Surg*. 1992;216:172–183.

49. Kortbeek JB, Haigh PI, Doig C. Duodenal versus gastric feeding in ventilated blunt trauma patients: A randomized controlled trial. *J Trauma*. 1999;46:992–998.

50. Taylor SJ, Fettes SB, Jewkes C, Nelson RJ. Prospective, randomized, controlled trial to determine the effect of early enhanced enteral nutrition on clinical outcome in mechanically ventilated patients suffering head injury. *Crit Care Med*. 1999;27:2525–2531.

51. Minard G, Kudsk KA, Melton S, Patton JH, Tolley EA. Early versus delayed feeding with an immune-enhancing diet in patients with severe head injuries. *JPEN*. 2000;24:145–149.

52. American Dietetic Association Evidence Analysis Library. Critical Illness Guidelines. Available at: www.adaevidencelibrary.org. Accessed January 2006.

53. Moore EE, Jones TN. Benefits of immediate jejunostomy feeding after abdominal trauma—A prospective, randomized study. *J Trauma*. 1986;26:874–881.

54. Biffl WL, Moore EE, Haenel JB. Nutrition support of the trauma patient. *Nutrition*. 2002;18:960–965.

55. Kozar RA, McQuiggan MM, Moore EE, et al. Postinjury enteral tolerance is reliably achieved by a standardized protocol. *J Surg Res.* 2002;104:70–75.

56. Sax HC, Illig KA, Ryan CK, Hardy DJ. Low dose enteral feeding is beneficial during total parenteral nutrition. *Am J Surg.* 1996;171:587–590.

57. Scaife CL, Saffle JR, Morris SE. Intestinal obstruction secondary to enteral feedings in burn trauma patients. *J Trauma.* 1999;47:859–863.

58. McIvor AC, Meguid MM, Curtas S, Kaplan DS. Intestinal obstruction from cecal bezoar: A complication of fiber-containing tube feedings. *Nutrition.* 1990;6:115–117.

59. Brown RO, Hunt H, Mowatt-Larssen CA, et al. Comparison of specialized and standard formulas in trauma patients. *Pharmacotherapy.* 1994;14:314–320.

60. Moore FA, Moore EE, Kudsk KA, et al. Clinical benefits of an immune-enhancing diet for early post-injury enteral feeding. *J Trauma.* 1994;37:607–614.

61. Kudsk KA, Minard G, Croce MA, et al. A randomized trial of isonitrogenous diets following severe trauma: An immune-enhancing diet reduces septic complications. *Ann Surg.* 1996;224:531–540.

62. Weimann A, Bastian L, Bischoff WE, et al. Influence of arginine, omega 3 fatty acids and nucleotide-supplemented enteral support on systemic inflammatory response syndrome and multiple organ failure in patients after severe trauma. *Nutrition.* 1998;14:165–172.

63. Mendez C, Jurkovich GJ, Garcia I, et al. Effects of an immune-enhancing diet in critically injured patients. *J Trauma.* 1997;42:933–940.

64. Beale RJ, Bryg DJ, Bihari DJ. Immunonutrition in the critically ill: A systematic review of clinical outcome. *Crit Care Med.* 1999;27:2799–2805.

65. Heys SD, Walker LG, Smith I, Eremin O. Enteral nutrition supplementation with key nutrients in patients with critical illness and cancer: A meta-analysis of randomized contolled clinical trials. *Ann Surg.* 1999;229:467–477.

66. Heyland DK, Novak F, Drover JW, et al. Should immunonutrition become routine in critically ill patients? A systematic review of the evidence. *JAMA.* 2001;286:944–953.

67. Consensus statement. Consensus recommendations from the U.S. summit on immune-enhancing enteral therapy. *JPEN.* 2001;25:S61–S62.

68. Souba W, Smith RJ, Wilmore DW. Glutamine metabolism by the intestinal tract. *JPEN.* 1985;9:609–617.

69. Long C, Borghesi L, Stahl R, et al. Impact of enteral feeding of a glutamine-supplemented formula on the hypoaminoacidemic response in trauma patients. *J Trauma.* 1996;40:97–102.

70. Jensen GL, Miller RH, Talabiska DG, Fish J, Gianferante L. A double-blind, prospective, randomized study of glutamine-enriched compared with standard peptide-based feeding in critically ill patients. *Am J Clin Nutr.* 1996;64:615–621.

71. Houdijk APJ, Rijnsburger ER, Jansen J, et al. Randomised trial of glutamine-enriched enteral nutrition on infectious morbidity in patients with multiple trauma. *Lancet.* 1998;352:772–776.

72. Hall JC, Dobb G, Hall J, et al. A prospective randomized trial of enteral glutamine in critical illness. *Intensive Care Med.* 2003;29:1710–1716.

73. Schulman AS, Willcutts KF, Claridge JA, et al. Does the addition of glutamine to enteral feeds affect patient mortality? *Crit Care Med.* 2005;33:2501–2506.

74. Bakalar B, Diska F, Pachl J, et al. Parenterally administered dipeptide alanyl-glutamine prevents worsening of insulin sensitivity in multiple-trauma patients. *Crit Care Med.* 2006;34:381–386.

75. Dechelotte P, Hasselmann M, Cynober L, et al. L-alanyl-L-glutamine dipeptide-supplemented total parenteral nutrition reduces infectious complications and glucose intolerance in critically ill patients: The French, controlled, randomized, double-blind, multicenter study. *Crit Care Med.* 2006;34:598–604.

76. Griffiths RD, Jones C, Palmer TEA. Six-month outcome of critically ill patients given glutamine-supplemented parenteral nutrition. *Nutrition.* 1997;13:295–302.

77. Goeters C, Wenn A, Mertes N, et al. Parenteral L-alanyl-L-glutamine improves 6-month outcome in critically ill patients. *Crit Care Med.* 2002;30:2032–2037.

78. Griffiths RD, Allen KD, Andrews FJ, Jones C. Infection, multiple organ failure, and survival in the intensive care unit: Influence of glutamine-supplemented parenteral nutrition on acquired infection. *Nutrition.* 2002;18:546–552.

79. Novak F, Heyland DK, Avenell A, Drover JW, Su X. Glutamine supplementation in serious illness: A systematic review of the evidence. *Crit Care Med.* 2002;30:2022–2029.

80. Garcia-de-Lorenzo A, Zarazaga A, Garcia-Luna PP, et al. Clinical evidence for enteral nutritional support with glutamine: A systematic review. *Nutrition.* 2003;19:805–811.

81. Heyland DK, Dhaliwal R, Drover JW, et al. Canadian clinical practice guidelines for nutrition support in mechanically ventilated, critically ill adult patients. *JPEN.* 2003;27:355–373.

82. McClave SA, Sexton LK, Spain DA. Enteral tube feeding in the intensive care unit: Factors impeding adequate delivery. *Crit Care Med.* 1999;27:1252–1256.

83. De Jonghe B, Appere-De-Vechi C, Fournier M. A prospective survey of nutritional support practices in intensive care unit patients: What is prescribed? What is delivered? *Crit Care Med.* 2001;29:8–12.

84. McClave SA, Lukan JK, Stefater JA, et al. Poor validity of residual volumes as a marker for risk of aspiration in critically ill patients. *Crit Care Med.* 2005;33:324–330.

85. Fuhrman MP. Diarrhea and tube feeding. *Nutr Clin Pract.* 1999;14:83–84.

86. Boosalis MG, Ott L, Levine AS, et al. Relationship of visceral proteins to nutritional status in chronic and acute stress. *Crit Care Med.* 1989;17:741–747.

87. Konstantinides FN, Radmer WJ, Becker WK, Herman VK, Warren WE, Solem LD, Williams JB, Cerra FB. Inaccuracy of nitrogen balance determinations in thermal injury with calculated total urinary nitrogen. *J Burn Care Rehabil.* 1992;13:254–260.

88. Demling RH. Comparison of the anabolic effects and complications of human growth hormone and the testosterone analog, oxandrolone, after severe burn injury. *Burns.* 1999;25:215–221.

89. Demling RH, Orgill DP. The anticatabolic and wound healing effects of the testosterone analog oxandralone after severe burn injury. *J Crit Care.* 2000;15:12–17.

90. Gervasio JM, Dickerson RN, Swearinger J, et al. Oxandralone in trauma patients. *Pharmacotherapy.* 2000;20:1328–1334.

91. Bulger EM, Jurkovich GJ, Farver CL, et al. Oxandralone does not improve outcome of ventilator dependent surgical patients. *Ann Surg.* 2004;240:472–480.

CHAPTER 10

Organ Transplantation

Jeanette Hasse, PhD, RD, LD, FADA, CNSD;
and Sara DiCecco, MS, RD, LD

INDICATIONS FOR AND TIMING OF TRANSPLANTATION

Transplantation is different from many surgeries in that the surgical procedure is just the beginning of the transplant journey. Following a successful surgical procedure is a lifelong commitment by the patient and medical team to continue medical therapies to prevent rejection and infection and to monitor for complications associated with surgery or medications. Transplantation is also unique in that it cannot be considered a purely emergent or elective surgery. Certainly, someone with fulminant liver failure who qualifies for transplantation needs an urgent transplant, but the opportunity for that surgery is dependent on an available donor organ. Unless a patient has a living donor (as is often the case with kidney transplantation), the surgery cannot be scheduled because of the lack of knowing when a matching donor will be found. Transplantation surgery is, at the least, life prolonging; at the most, it is life saving. Without a transplant, those with intestinal, kidney, and pancreas failure are destined to rely on therapies such as parenteral nutrition (PN), dialysis, and insulin therapy. On the other hand, those with heart, liver, or lung failure are destined to a short existence unless the diseased organ is replaced.

There are both medical and psychosocial indications and contraindications for transplantation. Medical indications usually encompass end-stage organ diseases (heart, intestine, kidney, liver, lung, or pancreas) that have already been maximally treated by other medical and surgical treatments (see Table 10–1). Medical and psychosocial contraindications include other comorbid diseases or social conditions that preclude long-term success with transplantation (see Table 10–2).

The appropriation of donor organs is regulated by the Organ Procurement and Transplantation Network (OPTN; *www.optn.org*) established by the U.S. Congress under the National Organ Transplant Act of 1984. The United Network of Organ Sharing (UNOS; *www.unos.org*) administers OPTN under contract with the Health Resources and Services Administration of the U.S. Department of Health and Human Services. Over 90,000 individuals are waiting for a transplant today (1). Unfortunately, there are not enough donors to make transplantation available for

Table 10–1 Common Disease Indications for Organ Transplantation in Adults

Organ	Disease Indications
Heart	• Cardiomyopathy (e.g., myocarditis, viral cardiomyopathy, amyloidosis, sarcoidosis) • Coronary artery disease • Congenital heart disease • Valvular heart disease • Retransplant/graft failure
Intestine	• Short-gut syndrome (e.g., resections due to volvulus, inflammatory bowel disease, mesenteric artery or venous thrombosis) • Functional bowel disease (e.g., Hirschsprung's disease, pseudo-obstruction, protein-losing enteropathy) • Retransplant/graft failure
Kidney	• Glomerular diseases • Diabetes • Polycystic kidney disease • Hypertensive nephrosclerosis • Congenital, rare familial, and metabolic diseases (e.g., congenital obstructive obstructive uropathy, Fabry's disease) • Tubular and interstitial diseases (e.g., acquired obstructive nephropathy, analgesic nephropathy, oxalate nephropathy, sarcoidosis, calcineurin-induced nephrotoxicity) • Neoplasms (e.g., incidental carcinoma, renal cell carcinoma, Wilms' tumor) • Retransplant/graft failure • Other (e.g., rheumatoid arthritis, familial nephropathy)
Liver	• Noncholestatic cirrhosis (e.g., alcoholic cirrhosis, viral hepatitis, autoimmune hepatitis, drug-induced liver failure) • Cholestatic liver disease/cirrhosis (e.g., biliary cirrhosis, sclerosing cholangitis) • Acute hepatic necrosis (e.g., viral hepatitis, drug-induced liver failure) • Metabolic diseases (e.g., alpha-1-antitrypsin deficiency, Wilson's disease, hemochromatosis) • Malignant neoplasms (e.g., hepatoma, cholangiocarcinoma) • Other (e.g., Budd-Chiari syndrome, parenteral nutrition-induced liver failure, polycystic liver disease)
Lung	• Congenital disease (e.g., Eisenmenger's syndrome) • Emphysema/chronic obstructive pulmonary disease • Cystic fibrosis • Primary pulmonary hypertension • Alpha-1-antitrypsin deficiency • Retransplant/graft failure • Other (e.g., sarcoidosis, bronchiectasis, pulmonary fibrosis)
Pancreas (or islet cells)	• Diabetes mellitus • Pancreatic cancer (whole pancreas only)

Source: (2)

Table 10–2 Contraindications for Transplantation

Usually Considered Absolute Contraindications for Transplantation	Usually Considered Relative Contraindications for Transplantation
Psychosocial • Lack of support system • Dementia or poor neurocognitive function (with the exception of reversible encephalopathy) • Active substance abuse	Psychosocial • History of medical noncompliance • Lack of understanding and commitment to transplant process
Medical • Active infection/uncontrolled sepsis • Other severe organ dysfunction not expected to improve with transplantation • Malignancy (outside of transplanted organ)	Medical • Advanced age • Morbid obesity • Severe cachexia • Multiple comorbid disease states (e.g., diabetes mellitus, cardiovascular disease)

Source: Adapted from various sources (3–9).

everyone. The medical community, along with other agencies, develops guidelines for each organ type to regulate how donor organs are appropriated. In general, once patients have been accepted for transplantation and placed on a transplant center's waiting list, the patients are registered with the UNOS Organ Center and placed into a computerized program. When an organ is available from a deceased donor, the computer program generates a list of potential recipients ranked according to the objective criteria specific for each organ (2). Examples of general objective data included are blood and tissue type, organ size, medical urgency of the recipient, time on the list, and distance between the donor and recipient (2). The procurement co-ordinator at UNOS Organ Center offers the available organ to the transplant surgeon with the top-ranked patient. If the organ is accepted, arrangements are made for donor and recipient surgeries.

IMMUNOSUPPRESSION

Transplantation is unique in that immunosuppressive medications are required (usually lifelong) to keep the transplanted organ from being rejected by the recipient. Over the last 20 years, new immunosuppressive medications have been added to the armamentarium of treatment options. While necessary to prolong graft life, immunosuppressants can increase risk of cardiovascular disease, opportunistic infections, and malignancy (10). With each drug and different combinations of drugs are specific nutrition interactions and influences. Table 10–3 highlights immuno-suppressive drugs and their interactions.

NUTRITION ASSESSMENT

A complete nutrition assessment should be a part of the transplant evaluation process. With the possibility of extended waiting time until transplantation, there is also the potential for significant, yet preventable, nutrition losses. Nutrition assessment should include an evaluation of a patient's medical history, a physical examination, biochemical and anthropometric measurements, and functional tests (see Table 10–4). Nutrition assessment in transplant recipients is often best achieved using the Subjective Global Assessment (SGA) method (11,12) because the interpretation of purely objective parameters may be affected by the symptoms of the organ failure. For example, fluid status (retention or dehydration) is the most common cause of misinterpretation of assessment parameters; alterations in body weight, hidden losses of muscle mass, and dilution or concentration of the levels of serum proteins and other nutrition-related laboratory values are affected by hydration status (13). SGA components include a review of the history from the perspective of weight changes, dietary intake relative to normal, gastrointestinal (GI) symptoms, functional capacity, and potential for disease-related changes in nutrient requirements as well as physical symptoms such as loss of muscle and/or fat stores, edema, and ascites. Based on a numerical grading of 1 = normal, 2 = mild to moderately affected or decreased, and 3 = severely affected, the individual is given a composite nutrition assessment score of 1 for well-nourished, 2 for suspected of or moderately malnourished, or 3 for severely malnourished (11). The decision about the type and level of pretransplant nutrition care will depend on this ranking, as well as the anticipated length of waiting period for transplantation. For example, patients with moderate or severe nutritional deficits and an expected long pretransplant wait may require tube feeding to improve their nutritional status. Meanwhile, a well-nourished or obese candidate may only require emphasis on good oral intake with regular nutrition follow-up visits.

PRETRANSPLANT NUTRITION ABNORMALITIES

Malnutrition in candidates for transplantation has been linked to effects on morbidity and mortality after transplantation for liver, kidney, lung, and heart transplant recipients (14–27). Malnutrition in organ transplant candidates has typically been defined as underweight and/or with a loss of muscle stores and a myriad of micronutrient abnormalities. Nutrient and tissues losses are commonly due to inadequate oral intake (for a variety of reasons) as well as increased metabolic demands and malabsorption. Improved nutritional status can be achieved for some patients and usually requires intensive oral supplementation (at a minimum) or EN or PN in other patients (28–30).

Table 10–3 Major Side Effects of Commonly Used Immunosuppressive Medications

	Antilymphocyte Serum	Azathioprine	Basiliximab	Daclizumab	Corticosteroids	Cyclosporine	Muromonab-CD3	Mycophenolate Mofetil	Sirolimus	Tacrolimus
Anorexia							✔			
Bone marrow suppression		✔						✔	✔	
Diarrhea	✔	✔					✔	✔		
Dysgeusia		✔								
Fever and chills	✔									
Gastrointestinal distress								✔	✔	✔
Hyperglycemia					✔	✔				✔
Hyperkalemia						✔				✔
Hyperlipidemia					✔	✔			✔	
Hyperphagia					✔					
Hypertension					✔	✔				✔
Hypomagnesemia						✔				✔
Impaired wound healing					✔				✔	
Macrocytic anemia		✔								
Nausea and vomiting	✔	✔					✔			✔
Nephrotoxicity						✔				✔
Neurotoxicity						✔				✔
Osteoporosis					✔					
Pancreatitis		✔			✔					
Sodium retention					✔					
Sore throat/mucositis		✔								
Ulcers					✔					
No known nutrition side effect			✔	✔						

Source: Adapted from Hasse J, Robien K. Nutrition support guidelines for therapeutically immunosuppressed patients. In: Pichard C, Kudsk KA, eds. *From Nutritional Support to Pharmacologic Nutrition in the ICU.* Berlin: Springer-Verlag; 2000:361–383.

Table 10–4 Components of Basic Nutrition Screening and Assessment

History	• Medical history
	• Surgical history
	• Psychosocial history
	• Diagnosis
	• Medications
	• Current dietary intake
Physical examination	• Assessment of muscle and fat stores
	• Presence of ascites and edema
Anthropometric measurements	• Height
	• Weight*
	• Skinfold and arm muscle measurements
	• Bioelectrical impedance analysis*
Biochemical measurements	• Serum albumin level*+
	• Serum transferrin level*+
	• Serum prealbumin level*+
	• Urinary measurements of creatinine and 3-methylhistidine*+
Functional tests	• Muscle strength/hand grip dynamometry
Immune function	• Skin testing§
	• Total lymphocyte count§

Note: A nutrition assessment of a transplant patient will not necessarily include all of these components because the validity of these tests can be affected by organ failure

* Affected by fluid retention

+ Affected by liver and renal failure

§ Affected by immunosuppression

Source: Adapted from Charney PJ. Nutritional screening and assessment. In: Skipper A, ed. *Dietitian's Handbook of Enteral and Parenteral Nutrition.* Gaithersburg, Md.: ASPEN Publishing, Inc; 1998:3–24.

Although the traditional assumption is that the pretransplant patient has the appearance of an underweight, cachectic individual, this is not always the case. Today, many patients presenting for transplantation are obese. The effect of obesity on transplant outcomes varies by type of organ transplanted. Obesity has been linked to morbidity and mortality in lung transplant recipients (31). Studies in liver transplantation suggest that obesity is associated with wound infections but not necessarily short-term survival (32–35). In other words, compared with nonobese liver recipients, obese liver transplant patients may have increased rates of short-term complications but survival is not significantly different between the two groups in the first few years after transplantation. Results are mixed in kidney transplant recipients. Many studies show that obesity affects wound healing and kidney graft function (36–44). Some studies suggest obesity affects kidney graft survival (45–48) while others haven't found an association between obesity and kidney survival (36,38,40,44,45,47,49–52). Many transplant programs will require, or at least recommend, weight loss prior to final acceptance of the patient for transplantation. Adequate weight loss may be difficult for many to achieve due to physical limitations from their disease (fatigue, respiratory failure) as well as psychosocial concerns. Bariatric surgery has been suggested for some patients to improve their candidacy for transplantation (53,54) but there is not enough experience to recommend this for all patients. Preliminary case reports have described significant weight loss after bariatric surgery in nine total patients who all went on to successful renal transplantation (53,54).

MODES OF NUTRITION THERAPY

The goals for nutrition therapy after transplantation surgery are to (55):

1. promote wound healing,
2. prevent infection,
3. promote anabolism or preserve lean body mass,
4. maintain hydration, and
5. provide energy for the patient to participate in physical therapy.

Goals for nutrient intake immediately after transplant are 30–35 calories per kg of dry weight or 130%–150% of basal energy expenditure (BEE by Harris Benedict equation using estimated dry weight). Recipients with fever, infection, or other complications may have increased calorie needs. A resting energy expenditure measurement, if possible, is warranted to document the degree of hypermetabolism. If indirect calorimetry is not available, the nutrition practitioner must estimate needs (such as just described) and then monitor the patient for clinical improvement (e.g., wound healing, recovery of physical activity, tolerance of nutrition support, etc.). Protein requirements are also elevated after transplant both due to the catabolic effect of the immunosuppressive medications and for wound healing. Patients should be encouraged to consume 1.2–2 g of protein per kg per day, with adjustments made for compromises in renal function and need for renal replacement therapy. Many patients will require intensive assistance with food choices, as well as encouragement to try a wider variety of tastes or textures and to eat smaller and more frequent portions. Nutrition supplement products are often necessary to achieve this level of intake but are not always well accepted. Tube feedings should be used to provide the adequate calories, protein, and other nutrients until the recipient's overall health and oral intake improve enough to meet their nutrient needs (55–58).

Oral Nutrition/Diet Orders

Oral diets can begin as soon as a patient is extubated and alert enough to safely chew and swallow. Although it is has been traditional to wait for a patient to have flatus before allowing oral intake, this is not necessarily required. However, the patient should be counseled to consume only small amounts as tolerated until their GI function returns to normal. Most renal and liver recipients will be able to start oral intake within the first 1–2 days after transplantation. If there has been significant manipulation of the bowel during surgery, the initiation of oral intake may be delayed until decompression via a nasogastric tube is no longer required. In the meantime, patients will need to be maintained on intravenous fluids with careful attention to fluid balance and electrolyte management (55–57). If heart and/or lung transplant patients remain intubated longer than 1–2 days, nutrition support should be initiated (58,59).

Intestinal graft recipients are not allowed an oral diet until graft function is assured. Once patients are able to consume oral intake, some transplant centers temporarily restrict sugar, fat, lactose, and caffeine to prevent diarrhea and malabsorption (60,61). However, some transplant programs do not restrict the diet in an effort to maximize oral nutrient intake. Regardless, small, frequent feedings should be offered.

Oral nutrition should be advanced from clear fluids to a regular diet as rapidly as tolerated, monitoring for symptoms of ileus. Most patients will need between-meal feedings or oral nutrition supplement products in order to achieve an adequate intake of calories, protein, and other nutrients. This can be determined best between the patient and transplant dietitian.

Restrictions of carbohydrate, sodium, or other nutrients should be avoided until good oral intake is established unless required to therapeutically treat a patient. A liberalized diet is often needed for the first 4–6 weeks to provide adequate intake needed to promote wound healing and begin repletion of muscle mass as well as vitamin and mineral stores. Once the recipient has begun to improve nutritionally, the patient and patient's caregivers should be taught nutrition concepts that promote a healthy diet and lifestyle. This is important to treat and prevent long-term side effects of the transplant and immunosuppressive medications. This would include strategies for weight control; lipid, blood pressure, and glucose management; and optimal bone health (see Table 10–5). Posttransplant diabetes is common and should be treated accordingly to prevent its deleterious effect on wound healing and susceptibility to infection.

Enteral Tube Feeding

Ideally, all patients would be fed via an oral diet within a few days after organ transplantation; however, this is not feasible in those who require prolonged mechanical ventilation, have an ileus, need reoperation, experience primary nonfunction of

Table 10–5 Long-Term Nutrition Complications Associated With Solid Organ Transplantation

Complication	Causes (Risk Factors)	Therapy
Obesity (59,62)	• Genetic predisposition • Hyperphagia from corticosteroids • Improved absorption after transplant	• Reduce caloric intake • Increase activity • Evaluate eating behaviors • Consider appetite-reducing medications
Diabetes mellitus (59,62–73)	• Obesity • Genetic predisposition • Medications (tacrolimus, cyclosporine, corticosteroids) • Hepatitis C infection • Certain ethnic groups (e.g., Native Americans, Hispanics, Asians) • Increasing age	• Reduce weight if overweight • Initiate self-glucose monitoring • Encourage carbohydrate-controlled diet • Prescribe insulin or oral hypoglycemic agent • Reduce calcineurin inhibitor and/or corticosteroid doses • Encourage exercise
Hypertension (59,62,65,71–76)	• High-sodium diet • Obesity • Calcineurin inhibitors	• Encourage low-sodium diet • Encourage weight loss if indicated • Prescribe antihypertensive medications • Encourage exercise
Hyperlipidemia (59,62,65,71–73,76–83)	• Cyclosporine, corticosteroids, rapamycin, tacrolimus (tacrolimus has least effect) • Loop diuretics • Weight gain • Diet	• Prescribe antihyperlipidemic drugs (usually statin drugs but also bile acid sequestrants, ezetimibe, fibrates) • Encourage low-saturated-fat diet • Encourage weight loss if indicated • Suggest use of stanol/sterol esters

(continues)

Table 10–5 Continued

Complication	Causes (Risk Factors)	Therapy
Osteoporosis (59,84–92)	• Corticosteroids and calcineurin inhibitors • Some pretransplant conditions such as renal failure, long-term parenteral nutrition, cholestatic liver disease, chronic corticosteroid use, etc.	• Provide adequate calcium and vitamin D intake (via diet and/or supplements) • Consider prescribing calcitonin or bisphosphonates • Consider prescribing estrogen therapy for postmenopausal women • Encourage weight-bearing exercise

Source: Adapted from various sources (see notes indicated in table).

the transplanted graft, or have received an intestinal transplant. Early enteral feeding should be initiated for those who will not begin oral intake in a timely fashion. In addition, enteral feedings should also be considered for those patients who are malnourished (as defined by the assessment tool specific for that transplant type) prior to transplantation so that adequate nutrient intake is ensured immediately after surgery. This may be achieved by the placement of an enteral feeding tube into the small bowel during the transplant operation. This procedure is more easily achieved in a liver transplant when the small bowel is exposed as opposed to a heart or lung transplant. If a feeding tube is not placed during the transplant operation, a tube may need to be placed at bedside or under fluoroscopy when tube feeding is required. Three randomized, prospective, controlled studies in liver transplant recipients showed that infectious complications were reduced when postoperative tube feedings were provided (93–95). Hasse et al. found a trend toward reductions in bacterial infections from 29% in nonfed patients to 14% in patients who received enteral feedings after liver transplantation (93). In two other studies, Rayes et al. showed a decrease in bacterial infections in patients who were enterally fed formulas containing fiber and/or *lactobacillus,* with the lowest infection rates in those who received feeds containing lactic acid bacteria and four types of fiber (94,95). Overall, patients will tolerate continuous pump-assisted feedings through small-bore tubes placed postpylorically. Postpyloric feedings are generally used instead of gastric feedings due to delayed gastric emptying often associated with the post-surgical period. Table 10–6 includes general recommendations for which enteral

Table 10–6 Tube Feeding Formula Considerations for Organ Transplant Recipients

Condition	Formula Recommendations
Normal postoperative course	• Standard (polymeric), high-nitrogen formula
Renal insufficiency	• Consider formula lower in potassium and/or phosphorus
	• Adjust fluid volume
Diarrhea/constipation	• Consider fiber-enriched formula
	• Maintain adequate fluid intake
Pancreatitis	• Consider low-fat, elemental formula if standard formula is not tolerated
Maldigestion	• Consider partially hydrolyzed formula with medium-chain triglycerides
Gastroparesis	• Place feeding tube into jejunum
Intestinal transplant	• Consider formula with low osmolality and medium-chain triglycerides

Source: Adapted from various sources (55,56,58,60).

formula types should be considered. The specific formula used will depend on formulary availability. Once patients begin to take a significant amount of oral intake, tube feeding can be changed to a cyclic nocturnal infusion. Tube feeding can be discontinued once oral intake consistently reaches 75% of calorie and protein requirements (13).

For intestinal transplant recipients, once any anastomotic leaks and/or postoperative ileus have resolved (often 1–2 weeks posttransplant), enteral and oral feedings may be started (60,61). Initial enteral feedings should be at a low rate with a gradual increase in volume to assess tolerance as well as begin to stimulate gut mucosa (60,61). Either nasoenteral or percutaneous enteral feedings tubes are used depending on the anticipated course of feeding and patient comfort as well as the individual's potential for complications. Once enteral tolerance has been established, parenteral nutrition can be tapered proportionally to avoid overfeeding; however, IV fluids may still be needed to maintain hydration if the stomal output is elevated. Eventually, oral intake is introduced; when oral intake is significant, the enteral feedings can be cycled to nocturnal administration and subsequently discontinued once the patient can meet his or her full nutrient requirements orally (96).

Parenteral Nutrition

PN should be resumed as soon as possible for those patients receiving an intestinal graft. In addition, PN is indicated for patients with a nonfunctional gut due to conditions such as intestinal obstruction or prolonged ileus. Due to the myriad of complications associated with parenteral nutrition, patients should be converted to enteral and/or oral nutrition as soon as possible (60,96). Parenteral solutions often need to be concentrated due to fluid overload situations due to intraoperative fluid requirements as well as postoperative cardiac instability or renal dysfunction, and is most commonly seen in heart, lung, or liver transplantation. A typical parenteral solution will provide 100% of the protein needs as amino acids with the balance of nonprotein calories as 30% lipids and 70% dextrose. A daily dose of vitamins and trace elements is usually adequate and does not require modifications for short-term feedings. Daily monitoring for serum electrolyte levels (especially potassium, phosphorus, and magnesium) as well as glucose and lipid management are required (55).

FOOD SAFETY ISSUES

Diets restricted in foods such as fresh fruits, raw vegetables, pepper, and cheeses are used by some transplant centers to minimize the risk of certain infections in addition to good food safety precautions. Common names for this type of diet may include: "Low Bacteria Diet," "Low Microbial Diet," "Neutropenic Diet," or "Diet for Immunosuppressed Patients." They may be used only during the hospitalization or for up to 100 days (3 months) following transplantation (97). Good scientific data of the efficacy of this type of diet is lacking. These restrictions, especially if used for a prolonged period of time, do not promote nutritional balance and may impede the oral intake from reaching an adequate amount to meet a patient's needs (97).

However, transplant patients must learn and practice good food safety practices because the relative increase in risk of food-borne illnesses due to their immunosuppressed state is unknown. Concern regarding illnesses from *salmonella, escherichia coli, listeria monocytogenes,* or other bacteria is both for their potential mortality as well as morbidity. Because the symptoms of most food-borne illnesses include nausea, vomiting, and/or diarrhea, any occurrence of these symptoms in transplant patients warrants monitoring of the patient's ability to stay hydrated as well as retain their immunosuppressive medications. Early detection/diagnosis as well as treatment and supportive care are crucial for ensuring both patient and graft survival. Basic food safety recommendations are included in Table 10–7.

NUTRITION MONITORING

After transplantation, the patient must be monitored closely for the rest of his or her life. While monitoring occurs daily in the immediate posttransplant phase, the frequency of laboratory and other tests as well as doctor visits decreases as the

Table 10–7 Food Safety Recommendations for Organ Transplant Patients

Avoid the following due to increased risk of food-borne illness contamination:
- All raw or undercooked meats (especially ground), poultry, fish, and game
- Sushi, raw seafood, and shellfish
- Raw or undercooked eggs and foods that contain them (i.e., Caesar dressing)
- All unpasteurized milk and dairy products, including cheeses
- All unpasteurized juices and cider
- All fresh sprouts (bean, alfalfa, etc.)
- Raw or spoiled food items or those with obvious mold
- Foods stored in bulk, self-serve containers in the grocery store
- Foods contaminated with food-borne illness
- Raw, unroasted nuts including nuts in a shell

Always practice the following:
- Use safe food-handling techniques
- Store food promptly and appropriately
- Wash all produce well, even those supposedly prewashed
- Reheat any deli-type lunch meats to steaming or eat sandwiches where the meat has been heated
- Eat leftovers within 1–2 days (freeze any additional portions)
- Be aware that buffets, salad bars, potlucks, etc. may be a source of food contamination
- Drink from safe water supplies
- Use a heat-processing method to do any home canning, food preservation, or smoking of meats

Source: Adapted from DiCecco SR, Francisco-Ziller N, Moore D. Overview and immunosuppression. In: Hasse JM, Blue LS, eds. *Comprehensive Guide to Transplant Nutrition*. Chicago: American Dietetic Association; 2002:1–30.

---

time from transplantation passes and stable organ function is achieved. Nutrition monitoring follows a similar course. Daily evaluation of nutrition may be required immediately following transplantation. However, as nutrition support is weaned or oral dietary intake is stabilized, the frequency and intensity of nutrition monitoring decreases. Table 10–8 describes common nutrition monitoring techniques that incorporate both objective and subjective measurements and criteria.

SPECIAL NUTRITION CONSIDERATIONS ASSOCIATED WITH TRANSPLANTATION

There are characteristics and complications associated with transplantation that make the nutrition therapy and nutrient requirements for these patients unique. The posttransplant complications most likely affecting nutrition include rejection, infection, renal failure, respiratory failure, GI complications, and hyperglycemia (98).

Table 10–8 Suggested Nutrition Parameters to Monitor Following Organ Transplantation

Category	Specific Tests	Rationale
Laboratory	• Values representing transplanted organ function	• To monitor transplanted organ function
	• Serum electrolyte levels	• To be able to respond with electrolyte replacement and changes in IV fluid or nutrition formulations
	• Serum glucose concentration	• Posttransplant hyperglycemia is common; insulin or oral hypoglycemic agent may be required
	• Hepatic transport proteins	• These are likely valid only when organ function is normal and patient is long-term posttransplant
	• Vitamin and mineral levels	• These should be monitored in those known to have abnormal pretransplant levels (e.g., long-term parenteral nutrition patients, patients with cholestatic liver disease, cystic fibrosis patients with known malabsorption, etc.)
		• If a deficiency is being treated, monitoring levels should help determine when treatment can be discontinued
Clinical	• Gastrointestinal function (such as bowel sounds, number/consistency of bowel movements)	• To evaluate for complications (such as diarrhea, constipation, esophagitis, gastroparesis, etc.) and subsequent interventions
	• Fluid intake and output records	• To evaluate need to withhold or supplement fluid
Nutritional	• Nutrient intake (e.g., calorie counts)	• To determine adequacy of nutrient intake (whether parenteral, enteral, or oral)
	• Body weight	• Weight change may reflect fluid retention vs. change in muscle and fat
	• Anthropometrics (e.g., mid-arm muscle circumference, tricep skinfolds)	• Anthropometric measurements likely only helpful over long term

Table 10–8 Continued

Category	Specific Tests	Rationale
Physical	• Muscle and fat stores	• Reflect long-term status of nutrition
	• Presence of ascites and edema	• Reflects fluid status
	• Physical activity	• Reflects ability to maintain muscle stores
	• Skin integrity and wounds	• To evaluate nutrient losses and/or additional nutrient requirements for healing
Other	• Bone density	• To evaluate for bone loss in those at high risk for osteoporosis (e.g., patients previously requiring hemodialysis or long-term parenteral nutrition; patients with potential vitamin D losses such as cholestatic liver disease or cystic fibrosis; patients on long-term corticosteroid therapy)
	• D-xylose or fecal fat excretion tests	• Occasionally performed to determine absorptive capability of a transplanted small intestine

Transplant Organ Dysfunction

Organ dysfunction can present as primary nonfunction (in which the organ never functions well), delayed graft function (from preservation injury associated with ischemia time and preservation solution), vascular thrombosis (of blood vessel to the newly transplanted organ), and acute rejection. Primary nonfunction requires retransplantation; nutrition support initiation may be interrupted by the need for retransplantation. Delayed graft function may require interventions to provide relief from organ dysfunction. For example, if a kidney recipient's transplanted organ has delayed function, he or she will likely need dialysis and possibly restriction of dietary fluid, phosphorus, and potassium. Repair of vascular anastomosis likely means interruption of nutrition for a period of NPO status. Acute rejection requires additional treatment with immunosuppressive medications. The nutritional side effects (see Table 10–3) can be magnified when doses of these medications are increased.

Infection

Because transplant patients are immunosuppressed, they are at increased risk of infection. Risk factors for infection in transplant patients include the presence of infection in either the donor or recipient as well as the type of organ transplanted, type and intensity of immunosuppression, patient age, and donor type (deceased vs. living donor) (99). Malnutrition also increases the chance of infection, and obesity is related to increased rates of wound infection (32–44). The most common infections in the first posttransplant month include bacterial and candida wound infection, pneumonia, and central line infections (100). Fungal infections may occur in the early (2–6 weeks) posttransplant period (usually *aspergillus, candida),* intermediate (1–6 months) period (usually *candida, aspergillus,* dimorphic fungal infections), and late (>6 months) posttransplant period (usually disseminated histoplasmosis, aspergillosis, and dermatophyte infections) (101). Infections with cytomegalovirus (CMV), Epstein Barr virus, and herpes simplex virus usually occur later. CMV can result in fever, malaise, leukopenia, and thrombocytopenia (102) and can affect many organs including the lungs, intestines, liver, and skin (99). Prophylaxis against microbes is common; any time infection is suspected, antimicrobial drugs are initiated. Antimicrobial agents may cause GI distress (diarrhea, dysguesia, dyspepsia, nausea, and vomiting). Interventions should aim to reduce and treat these side effects to optimize nutrient intake. Such interventions could include providing foods tolerated by the patient and prescribing medications designed to reduce GI side effects such as H2 blockers or proton-pump inhibitors, antiemetics, and antidiarrheal medications (once an infectious cause is ruled out).

Renal Failure

Because many immunosuppressive drugs are nephrotoxic, renal insufficiency occurs frequently following transplantation. If a patient is anuric or has severe electrolyte or acid-base abnormalities, renal replacement therapy may be necessary. Nutrition therapy may need to be altered to restrict fluid, phosphorus, or potassium, although the type of dialysis dictates if these nutrients must be restricted or supplemented. For example, with conventional hemodialysis, serum phosphorus levels tend to rise. With continuous dialysis modes (such as continous venovenous hemodialysis), serum phosphorus levels may drop. Adequate protein intake is necessary when dialysis is required. Patients should be counseled to eat high-protein foods but may require the addition of nutrition supplements to meet protein requirements.

Respiratory Failure

Patients with graft dysfunction, sepsis, pneumonia, fluid overload, and acute respiratory distress syndrome may require prolonged ventilatory support. Obviously, nutrition support is required for ventilated patients because an oral diet is precluded. Tube feeding is used unless contraindicated by GI dysfunction. Once a patient is extubated after a prolonged intubation period, he or she should be evaluated by a speech pathologist for dysphagia.

GI Complications

GI complications include oral lesions, esophagitis, peptic ulcers, ileus, constipation, and diarrhea (103). Oral lesions are often caused by immunosuppressive drugs or infection; esophagitis is often fungal in origin but occurs most often in patients receiving mycophenolate mofetil (103). Viral infections such as cytomegalovirus and herpes simplex contribute to other GI symptoms such as nausea, vomiting, gastroparesis, and bleeding (103). Ileus or constipation can occur in the postoperative period. Stool softeners, laxatives, or enemas may be required to help resolve constipation. After infectious causes of diarrhea are ruled out, antidiarrheal medications may be added to a patient's treatment. In addition, current medications must be reviewed to check for any that may be causing diarrhea. For example, a major side effect of mycophenolate mofetil is diarrhea; sometimes dose adjustments improve diarrhea. Adequate fluid is required to help reduce constipation or reduce losses associated with diarrhea. Fiber may also be useful with ameliorating constipation or diarrhea, although no specific type or amount of fiber has been evaluated with this patient population.

Intestinal transplant patients may display signs of gastric atony or altered transit time (104). Acute rejection in a transplanted bowel may cause fever, nausea, vomiting, abdominal pain, and increased ostomy output (61). These complications may require initiation or continuation of PN until the complication is resolved. Other unique GI complications related to small bowel transplantation include extrinsic denervation, disrupted neural activity, and interrupted lymphatic drainage that can cause chylous ascites (61,104). A low-fat diet may be necessary as chylous ascites resolves.

Hyperglycemia

Hyperglycemia occurs frequently following transplantation. Corticosteroids cause insulin resistance and alter metabolic responses to neurohormonal and cytokine-mediated stimuli (63). Calcineurin inhibitors inhibit pancreatic islet cell function, hamper insulin secretion, and cause insulin resistance (63). Of the two calcineurin inhibitors, tacrolimus is considered more diabetogenic than cyclosporine (64). The incidence of new onset diabetes mellitus (differentiated from transient postoperative hyperglycemia) among all solid organ transplant recipients is approximately 13.4% (64).

Postoperative hyperglycemia has been found to be related to risk of kidney transplant rejection. Thomas et al. retrospectively evaluated 230 cyclosporine-treated kidney transplant recipients without a history of diabetes mellitus (105). Patients with an early postoperative serum glucose level >144 mg/dL had a 71% rate of rejection compared with a 42% rate in patients whose glucose level was <144 mg/dL.

The same trend was true in kidney recipients with preexisting diabetes mellitus (106). Those with a 100-hour posttransplant serum glucose level <201 mg/dL had an 11% rate of acute rejection; the rate was 58% among those with a 100-hour posttransplant serum glucose level >201 mg/dL.

Posttransplant hyperglycemia should be treated with insulin or oral hypoglycemic agents. Some centers use continuous insulin infusions to treat hyperglycemia in the early postoperative phase; the threshold for the criteria (i.e., glucose level) at which to start insulin drip is debatable. If hyperglycemia persists as the patient approaches discharge, he or she should be taught how to self-monitor glucose levels. Those whose blood glucose does not return to normal should be referred to diabetes professionals for education and treatment.

CONCLUSION

The evaluation of nutritional status and nutrient needs of transplant recipients is crucial to provision of adequate and appropriate nutrition to help promote optimal transplant outcomes. Those providing care to these patients should be familiar with the transplant process, immunosuppressive drugs and their side effects, nutrition assessment techniques for transplant patients, appropriate nutrition support methods, and adjustments in nutrition therapy for complications following transplantation. Transplant science is changing rapidly; transplant nutrition guidelines will need to adapt to match the advances in the field.

REFERENCES

1. United Network of Organ Sharing. Available at www.unos.org. Accessed 11/18/05.

2. Organ Procurement and Transplantation Network. Available at www.optn.org.

3. Cupples SA, Boyce SW, Stamou SC. Heart transplantation. In: Cupples SA, Ohler L, eds. *Solid Organ Transplantation. A Handbook for Primary Health Care Providers.* New York, NY: Springer Publishing Company, Inc.; 2002:146–188.

4. Bartucci MR, Hricik DE. Kidney transplantation. In: Cupples SA, Ohler L, eds. *Solid Organ Transplantation. A Handbook for Primary Health Care Providers.* New York, NY: Springer Publishing Company, Inc.; 2002:189–222.

5. Dimercurio B, Henry L, Kirk AD. Simultaneous Kidney-pancreas transplantation. In: Cupples SA, Ohler L, eds. *Solid Organ Transplantation. A Handbook for Primary Health Care Providers.* New York, NY: Springer Publishing Company, Inc.; 2002:223–239.

6. Nathan S, Ohler L. Lung and heart-lung transplantation. In: Cupples SA, Ohler L, eds. *Solid Organ Transplantation. A Handbook for Primary Health Care Providers.* New York, NY: Springer Publishing Company, Inc.; 2002:240–260.

7. Pirsch JD, Douglas MJ. Liver transplantation. In: Cupples SA, Ohler L, eds. *Solid Organ Transplantation. A Handbook for Primary Health Care Providers.* New York, NY: Springer Publishing Company, Inc.; 2002:261–291.

8. Williams L, Horslen SP, Langnas AN. Intestinal transplantation. In: Cupples SA, Ohler L, eds. *Solid Organ Transplantation. A Handbook for Primary Health Care Providers.* New York, NY: Springer Publishing Company, Inc.; 2002:292–333.

9. Ohler L, Harlan D. Islet cell transplantation. In: Cupples SA, Ohler L, eds. *Solid Organ Transplantation. A Handbook for Primary Health Care Providers.* New York, NY: Springer Publishing Company, Inc.; 2002:334–342.

10. Lechler RI, Sykes M, Thomson AW, Turka LA. Organ transplantation—how much of the promise has been realized. *Nature Med.* 2005;11:605–613.

11. Detsky AS, McLaughlin JR, Baker JP, Johnston N, et al. What is subjective global assessment of nutritional status? *JPEN J Parenter Enteral Nutr.* 1987;11:8–13.

12. Hasse J, Strong S, Gorman MA, Liepa G. Subjective global assessment: alternative nutrition-assessment technique for liver-transplant candidates. *Nutrition.* 1993;9:339–343.

13. Hasse JM, DiCecco SR. Solid organ transplantation. In: Skipper A, ed. *Dietitian's Handbook of Enteral and Parenteral Nutrition.* Gaithersburg MD: ASPEN Publishing, Inc. 1998:295–323.

14. Harrison J, McKiernan J, Neuberger JM. A prospective study on the effect of recipient nutritional status on outcome in liver transplantation. *Transpl Int* 1997;10:369–374, 1997.

15. Selberg O, Böttcher J, Tusch G, et al. Identification of high- and low-risk patients before liver transplantation: A prospective cohort study of nutritional and metabolic parameters in 150 patients. *Hepatology* 1997;25:652–657.

16 Lautz HU, Selberg O, Körber J, et al. Protein-calorie malnutrition in liver cirrhosis. *Clin Invest* 1992;70:478–486.

17. Figueiredo F, Dickson ER, Pasha T, et al. Impact of nutritional status on outcomes after liver transplantation. *Transplantation* 2000;70(9):1347–1352.

18. Tritt L. Nutritional assessment and support of kidney transplant recipients. *J Infusion Nursing.* 2004;27:45–51.

19. Miller DG, Levine SE, D'Elia JA, Bistrian BR. Nutritional status of diabetic and nondiabetic patients after renal transplantation. *Am J Clin Nutr.* 1986;44:66–69.

20. Plochl W, Pezawas L, Artemiou O, Grimm M, Klipetko W, Hiesmayr M. Nutritional status, ICU duration and ICU mortality in lung transplant recipients. *Intensive Care Med.* 1996;22:1179–1185.

21. Madill J, Maurer JR, de Hoyes A. A comparison of preoperative and postoperative nutritional states of lung transplant recipients. *Transplantation.* 1993:56:347–350.

22. Schwebel C, Pin I, Barnoud D, et al. Prevalence and consequences of nutritional depletion in lung transplant candidates. *Eur Respir J.* 2000:16:1050–1055.

23. Grady K, White Williams C, Naftle D, et al. Are preoperative obesity and cachexia risk factors for post-heart transplant morbidity and mortality: a multi-institutional study of preoperative weight-height in disease? *J Heart Lung Transplant.* 1999;18:750–763.

24. Frazier O, VanBuren C, Pointdexter S, Waldenberger F. Nutritional management of the heart transplant recipient. *Heart Transplant.* 1985;4:450–452.

25. Pikul J, Sharpe MD, Lowndes R, Chent CN. Degree of preoperative malnutrition is predictive of postoperative morbidity and mortality in liver transplant recipients. *Transplantation.* 1994;57:469–472.

26. Hasse JM, Gonwa TA, Jennings LW, et al. Malnutrition affects liver transplant outcomes [Abstract]. *Transplantation.* 1998;66(8):S53.

27. Hade AM, Shine AM, Kennedy NP, McCormick PA. Both under-nutrition and obesity increase morbidity following liver transplantation. *Irish Medical J.* 2003;96:140–142.

28. Plank LD, McCall JL, Gane EJ, et al. Pre- and postoperative immunonutrition in patients undergoing liver transplantation: a pilot study of safety and efficacy. *Clin Nutr.* 2005;24:288–296.

29. Forli L, Bjortuft O, Vatn M, Kofstad J, Boe J. A study of intensified dietary support in underweight candidates for lung transplantation. *Ann Nutr Metab.* 2001;45:159–168.

30. Mullen JL, Buzby G, Matthews D, Smale B, Rosato EF. Reduction of operative morbidity and mortality by combined preoperative and postoperative nutritional support. *Ann Surg.* 1980;192:604–613.

31. Madill J, Gutierrez C, Grossman J, et al. Nutritional assessment of the lung transplant patient: body mass index as a predictor of 90-day mortality following transplantation. *J Heart Lung Transplant.* 2001;20:288–296.

32. Keefe EB, Getts C, Esquivel CO. Liver transplantation in patients with severe obesity. *Transplantation.* 1994;57:309–311.

33. Braunfeld MYY, Chan S, Pregler J, et al. Liver transplantation in the morbidly obese. *J Clin Anesth.* 1996;8:585–590.

34. Sawyer RB, Pelletier SJ, Pruett TL. Increased early morbidity and mortality with acceptable long-term function in severely obese patients undergoing liver transplantation. *Clin Transplant.* 1999;13:126–130

35. Nair S, Verma S, Thuluvath PJ. Obesity and its effect on survival in patients undergoing orthotopic liver transplantation in the United States. *Hepatology.* 2002;35:105–109.

36. Johnson DW, Isbel NM, Brown AM, et al. The effect of obesity on renal transplant outcomes. *Transplantation.* 2002;74:675–680.

37. Marks WH, Florence LS, Chapman PH, Precht AF, Perinson DT. Morbid obesity is not a contraindication to kidney transplantation. *Am J Surg.* 2004;187:635–638.

38. Bennett WM, McEvoy KM, Henell KR. Valente JF, Douzdjian V. Morbid obesity does not preclude successful renal transplantation. *Clin Transplant.* 2004;18:89–93.

39. Moreso F, Seron D, Anunciada AI, et al. Recipient body surface area as a predictor of posttransplant renal allograft evolution. *Transplantation.* 1998;65:671–676.

40. Pirsch JD, Armbrust MJ, Knechtle SJ, et al. Obesity as a risk factor following renal transplantation. *Transplantation.* 1995;59:631–633.

41. Holley JL, Shapiro R, Lopatin WB, Tzakis AG, Hakala TF, Starzl TE. Obesity as a risk factor following cadaveric renal transplantation. *Transplantation.* 1990;49:387–389.

42. Drafts HH, Anjum MR, Wynn JJ, Mullow LL, Bowley JN, Humphries AL. The impact of pretransplant obesity on renal transplant outcomes. *Clin Transplantation.* 1997;11:493–496.

43. Bumgardner GL, Henry, ML, Elkhammas E, et al. Obesity as a risk factor after combined pancreas/kidney transplantation. *Transplantation.* 1995;60:1426–1430.

44. Orofino L, Pascual J, Quereda C, Burgos J, Marcen R, Ortuno J. Influence of overweight on survival of kidney transplant. *Nephrol Dial Transplant.* 1997;12:855.

45. Gill IS, Hodge EE, Novick AC, Steinmuller DR, Garred D. Impact of obesity on renal transplantation. *Transplant Proc.* 1993;25:1047–1048.

46. Wilson GA, Bumgardner GL, Henry ML, et al. Decreased graft survival in obese pancreas/kidney recipients. *Transplant Proc.* 1995;27:3106–3107.

47. Halme L, Eklund B, Kyllönen L, Salmela K. Is obesity still a risk factor in renal transplantation? *Transpl Int.* 1997;10:284–288.

48. Meier-Kriesche H-U, Vaghela M, Thambuganipalle R, Friedman G, Jacobs M, Kaplan G. The effect of body mass index on long-term renal allograft survival. *Transplantation.* 1999;68: 1294–1297.

49. Modlin CS, Flechner SM, Gooormastic M, et al. Should obese patients lose weight before receiving a kidney transplant? *Transplantation.* 1997;64:599–604.

50. Drafts JJ, Anjum MR, Wynn JJ, Mulloy LL, Bowley JN, Humphries AL. The impact of pretransplant obesity on renal transplant outcomes. *Clin Transplant.* 1997;11:493–496.

51. Rogers J, Chavin KD, Baliga PK, et al. Influence of mild obesity on outcome of simultaneous pancreas and kidney transplantation. *J Gastrointest Surg.* 2003;7:1096–1101.

52. Howard RJ, Thai VB, Patton PR, et al. Obesity does not portend a bad outcome for kidney transplant recipients. *Transplantation.* 2002;73:53–55.

53. Newcombe V, Blanch A, Slater GH, Szold A, Fielding GA. Laparoscopic adjustable gastric banding prior to renal transplantation. *Obesity Surgery.* 2005;15:567–570.

54. Alexander JW, Goodman HR, Gersin K, et al. Gastric bypass in morbidly obese patients with chronic renal failure and kidney transplant. Transplantation. 2004;78:469–474.

55. Hasse JM. Adult Liver Transplantation. In: Hasse JM, Blue LS, eds. *Comprehensive Guide to Transplant Nutrition.* Chicago: American Dietetic Association. 2002;58–89.

56. Blue LS. Adult Kidney Transplantation. In: Hasse JM, Blue LS, eds. *Comprehensive Guide to Transplant Nutrition.* Chicago: American Dietetic Association. 2002;44–57.

57. Obayashi PAC. Adult Pancreas Transplantation. In: Hasse JM, Blue LS, eds. *Comprehensive Guide to Transplant Nutrition.* Chicago: American Dietetic Association. 2002;90–105.

58. Pahwa N, Hedberg AM. Adult Heart and Lung Transplantation. In: Hasse JM, Blue LS, eds. *Comprehensive Guide to Transplant Nutrition.* Chicago: American Dietetic Association. 2002; 31–43.

59. Tynan C, Hasse JM. Current nutrition practices in adult lung transplantation. *Nutr Clin Pract.* 2004;19:587–596.

60. Weseman RA. Adult Small Bowel Transplantation. In: Hasse JM, Blue LS, eds. *Comprehensive Guide to Transplant Nutrition.* Chicago: American Dietetic Association. 2002;106–123.

61. Weseman RA, Gilroy R. Nutrition management of small-bowel transplant patients. *Nutr Clin Pract.* 2005;5:509–516.

62. Ducloux D, Kazory A, Simula-Faivre D, Chalopin J-M. One-year post-transplant weight gain is a risk factor for graft loss. *Am J Transplant.* 2005;5:2922–2928.

63. Jindal RM, Sidner RA, Milgrom ML. Post-transplant diabetes mellitus. The role of immunosuppression. *Drug Safety.* 1997;16:242–257.

64. Heisel O, Heisel R, Balshaw R, Keown P. New onset diabetes mellitus in patients receiving calcineurin inhibitors: a systematic review and meta-analysis. *Am J Transplant.* 2004;4:583–595.

65. Fellstrom B. Risk factors for and management of post-transplantation cardiovascular disease. *BioDrugs.* 2001;15:261–278.

66. Marchetti P. New-onset diabetes after liver transplantation: from pathogenesis to management. *Liver Transplant.* 2005;11:612–620.

67. Heisel O, Heisel R, Balshaw R, Keown P. New onset diabetes mellitus in patients receiving calcineurin inhibitors: a systematic review and meta-analysis. *Am J Transplant.* 2004;4:583–595.

68. Davidson J, Wildinson A, Dantal J, et al. New-onset diabetes after transplantation: 2003 international consensus guidelines. *Transplantation.* 2003;75(Suppl):SS3–SS24.

69. Kahn J, Rehak P, Schweiger M, Wasler A, Wascher T, Tscheliessnigg KH, Müller H. The impact of overweight on the development of diabetes after heart transplantation. *Clin Transplant.* 2005;DOI: 10.111/j.1300-0012.2005.00441.x

70. Parikh CR, Klem P, Wong C, Yalavarthy R, Chan L. Obesity as an independent predictor of post-transplant diabetes mellitus. *Transplant Proc.* 2003;35:2922–2926.

71. Rabkin JM, Rosen HR, Corless CL, Olyaei AJ. Tacrolimus is associated with a lower incidence of cardiovascular complications in liver transplant recipients. *Transplant Proc.* 2002;34:1557–1558.

72. Liindenfeld J, Page RL, Zolty R, Shakar SF, Levi M, Lowes B, Wolfel EE, Miller GG. Drug therapy in the heart transplant recipient. Part III: common medical problems. *Circulation.* 2005;111: 113–117.

73. Armstrong KA, Campbell SB, Hawley CM, Johnson DW, Isbel N. Impact of obesity on renal transplant outcomes. *Nephrology.* 2005;10:405–413.

74. Textor SC, Taler SJ, Canzanello VJ, Schwartz L, Augustine JE. Posttransplantation hypertension related to calcineurin inhibitors. *Liver Transpl.* 2000;6:521–530.

75. Neal DAJ, Gimson AES, Gibbs P, Alexander GJM. Beneficial effects of converting liver transplant recipients from cyclosporine to tacrolimus on blood pressure, serum lipids, and weight. *Liver Transplant.* 2001;7:533–539.

76. Johnston SD, Morris JK, Cramb R, Gunson BK, Neuberger J. Cardiovascular morbidity and mortality after orthotopic liver transplantation. *Transplantation.*2002;73:901–906.

77. Zachoval R, Gerbes AL, Schwandt P, Parhofer KG. Short-term effects of statin therapy in patients with hyperlipoproteinemia after liver transplantation: results of a randomized cross-over trial. *J Hepatol.* 2001;35:86–91.

78. Morrisett JD, Abdel-Fattah G, Kahan BD. Sirolimus changes lipid concentrations and lipoprotein metabolism in kidney transplant recipients. *Transplant Proc.* 2003:35(Suppl A):143S–150S.

79. Zachoval R, Gerbes AL, Schwandt P, Parhofer KG. Short-term effects of statin therapy in patients with hyperlipoproteinemia after liver transplantation: results of a randomized cross-over trial. *J Hepatol.* 2001;35:86–91.

80. Wenke K, Meiser B, Thiery J, Reichart B. Impact of simvastatin therapy after heart transplantation. *Herz.* 2005;30:431–432.

81. Jardine AG, Fellström B, Logan JO, Cole E, Nyberg G, Grönhagen-Riska C, Madsen S, Neumayer H-H, Maes B, Ambühl P, Olsson AG, Pedersen T, Holdaas H. Cardiovascular risk and renal transplantation: post hoc analyses of the assessment of lescol in renal transplantation (ALERT) study. *Am J Kid Dis.* 2005;46:529–536.

82. Zaffari D, Losekann A, Santos AF, Manfroi WC, Bittar AE, Keitel E, Souza VB, Costa M, Prates VC, Kroth L, Braun ML. Effectiveness of diet in hyperlipidemia in renal transplant patients. *Transplant Proc.* 2004;35:889–890.

83. Vorlat A, Conraads VM, Vrints CJ. Regular use of margarine-containing stanol/sterol esters reduces total and low-density lipoprotein (LDL) cholesterol and allows reduction of statin therapy after cardiac transplantation: preliminary observations. *J Heart Lung Transplant.* 2003;22:1059–1062.

84. Keogh JB, Tsalamandris C, Sewell RB, Jones RM, Angus PW, Nyulasi IB, Seeman E. Bone loss at the proximal femur and reduced lean mass following liver transplantation: a longitudinal study. *Nutrition.* 1999;15:661–664.

85. Leidig-Bruckner G, Hosch S, Dodidou P, Ritschel D, Conradt C, Lose C, Otto G, Lange R, Theilmann L, Zimmerman R, Pritsch M, Ziegler R. Frequency and predictors of osteoporotic fractures after cardiac or liver transplantation: a follow-up study. *Lancet.* 2001;3:342–347.

86. Trautwein C, Possienke M, Schlitt H-J, et al. Bone density and metabolism in patients with viral hepatitis and cholestatic liver diseases before and after liver transplantation. *Am J Gastroenterol.* 2000;95:2343–2351.

87. Hay JE, Malinchoc M, Dickson ER. A controlled trial of calcitonin therapy for the prevention of post-liver transplantation atraumatic fractures in patients with primary biliary cirrhosis and primary sclerosing cholangitis. *J Hepatol.* 2001;34:292–298.

88. Isoniemi H, Appelberg J, Nilsson C-G, Mäkelä P, Risteli J, Höckerstedt K. Transdermal oestrogen therapy protects postmenopausal liver transplant women from osteoporosis. A 2-year follow-up study. *J Hepatol.* 2001;34:299–305.

89. Reeves HL, Francis RM, Manas DM, Hudson M, Day CP. Intravenous bisphosphonate prevents symptomatic osteoprortic vertebral collapse in patients after liver transplantation. *Liver Transpl Surg.* 1998;4:404–409.

90. Ninkovic M, Love S, Tom BDM, Bearcroft PWP, Alexander GJM, Compston JE. Lack of effect of intravenous pamidronate on fracture incidence and bone mineral density after orthotopic liver transplantation. *J Hepatol.*2002;37:93–100.

91. Hussaini SH, Oldroyd B, Stewart SP, Roman F, Smith MA, Pollard S, Lodge P, O'Grady JG, Losowsky MS. Regional bone mineral density after orthotopic liver transplantation. *Eur J Gastroenterol Hepatol.* 1999;11:157–163.

92. Ninkovic M, Skingle SJ, Bearcroft PWP, Bishop N, Alexander GJM, Compston JE. Incidence of vertebral fractures in the first three months after orthotopic liver transplantation. *Eur J Gastroenterol Hepatol.* 2000;12:931–935.

93. Hasse JM, Blue LS, Liepa GU, et al. Early enteral nutrition support in patients undergoing liver transplantation. *JPEN J Parenter Enteral Nutr.* 1995;19:437–443.

94. Rayes N, Seehofer D, Hansen S, et al. Early enteral supply of lactobacillus and fiber versus selective bowel decontamination: a controlled trial in liver transplant recipients. *Transplantation.* 2002;74:123–128.

95. Rayes N, Seehofer D, Theruvath T, et al. Supply of pre- and probiotics reduces bacterial infection rates after liver transplantation–A randomized, double-blind trial. *Am J Transplant.* 2005;5: 125–130.

96. Rovera GM, Graham TO, Hutson WR, et al. Nutritional management of intestinal allograft recipients (abstract). Presented at: Fifth International Symposium on Intestinal Transplantation; July 1997; Cambridge, UK.

97. Moore C, Chowdhury Z, Young JB. Heart transplant nutrition programs: a national survey. *J Heart & Lung Transplantation.* 1991;10:50–55.

98. Hasse JM, Chinnakotla S. Solid organ transplantation. In: Cresci G, ed. *Nutrition Support for the Critically Ill.* Boca Raton, FL: CRC Press. 2005:457–477.

99. Preiksaitis JK, Brennan DC, Fishman J, Allen U. Canadian Society of Transplantation Consensus Workshop on cytomegalovirus management in solid organ transplantation final report. *Am J Transplant.* 2005;8:218–227.

100. Rao VK. Posttransplant medical complications. *Surg Clin North Am.* 1998;78:113–132.

101. Venkatesan P, Perfect JR, Myers SA. Evaluation and management of fungal infections in immunocompromised patients. *Derm Therapy.* 2005;18:44–57.

102. Hodson EM, Jones CA, Webster AC, Strippoli GFM, Barclay PG, Kable K, Vimalachandra D, Craig JC. Antiviral medications to prevent cytomegalovirus disease and early death in recipients of solid-organ transplants: a systematic review of randomised controlled trials. *Lancet.* 2005; 365:2105–2115.

103. Ponticelli C, Passerini P. Gastrointestinal complications in renal transplant recipients. *Transplant Int.* 2005;18:643–650.

104. Rovera GM, Schoen RE, Goldbach B, Janson D, Bond G, Rakela J, Graham TO, O'Keefe S, Abu-Elmagd K. Intestinal and multivisceral transplantation: dynamics of nutritional management and functional autonomy. *JPEN J Parenter Enteral Nutr.* 2003;27:252–259.

105. Thomas MC, Moran J, Mathew TH, Russ GR, Rao MM. Early peri-operative hyperglycaemia and renal allograft rejection in patients without diabetes. *BMC Nephrology.* 2000;1:1.

106. Thomas MC. Mathew TH, Russ GR, Rao MM, Moran J. Early peri-operative glycaemic control and allograft rejection in patients with diabetes mellitus: a pilot study. *Transplantation.* 2001;72: 1321–1324.

CHAPTER 11

Inflammatory Bowel Disease

Peter Beyer, MS, RD

INTRODUCTION

Inflammatory bowel disease (IBD) typically refers to two primary forms of chronic, relapsing inflammatory disease of the gastrointestinal tract, Crohn's disease (CD), and ulcerative colitis (UC). Each manifests varying degrees of activity and severity, and each commonly requires surgery during its course. Inflammatory bowel disease can significantly compromise nutrition, overall health, and quality of life. Diet and nutrition play important roles in the underlying pathology as well as in the overall management of the disease. Recent studies imply that IBD is more heterogeneous than originally thought, although the division of IBD into two major types is justifiable. Each form may present with different clinical manifestations and treatment requirements (1,2). The heterogeneity in genotype results in different disease presentation, location, and clinical course, and may help explain the disparity in effectiveness of medical, surgical, and nutritional interventions among populations and individuals.

OVERVIEW OF IBD

Incidence and Prevalence

The incidence of IBD in North America ranges from about four to seven new cases per 100,000 persons per year for CD and two to eleven cases for UC. Approximately 1 million Americans have IBD (3–5). Worldwide, incidence rates may vary from less than 2 to greater than 20 cases per 100,000 people (3,4). The incidence rates correspond to a lifetime risk for either one of the two diseases of between 0.5% and 1% (4). The prevalence (i.e., the number of existing cases per 100,000 persons) of IBD in North America depends on the region surveyed. Prevalence of UC ranges from approximately 40 to 250 cases per 100,000 persons, and for CD, about 30 to 200 cases per 100,000 (3). Although IBD is still relatively uncommon, health care professionals may frequently encounter persons with symptoms and complications related to the disease.

Complications

Symptoms attributed to both CD and UC include anorexia, growth failure, weight loss, fatigue, various anemias, fever, diarrhea, several forms of gastrointestinal (GI) distress, frequent reports of food intolerances, increased risk of cancer, systemic inflammatory manifestations, and the eventual likelihood of surgery (1,2,5,6). Although individuals with UC may suffer significant morbidity, including malnutrition, those with CD are at greater lifetime risk for fistulas, mucosal thickening, strictures and small bowel obstruction, small bowel resections, malabsorption, and macro- and micronutrient malnutrition (see Table 11–1 through Table11–3).

Table 11–1 Complications of CD *and* UC

- Weight loss, growth failure, fatigue
- Diarrhea
- Crampy abdominal pain
- Fever
- Various anemias related to blood loss and nutrient inadequacies/losses
- Increased risk of malignancy
- Presence of extraintestinal manifestations involving joints, eyes, skin
- Surgery likely (during a lifetime)

Table 11–2 Characteristics Typical of Crohn's Disease

- May occur in any area of the GI tract
- Most commonly involves the distal small bowel and colon
- Areas of normal bowel are adjacent to diseased segments
- Typically transmural rather than mucosal involvement
- 70% of patients undergo surgery that does not guarantee a cure
- Strictures, partially obstructed segments more common
- Abscesses, sinus tracts, fistulas not uncommon

Table 11–3 Characteristics Typical of Ulcerative Colitis

- Confined to colon
- Disease continuous throughout bowel, typically involving rectum
- Typically mucosal rather than transmural involvement
- GI bleeding more common than with CD
- Fistulas and strictures rare
- Ulcerations present on inflamed mucosa

Figure 11–1 depicts a low power view of active CD with transmural acute and chronic inflammation. Figure 11–2 illustrates multiple noncaseating granulomas, classically seen in CD. Figure 11–3 exhibits a low power view of UC, with marked acute and chronic inflammation limited to the mucosa with inflammatory polyp formation. Lastly, Figure 11–4 depicts a higher magnification of UC, highlighting cyptitis and crypt abscesses classically seen in the disease.

Etiology

Although the cause of IBD is not known, dysregulation of the mucosal immune system, inflammation, increased permeability, and autoimmune activity appear to be primary features. Each form of IBD appears to involve genetic mutations that increase the risk of abnormal interactions between the host GI mucosa immune system and the luminal environment. Several genes are likely involved in the susceptibility to CD. In 2001, mutations of a gene on Chromosome 16 known as nucleotide oligomerization domain (NOD2) were identified as risk factors for CD. This gene was later named caspase activating and recruitment domain protein 15

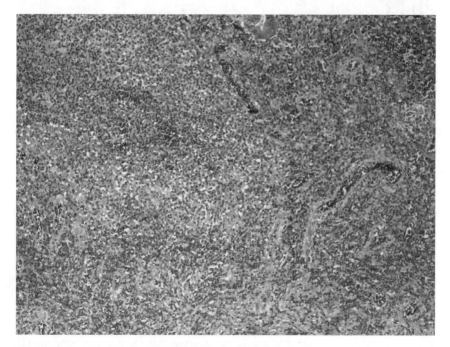

Figure 11–1 A Low Power View of Active Crohn's Disease

Source: Used with permission and courtesy of Ossam Tawfik, MD, Professor of Pathology, University of Kansas Medical Center.

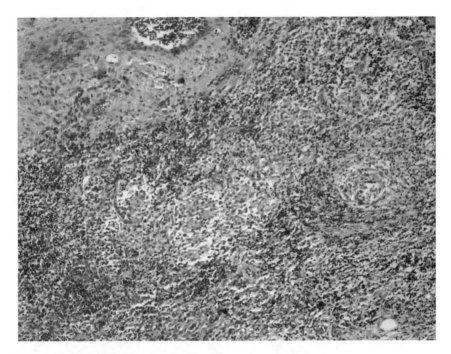

Figure 11–2 Multiple Noncaseating Granulomas

Source: Used with permission and courtesy of Ossam Tawfik, MD, Professor of Pathology, University of Kansas Medical Center.

(CARD15). Since that discovery, mutations in several other genes have been identified that result in abnormal recognition of luminal bacteria, activation of the immune response, membrane transport, and GI permeability (7,8,9).

Additional genetic links that may explain the differences in susceptibility, presenting symptoms, location, severity, progression, and response to treatments continue to be discovered. Environmentally, certain intestinal microbes or fragments of microbial cells have been the target of considerable scrutiny and appear to be the source of the inflammatory interaction with the host immune system (8,10,11).

In the normal individual, a remarkable coexistence develops between the host GI immune system and the contents of the GI lumen. The host's genome, the mucosal immune system, and physical barrier of the gut wall must provide a defense against invading pathogens without adversely affecting host tissues. Appropriate mechanisms must be in place to provide regulatory and anti-inflammatory mechanisms that allow tolerance to the 400 species of microorganisms that populate the GI lumen, plus the thousands of potential dietary antigens ingested over one's lifetime. The host's genetic profile, myriad dietary substances, the commensal microflora, intestinal pathogens, and the molecules and cell fragments produced from them can impact innate and adaptive immunity (12–15).

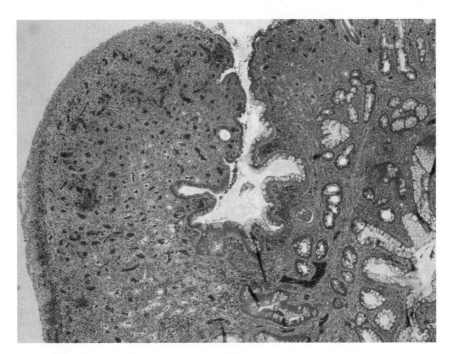

Figure 11–3 Low Power View of Ulcerate Colitis

Source: Used with permission and courtesy of Ossam Tawfik, MD, Professor of Pathology, University of Kansas Medical Center.

In addition to an abnormal immune response to enteric microflora, a number of environmental and endogenous triggers may be involved in the initiation of IBD, including microbial and viral pathogens, smoking (CD), increased hygiene, and diet (1,3,4,11). Diet may play a role in that the foods and nutrients consumed (or lacking) may alter the immune response, change the ratio of microbial species produced in the GI tract, serve as a source of microbes, serve as a source of antigens, or alter symptoms produced in the course of the disease.

Dietary factors that have been associated with the onset or prevalence of IBD include sugar and refined carbohydrates, meat, alcohol, certain dietary lipids, increased homocysteine levels, inorganic microparticles (e.g., abrasives in toothpaste, talc, silicates), and dietary antigens (16–20). Dietary factors considered protective against IBD include fruit and vegetable intake, dietary fiber intake, n-3 fatty acids, breast feeding, prebiotic foods, foods containing probiotic microorganisms, and adequate vitamin D, calcium, and folate intake. The dietary factors have been linked primarily by epidemiologic associations and a few case-controlled studies but in some cases by mechanistic evidence, cohort studies, or controlled trials. Evidence-based dietary factors and recommendations for management of IBD will be addressed later in the chapter.

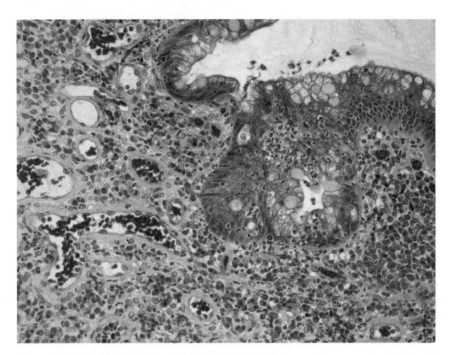

Figure 11–4 Higher Magnification of Ulcerative Colitis

Source: Used with permission and courtesy of Ossam Tawfik, MD, Professor of Pathology, University of Kansas Medical Center.

Treatment

The pathology of IBD involves an aberrant interaction between the host immune state, intestinal microflora, and the external environment (including components of the diet and tobacco). Treatment includes efforts to control the immune and inflammatory response, alter the microbial flora, change dietary practices, and, at least for CD, modify tobacco use. Medications, diet, and surgical interventions are used to manage symptoms and complications associated with the disease (5,6,11,21,22).

Medical management includes attenuating the primary immune response and inducing remission, treating complications, and preventing exacerbations. Medications generally fall in the categories of anti-inflammatory, immunosuppressive, and/or antibiotics. Newer categories include drugs designed to block specific inflammatory cytokines or enhance those that suppress acute phase reactions (see Table 11–4). Antimotility and antisecretory agents may also be used to treat diarrhea and malabsorption.

Surgery is generally reserved for patients with medically refractory, fulminant UC or CD, severe complications, or evidence of cancer.

Table 11–4 Medical Management of IBD

- Anti-inflammatory drugs: corticosteroids, sulfasalazine, 5-ASA
- Immune modulators or suppressants: 6-mercaptopurine, cyclosporine, methotrexate, azothioprine
- Antibiotics: e.g., metronidazole ciprofloxacin
- Monoclonal antibody to tumor necrosis factor alpha
- Recombinant human interleukin 10, 11

DISEASE MANAGEMENT

Ulcerative Colitis

In UC, surgery decreases the long-term risk of cancer and abolishes the disease. The timing for surgery is based on indicators of the severity of disease, presence of complications such as profuse bleeding, unrelenting diarrhea, perforation, toxic megacolon, or evidence of premalignant lesions. In emergent cases, it may save the patient's life. About 20% of patients with UC have surgery in their lifetime (1). When a colectomy is performed, surgical management options that are considered include creation of a traditional ileostomy, an ileoanal anastomosis, or several versions of pouches formed from segments of ileum to serve as fecal reservoirs.

Crohn's Disease

Surgery does not abolish CD. About 40%–80% of patients with CD ultimately have surgery, and those who undergo surgery typically have at least one subsequent surgical procedure (1,21,22) Surgical procedures for CD may be significantly more diverse and include repair of strictures, removal of obstructed or dysfunctional segments, drainage of abscesses, and repair of fistulas. Resections of severely diseased segments of bowel can be significant in some cases, and CD has become a primary cause of short bowel syndrome (SBS) in adults.

Nutrition and Diet

Nutrition and diet are vitally important in all stages of IBD. Patients are at increased risk for overall and specific forms of malnutrition. The presenting symptoms of IBD (e.g., bloating, obstruction, abdominal pain, diarrhea, fistulas) can limit both the quantity and types of foods consumed and even the desire to eat. Malnutrition may further compromise the health of the patient by increasing the number of complications and the duration and intensity of required treatment.

Patients are often confused or frustrated about the information provided regarding the role of foods, diets, and dietary supplements in the management of IBD. Questions about diet are among the most common topics in hospital and clinic visits, support groups, and Internet chat rooms. The information offered regarding special foods, diets, and supplements may be contradictory, unsound, or not sufficiently tailored to individual situations. Patients may present with a tremendous range of past medical, surgical, and nutrition profiles; therefore, nutrition care must be tailored to individual needs.

New information provides clues that diet may be related to the course and underlying pathology of the disease. Dietary factors may exacerbate or attenuate the inflammatory response by modifying the enteric microflora or its relationship with the host; altering the expression of cytokines, adhesion molecules, eicosanoids, and reducing oxidative stress; and altering GI permeability and mucosal barrier functions. Most of the time, individuals with IBD lead active, productive lives and strive to maintain their health and avoid unnecessary medical and surgical interventions. Good nutrition care may reduce the risks associated with surgery, shorten recovery time, decrease complications and symptoms related to the disease, and increase the patient's satisfaction and confidence with health care team members.

Risk of Malnutrition

Macronutrient (protein, lipids, fluid, and energy) and micronutrient (vitamins, minerals, trace elements, and electrolytes) deficiencies are common in IBD (6,23–26). Malnutrition may result from poor dietary intake due to food intolerance(s) and/or to the abnormal metabolic state resulting from the inflammatory process. The overall quality of the dietary intake in the United States is poor, and a diagnosis of IBD may further limit intake and worsen nutritional status. Patients may eliminate entire categories of foods (e.g., dairy products, fruits, vegetables, and whole grains) as a result of perceived food intolerance, and/or advice from health professionals, the media, or well-intentioned associates.

The inflammatory response from any physiologic stressor contributes to anorexia. Significant food associations and aversions may develop during acute stages of illness, with elimination of favorite foods. Self-appointed food faddists may steer patients to diet regimens that are more austere than necessary or are completely contraindicated. Maldigestion or malabsorption resulting from the disease state plus surgical resections or drug-nutrient interactions can further contribute to malnutrition (see Table 11–5).

Nutrition Assessment

Nutrition assessment serves several functions. It identifies the degree of nutrition risk, provides the evidence for the nutrition diagnoses, identifies the need for further evaluation, and finally, provides justification for appropriate nutrition interventions. Key components in a nutrition assessment include qualitative and quantitative review of the patient's diet history, medical and surgical history, and appropriate laboratory/biochemical, physical, and psychosocial data (see Table 11–6).

Table 11–5 Factors Leading to Poor Intake and Risk for Malnutrition

- Disease symptoms—pain, nausea, bloating, diarrhea
- Anorexia from disease, cytokines
- Malabsorption (resections, inflammation)
- Dietary limitations (iatrogenic and self-imposed)
- Food intolerances, associations made with symptoms
- Fear of eating/symptoms
- Drug-nutrient interactions

Dietary Intake

The dietary assessment typically includes an estimate of how well (or poorly) the patient has eaten during a defined period. An estimate of the quality and quantity of the patient's diet can be made using a food frequency tool. The tool can assist with identification of degree of malnutrition and of foods that may be affecting symptoms. Foods and nutrients of special interest (lipid, fiber, protein, energy, sugars, caffeine, dietary supplements, and dairy products) can be listed in boxes for easy completion and review. Assessment of patients' perceptions and concerns regarding food intake, the role of nutrition, food aversions, and intolerances is also appropriate at this stage.

Physical Exam, Signs, and Symptoms

Nutritional physical assessment and the notation of signs and symptoms that may be related to diet or affect dietary management are a crucial part of nutrition assessment. Anthropometric measures such as weight history, weight changes over

Table 11–6 Elements of Nutrition Assessment

- Dietary quality and quantity, and duration of dietary patterns
- Anthropometric/body composition/physical exam
- Location, severity and duration of disease of surgical resections, strictures, obstructions
- Medications with nutrition implications including over the counter medications and supplements
- Hydration status, fluid intake and output
- Laboratory indicators of severity of disease
- Knowledge of disease, nutritional implications, options, guidelines, and mechanisms
- Psychosocial status, e.g., resources, support systems, degree of self-sufficiency

time, BMI (body mass index), skinfold thickness, and arm muscle circumference may give reasonable estimates of energy balance and lean and fat mass. Dual energy absorptiometry (DEXA) provides a good assessment of fat and lean mass and of bone density. Presence of physical features consistent with energy and protein wasting, dehydration, loss of physical strength, or pallor aid in confirmation of other observations in the assessment. Assessment of each measure should include the degree to which the observation departs from the normal range. Descriptions of the severity and duration of complaints such as bloating, distention, nausea, vomiting, diarrhea, and anorexia help in determining the reason for nutrition problems and predicting the route of nutrition intervention. Presence and location of fistulae, ostomies, and of enteral nutrition (EN) and parenteral nutrition (PN) administration sites and access devices should be documented.

Medical and Surgical History

The clinician should collect data about the location, severity, duration of disease; location and presence of narrowed or strictured bowel; presence of nutrition-related comorbidities such as diabetes; use of medications that have implications for diet/nutrition such as steroids, broad spectrum antibiotics, antimotility or antidiarrheal agents; and presence of gastrointestinal resections, pouches, or roux limbs.

Appropriate biochemical indicators (levels of cytokines and acute phase proteins, and changes in white blood cell count) may reflect the severity of inflammation, disease, or its complications. As appropriate (e.g., with significant malabsorption, diarrhea, or poor dietary intake), laboratory tests may be ordered to detect common nutrition problems such as anemia (iron, folate, B_{12}), altered serum electrolytes and hydration status, and status of specific micronutrients (e.g., magnesium, phosphorus, and zinc).

NUTRITION IN THE MANAGEMENT OF IBD

Perioperative Nutrition

Many of the complications associated with IBD increase the risk of vitamin-mineral malnutrition, protein-calorie malnutrition, and significant fluid and electrolyte deficits. Abdominal pain, diarrhea, strictures, obstructions, bloating, cramping, maldigestion, malabsorption, diarrhea, steatorrhea, blood, and protein loss may result in poor intake and/or increased losses of nutrients and fluid. Net fluid needs may exceed several liters per day as a result of diarrhea, steatorrhea, vomiting, and/or fistula output.

At the least, appropriate fluid and electrolyte replacement should be provided. To the degree possible, macro- and micronutrient deficits should be restored before surgery. Whether and what to feed preoperatively in patients with IBD may be somewhat more complicated than with other surgical candidates. If the patient cannot eat and the GI tract is working sufficiently, then EN is preferred to PN in most situations. If the patient is malnourished and the GI tract is not sufficiently functional or is obstructed, PN may be warranted. Evidence suggests that perioperative nutrition support in malnourished patients is beneficial in terms of fewer complications, fewer hospital days, less patient discomfort, and lower overall costs (26–33).

Parenteral Nutrition

PN was once considered a routine or even primary treatment for IBD because it was thought to rest the gut would be beneficial while other therapeutic interventions were provided. Although the use of PN has resulted in attenuation of symptoms or remission of clinical features of IBD in some cases, it is not considered to be as effective as corticosteroids, does not induce permanent remission of the disease, and may not be as effective as EN when the GI tract can be used (6,34–38). The roles of PN are limited to restorative and supportive functions, in defined circumstances.

PN is generally indicated as a means of providing nutrition restoration and maintenance when it is known or anticipated that oral nutrition or EN cannot meet the patient's needs. Examples include patients with high-output fistulas in the proximal to mid small bowel, GI obstruction, unrelenting disease requiring fluid and nutrition resuscitation, and short bowel syndrome refractory to administration of EN. Because patients with IBD may be significantly depleted, they may develop refeeding syndrome. Because practitioners may be anxious to restore nutrition status or growth, overfeeding may also be a temptation (39). Especially during initiation of PN, close attention to markers of homeostasis (e.g., serum phosphorus, potassium, magnesium, blood sugar, pCO_2, respiratory quotient, and hydration) are warranted. Energy goals for adults may range from 15–25 calories per kilogram body weight initially in depleted patients to 30–35 kcal per kilogram for restoration of body mass. Children require much more, adjusted to age and requirement for growth. Protein requirements typically range from 1.0 to 1.5 grams per kilogram of body weight. Rarely, such as in cases of protein-losing enteropathies, larger amounts of protein may be needed.

Enteral Nutrition

EN was initially provided to IBD patients for sustenance or preoperative restoration of nutritional status. However, it was noted that indicators of the severity of illness seemed to abate in many of the patients with CD treated with elemental diets (40). Whether, and the degree to which, EN is considered a treatment for IBD has continued to be evaluated (6,24–26,37,41–49). In some parts of the world, EN is considered a primary form of therapy for IBD, especially for children with CD (6,24,44). Results of several pooled studies show response rates ranging from 50% to 75% of patients compared to approximately 85% response rate to corticosteroids.

Although response rates from EN are not as great as with corticosteroids and a 60%–70% relapse is noted within 12 months of resumption of a normal diet, the side effects of steroids and other medical and surgical interventions are avoided or delayed and nutritional status improves (6,17,24–26). In children, restoration of growth and bone mineralization may occur. In several of the trials, different enteral formulations were reported to improve symptoms, reduce gastrointestinal permeability, decrease biomarkers of inflammation, and in some cases, result in endoscopic evidence of mucosal healing (41–49). Many of the enteral formulations are considered elemental or semielemental, meaning that protein is provided in the form of amino acids or peptides and carbohydrate is provided in oligosaccharides. From an immunologic standpoint, avoidance of intact proteins and large peptides may have a theoretical advantage. However, some polymeric diets have been shown to be effective in management of IBD. Patients with IBD may suffer some degree of malabsorption due to bowel resections and the inflammatory state, but rarely are unable to digest proteins.

The reasons why certain defined enteral formulations may be effective in some IBD patients is not completely explained. Possibilities include:

1. *To replace nutrients and restore normal immunologic and protective functions.* One of the most valuable and rarely disputed justifications for EN is to restore nutrition and prevent weight loss when foods cannot. Patients' nutrition intake may have been inadequate in a number of nutrients and insufficient in quantity for the many reasons mentioned previously. EN might provide energy, protein, and/or missing micronutrients to not only restore basic needs, but also correct the host's normal immune and regulatory functions and repair physiologic barriers of the gastrointestinal tract (6,7,13,15, 20,47,48). The formulations contain simple carbohydrates, are lactose free, and contain no polyols. Some contain dietary fiber.

2. *To reduce antigenic load from food and microbes.* A normal diet, even one that is clean, still provides a tremendous number of potential antigens in the form of proteins, peptides, and a wide variety of microorganisms that may remain in or on foods. In contrast to the thousands of different foods consumed in a normal diet, an enteral formula normally contains only one or two sources protein, carbohydrates, and fats, and the diets are essentially sterile.

   Although little information is available regarding ability of EN to change host microflora to a less toxic milieu, it has been mentioned as a possible explanation for the improved tolerance to EN compared to normal diets (6,17–20).

3. *To provide food in a form that can be easily consumed.* Liquid diets are not likely to cause obstruction, and if introduced at reasonable rates, are normally well tolerated.

4. *To provide therapeutic nutraceuticals and conditional nutrients.* Some of the products may be in elemental (amino acids or small peptides) form, while

some may contain a source of fiber, and/or or additional nutraceutical or conditional elements such as glutamine, arginine, antioxidants, and/or n-3 fatty acids. Although there are theoretical and mechanistic advantages for those that are low in fat and contain n-3 fatty acids, distinctions in the effectiveness of the products are not always clear (6,7,12,41).

The specific formula and route of administration should be based on the age and status of the patient. For example, EN may be infused initially at 15–25 mL per hour in diluted fashion to restore enteric function during transition from PN or to stimulate enteral growth after significant bowel resections. EN can be advanced as appropriate to provide adequate fluid, electrolytes, energy, and protein. Supplemental micronutrients, electrolytes, and fluid may be needed, depending on the nutrition history of the patient and whether digestive and absorptive functions have been compromised. Adults may eventually need 30–35 kcal and 1–2 grams protein per kilogram body weight; children need more for growth, depending on age and weight history. In general, during restoration, normal age-specific energy and protein requirements for children can be used and adjusted as needed.

Use of EN requires considerable commitment from patients and providers. The products generally must be consumed as the exclusive source of nutrition, and favorite foods, even those considered by the patients as well tolerated and innocuous, must be eliminated. Often, tube feeding is the most effective manner to deliver EN. Elemental enteral formulations can be used at the patient's home but typically must be used for 4–8 weeks. Noncompliance is a significant concern. Return to usual food intake often results in return of symptoms and markers of disease.

OTHER DIETARY FACTORS AS POTENTIAL THERAPEUTIC TOOLS

Dietary Lipids

For the last 2 decades, the predominant form of polyunsaturated fats in the western diet has been n-6 fatty acids in the form of oils such as corn, safflower, and cottonseed. Consumed in considerably smaller amounts are n-3 fatty acids. The western diet contains a high ratio of n-6 fatty acids to n-3 fatty acids. According to dietary surveillance data, (78) Americans are consuming at least sufficient amounts of the dietary references intake(s) (DRI) for linoleic acid, the predominant dietary n-6 fatty acid, but relatively less of the n-3 fatty acids (50,51). Although no DRI has been established for other n-3 fatty acids including eicosapentaenoic acid (EPA) and docosahexaenoic acid (DHA), their consumption is equally important. Omega-3 fatty acids play an important role in the modulation of the inflammatory response, which has attracted substantial attraction for the potential of playing a therapeutic role in the management of IBD. Eicosanoids produced from n-6 fatty acids are generally proinflammatory. They stimulate production and chemotaxis of white cells, stimulate the production of acute phase proteins, increase platelet aggregation, stimulate secretion of proinflammatory cytokines, increase vascular permeability, and increase the thrombotic potential. Omega-3 fatty acids, on the other hand, tend to be anti-inflammatory (see Table 11–7). In animal studies and in some human trials, n-3 fatty acids have been shown to inhibit the production of n-6 eicosanoids, decrease the production of certain proinflammatory cytokines, decrease chemotaxis, and decrease platelet aggregation (52–54).

Clinical studies in which n-3 fatty acids were added to the diets of patients with inflammatory bowel disease are encouraging but somewhat conflicting (52,55). Even in studies reporting positive results, the outcomes are seldom dramatic when n-3 supplements were used as a single clinical intervention. Summaries of the trials investigating the impact of supplemental n-3 fatty acids in animal models of inflammatory bowel disease and some human studies have suggested a positive effect, especially when the diet is relatively low in total fat or low in n-6 fatty acids. Examples of reported benefits include lowered proinflammatory cytokine levels, decreased acute phase proteins, improved (decreased) GI permeability, and prolonged remissive states. Reviewers cite differences in doses (1–8 grams daily) and form in which the lipid is fed (linolenic acid or combinations of DHA and EPA, and/or mixed fish oils, enteric coated, with or without antioxidant) as possible variables in response rates (52–56). The role of n-3 fatty acids is likely to be complementary rather than primary.

Table 11–7 Omega-6 Versus Omega-3 Fatty Acids

n-6 fatty acids
- Predominate in western diet
- Result in eicosanoids which are primarily proinflammatory, increase leukocyte adhesion and migration
- Indirectly increases production of, and potentiates inflammatory cytokines, proteolytic enzymes, and oxygen radicals
- Subject to peroxidation

n-3 fatty acids
- Intake is generally marginal in typical western diet
- Low-fat intake decreases likelihood of adequate consumption
- Eicosanoids produce less inflammation
- Decrease platelet aggregation and adhesion
- Even more labile to peroxidation
- Have been tried in various forms in patients with IBD with varying degrees of success
- Some forms taste "fishy"

PROBIOTICS

The term *probiotics* refers to live microbial populations that confer beneficial health effects to the host. Probiotics may serve to replace, reduce, or compete with the harmful bacteria. The issue is to identify the most effective probiotic bacteria that will result in a more favorable relationship with other microbes and the host's immune mechanisms.

The underlying cause of CD, UC, and probably pouchitis appears to be dysregulation of the normal immune response to commensal enteric bacteria in genetically predisposed individuals (7,18,19,57,58). Efforts to use selected antibiotics to reduce bacterial counts and use pro- and prebiotics to change and maintain a different milieu make at least theoretical sense. There are, however, hundreds of resident species of microbes in the GI tract and other transients are ingested; identification of the offending microbe(s) or the antigens they produce is difficult.

Several probiotics, at least in some patients, show evidence of tempering the disease and delaying or preventing relapse. Because of the tremendous numbers and concentrations of microbial species in the GI tract, the heterogeneity of IBD, the individual patient's genome, and the relationships created with established and transient microbial populations, it is not likely that a single strain will be successful for either disease or for every patient. More likely, different combinations of strains will be applied and eventually be tailored to the type of disease (57–59).

In general, the use of probiotics has yielded mixed results in reducing symptoms, severity of disease indicators, and prolonging remission. The most positive applications appear to be with treatment of pouchitis with VSL-3, a mixture of eight probiotics and prebiotics, and S boulardii, VSL No. 3, and *E coli* Nissle 1917 in the management of CD and UC (57–60). Typically, patients are treated with antibiotics, with or without probiotics, and occasionally with prebiotic supplements as well. Although they are good sources of many nutrients and should be well tolerated by persons with IBD, commonly used commercial yogurts may not normally have sufficient concentrations of therapeutic cultures to escape the effects of gastric acid, digestive enzymes, and bile.

Another recent application for probiotics (often combined with prebiotics) is to prevent or treat antibiotic associated diarrhea (e.g., due to *Clostridium difficile*), prevent growth of opportunistic organisms, and treat/prevent small bowel microbial overgrowth. Accumulating evidence shows potential for several products but not all have been positive. The prebiotics used to prevent antibiotic-associated diarrhea may not be effective for primary treatment of IBD.

PREBIOTICS

Prebiotics are fermentable forms of dietary fiber and starches resistant to digestion in the proximal GI tract. Consumption of a diet rich in prebiotic material results in a more acid milieu that favors the growth and maintenance of lactic acid bacteria (e.g., lactobacillus and bifidobacterium). The resultant microflora may be more stable and protect against the proliferation of organisms that may contribute to the inflammatory process. Research supports the use of prebiotics in the prevention of some forms of opportunistic infections. Many commercial enteral products now contain at least one source of prebiotic fiber. Studies in animal models and some human studies of IBD and pouchitis have demonstrated that consumption of pre-biotics may result in increased decreased pH, increased butyrate, decreased indi-cators of inflammation, decreased volume of diarrhea, prolonged remissive states, and altered relationship with the host immune mechanisms (57,61–63). Additional study is needed to identify the types, amounts of prebiotics that may best provide protection of flora, how they interface with probiotics (as synbiotics), and in what form(s) they should be consumed (e.g., as supplement combinations, whole food-stuffs, or in other forms). Sources of prebiotic material include fruits, vegetables, legumes, nuts, and seeds. Examples of foods or specific oligosaccharides from those foods that have been used in IBD trials include inulin, fructooligosaccharides, psyllium, chicory, banana flakes, oats, plantago ovata, soy polysaccharide, germi-nated barley, and mixtures of foodstuffs. See Table 11–8 for further information.

MANAGEMENT OF LONG-TERM NUTRITION-RELATED COMPLICATIONS

Nutrition is involved in many aspects of IBD and its surgical interventions. Nutri-tional status and dietary selections can significantly impact the symptoms and qual-ity of life related to the disease and its treatment.

Anemia

Patients with IBD may suffer from several types of anemia, related to blood loss, poor intake of nutrients, malabsorption, or microbial use (25,26) Microcytic anemia is likely due to blood loss but inadequate intake or poor tolerance to iron-containing foods may contribute. Premenopausal females and children are at greater risk. Oral iron supplements are tolerated in most individuals but in refractory cases intra-venous iron and/or erythropoietin may be necessary (26,27,64–66).

Table 11–8 Prebiotics

- Carbohydrate polymers that are not digested or completely digested but are fermented to varying degrees to short chain fatty acids and gases
- Examples include fructooligosaccharides, inulin, pectin, gums, resistant starch
- Reduce toxicity of many drugs
- May change the type/ratios of microorganisms in the colon to a more protective state
- Have been shown to prevent overgrowth of opportunistic microbes

Folate intake is inadequate in a large segment of the U.S. population. Fresh fruits and vegetables are often restricted by patients with IBD. Medications (e.g., sulfasalazine, methotrexate) may also increase the need for folate. Vitamin B_{12} deficiency may result from inadequate intake, increased utilization by intestinal microbes, and/or inadequate utilization because of loss or dysfunction of ileal sites for absorption of intrinsic factor/B_{12} (66).

Evaluation of anemias should include dietary intake of iron, folate, and vitamin B_{12}; serum hemoglobin and hematocrit, mean corpuscular volume, mean corpuscular hemoglobin, red cell folate, and serum B_{12} levels; the status of the terminal ileum; and the use of any medications with interactions with the nutrients listed. Higher homocysteine levels have been noted in adult and pediatric patients with IBD. Inadequate B_{12} and/or folate intake may contribute to the hyperthrombinemia often seen in IBD. For restoration and maintenance, appropriate oral supplements are appropriate. In cases of malabsorption or maldigestion, or if the GI tract cannot be used, intramuscular or parenteral nutrient administration may be needed.

The complications and therapeutic interventions associated with IBD increases the risk for several forms of malnutrition. Nutrition and diet may play a number of roles in the presenting complications and symptoms, the resolution, and perhaps even the underlying causes of IBD. In the future, dietary and medical interventions may be better tailored toward the individual patient based on the subject's age genome, as well as the presentation, duration, and location of the disease and genome.

Diarrhea

Diarrhea may be secretory (related to GI infection or the inflammatory state), osmotic (from overconsumption of small molecular weight carbohydrates), or functional (due to inadequate bowel absorptive capacity/surface area). During acute exacerbations of IBD, fluid output may exceed 2 or more liters daily for several days. Appropriate fluid and electrolyte replacement should be initiated. Standard oral rehydration solutions recommended by the World Health Organization (WHO) and the American Academy of Pediatrics (AAP) contain 2% glucose (20 g/L), 45 to 90 mEq/L of sodium, 20 mEq/L of potassium, and a citrate base (see Table 11–9). Although newer, reduced osmolarity (130 to 200 mOsm/L) solutions might be preferred in some forms of diarrhea in children, they may not resolve hyponatremia (67,68). Patients with severe diarrhea, malabsorption, and short bowel syndrome may require 200 mm or more of sodium daily.

Commercial solutions (sold under brand names such as Pedialyte, Infalyte, Lytren, Equalyte, and Rehydralyte) typically contain less glucose and slightly less salt and are available in pharmacies, some without prescription. Standard sports drinks may not provide sufficient amounts or ratios of electrolytes and should not be used as replacements for oral rehydration fluids or tailored therapy. Fluid and electrolyte intake, output, and hydration status should be carefully assessed and subsequently monitored for several days after resolution of the underlying problems.

Table 11–9 Composition of Oral Rehydration Solutions (ORS)

Composition	WHO Formulation	Pedialyte	CereLyte90	Rehydralyte	Equalyte	Sport Drink (Typical)
Sodium (mm/L)	90	45	90	75	78	4–20
Potassium (mm/L)	20	20	20	20	22	3–4
Chloride (mm/l)	80	35	80	65	68	NA
Bicarbonate (mm/L)	30	20	—	—	—	NA
Citrate (mm/L)	—	10	30	30	30	NA
Carbohydrate (g/L)	20	25	40	25	25	45–80

With osmotic diarrhea, as in short bowel syndrome, reduction of total dietary sugars, especially those that are poorly digested or absorbed (lactose, fructose, and the alcohol/polyol sugars sorbitol, mannitol, and xylitol) is appropriate (69,70). With short bowel syndrome, rapid GI transit and small intestinal bacterial contamination, even sucrose may be poorly tolerated.

Obstruction/Partial Obstruction, Dysmotility, Small Bowel Bacterial Overgrowth

One of the complications of IBD is narrowed, scarred, strictured, or otherwise dysfunctional segments of small bowel. The particle size of dietary fiber or consumption of fiber supplements in bolus form is of concern in the presence of these issues. Dietary fiber is not significantly digested in the upper GI tract and the size of particles consumed may still be large enough to impede or partially obstruct the GI tract at the narrowed or dysfunctional sites. Complete restriction of dietary fiber is not necessarily required, but particle size may need to be limited. In early studies of the effects of fiber on GI function, it was shown that healthy, young subjects with good dentition passed relatively intact and recognizable hulls of corn and peas, segments of potato skins several centimeters in diameter, and pieces of peanuts a centimeter in length (71). Patients with suspected narrowing and strictures and at least partial obstruction should chew foods well and consume fibrous foods in very small particles or in blended form until the potential for obstruction is resolved.

Small intestinal bacterial overgrowth occurs more commonly in patients with strictures, partial obstruction, surgically created loops, segments of bowel with dysmotility, and in patients who take gastric acid suppressive agents (72–75).

Small bowel bacterial contamination occurs more commonly with dysfunction or loss of the ileocecal valve. Patients may experience postprandial bloating, increased gas, and subsequent loose stools or diarrhea, especially after consumption of refined carbohydrates or sugars, notably polyols. Sucrose or high-fructose corn syrup may also contribute to symptoms. Opportunistic organisms may ferment unabsorbed carbohydrates resulting in increased production of gases, higher concentrations of organic acids, and more acidic luminal contents. Small bowel bacterial overgrowth may increase degradation of conjugated bile acids, which, in turn, results in decreased lipid and fat soluble nutrient absorption. Small intestinal bacterial overgrowth may also increase the microbial use of vitamin B_{12} and lead to deficiencies (72–75). Treatment may include nonabsorbable antibiotics, probiotics, and prebiotics.

Osteoporosis

Osteoporosis is relatively common in persons with IBD. Risk factors for osteoporosis and fractures include activity, severity and duration of disease, use of corticosteroids, underweight, weight loss, bowel resection, malabsorption, and insufficient intake/utilization of nutrients associated with bone metabolism. Intake and utilization of vitamin D, calcium, vitamin K, magnesium, and zinc have been associated with decreased bone mineral density in IBD. Nutrition treatment and prevention include maintaining/replacing nutrient stores using oral or parenteral supplements as indicated. Bisphosphonate medications and appropriate hormone therapy may be required (76–78).

MAINTENANCE DIET AND NUTRITION

The diet of Americans is marginal in a number of nutrients valuable not only for maintaining normal nutrition status and health but also for possible protection against common symptoms and the underlying pathology of IBD. Intake of calcium, magnesium, potassium, folate, vitamin A, and vitamin D are less than adequate for a large percent of the U.S. population despite the availability of healthy foods (50,79).

Individuals with IBD are at greater risk for nutrient deficiencies as a result of increased nutritional requirements, decreased nutrient absorption, and drug-nutrient interactions. Although the relationships between dietary factors and IBD may not be causal, there are sufficient data to suggest that poor dietary practices can worsen symptoms and that proper diet can at least attenuate some of the presenting features. Most of the same dietary recommendations made for prevention of heart disease, hypertension, osteoporosis, diabetes, and cancers would also be appropriate for maintaining good health for an individual with IBD. Health care practitioners should encourage patients to practice lifelong health maintenance through good nutrition. Diets rich in fruits, vegetables, whole grains, legumes, and nuts contain a host of nutrients and phytochemicals that have antioxidant, anti-inflammatory, immunoregulatory, antithrombotic, and anticancer properties. Foods containing dietary fiber and resistant starches also serve as prebiotics and have been shown to favorably alter/stabilize microbial populations and to resist proliferation or establishment of pathogens and normalize bowel function. Whole foods offer the most complete nutrition but when appropriate and with sufficient evidence, dietary supplements and nutraceuticals may be added to the diet to maintain or improve nutritional status.

CONCLUSION

IBD increases the risk for a number of nutrition problems related to the symptoms and complications of the disease and to the nutritional effects of medications and surgical interventions. Nutrition and diet may play a number of roles in the presenting complications and symptoms, the resolution, and perhaps even the underlying causes of IBD. In the future, dietary and medical interventions may be better tailored toward the individual patient based on the subject's age; presentation, duration, and location of the disease; and genome.

REFERENCES

1. Bamias G, Giorgios MD, Nyce M, et al. New concepts in the pathophysiology of inflammatory bowl disease. *Ann Intern Med.* 2005;143:895–904.

2. Sand BE. From symptom to diagnosis: Clinical distinction among various forms of intestinal inflammation. *Gastroenterology.* 2004;126:1518–1532.

3. Loftus EV. Clinical epidemiology of inflammatory bowel disease: Incidence, prevalence, and environmental influences. *Gastroenterology.* 2004;126:1504–1517.

4. Ekbom A. The epidemiology of IBD: A lot of data but little knowledge. How shall we proceed? *Inflamm Bowel Dis.* 2004;10(suppl):32–34.

5. Crohn's Colitis Foundation of America. About Crohn's Disease. Available at: www.ccfa.org/info/about/crohns. Accessed October 22, 2006.

6. Kim SC, Perry GD. Inflammatory bowel diseases in pediatric and adolescent patients: Clinical, therapeutic, and psychosocial considerations. *Gastroenterology.* 2004;126:1550–1560.

7. MacDonald TT, DiSabatino A, Gordon JN. Immunopathogenesis of Crohn's disease. *JPEN.* 2005;29:118–125.

8. Ahmad T, Tamboli CP, Jewell D, et al. Clinical relevance of advances in genetics and pharmacogenetics of IBD. *Gastroenterology.* 2004;126:1533–1549.

9. Mathew CG, Lewis CM. Genetics of inflammatory bowel disease: Progress and prospects. *Human Molecular Genetics.* 2004;13:161–168.

10. Freeman HJ. Long-term clinical behavior of jejunoileal involvement in Crohn's disease. *Can J Gastro.* 2005;19:575–578.

11. Rook GW, Brunet LR. Microbes, immunoregulation, and the gut. *Gut.* 2005;54:317–320.

12. Seibold F. Food-induced immune response as origin of bowel disease? *Digestion.* 2005;71:251–260.

13. Tlaskalova-Hogenova H, Stepankova R, Kozakova H, et al. Commensal bacteria (normal microflora), mucosal immunity and chronic inflammatory and autoimmune diseases. *Immunology Letters.* 2004;93:97–108.

14. Gill HS, Guarner F. Probiotics and human health: A clinical perspective. *Postgrad Med J.* 2004;80:516–526.

15. Bourlioux P, Koletzko B, Guarner F, Braesco V. The intestine and its microflora are partners for the protection of the host: Report on the Danone Symposium, The Intelligent Intestine, held in Paris, June 14, 2002. *Am J Clin Nutr.* 2003;78:675–683.

16. Cashman KD, Shanahan F. Is nutrition an aetiological factor for inflammatory bowel disease? *Eur J Gastroenterology Hepatology.* 2003;6:607–613.

17. Cantorna MT, Zhu Y, Froicu M, Wittke A. Vitamin D status, 1,25-dihydroxyvitamin D3, and the immune system. *Am J Clin Nutr.* 2004;80:1717–1720.

18. Jowett SL, Seal SJ, Pearce MS, et al. Influence of dietary factors on the clinical course of ulcerative colitis: A prospective cohort study. *Gut.* 2004;53:1479–1484.

19. Danese S, Silvio MD, Sgambato A, et al. Homocysteine triggers mucosal microvascular activation in inflammatory bowel disease. *Am J Gastroenterology.* 2005;4:886–895.

20. Lomer MC, Hutchinson C, Volkert S, et al. Dietary sources of inorganic microparticles and their intake in healthy subjects and patients with Crohn's disease. *Br J Nutr.* 2004;9:947–955.

21. Krupnick AS, Morris JB. The long-term results of resection and multiple resections in Crohn's disease. *Semin Gastrointest Dis.* 2000;11:41–51.

22. Cima RR, Pemberton JH. Medical and surgical management of chronic ulcerative colitis. *Arch Surg.* 2005;140:300–310.

23. Goh J, O'Morain CA. Review article: Nutrition and adult inflammatory bowel disease. *Aliment Pharmacol Ther.* 2003;17:307–320.

24. Graham TO, Kandil HM. Nutritional factors in inflammatory bowel disease. *Gastroenterol Clin N Am.* 2002;31:203–218.

25. Campos FG, Waitzberg DL, Teixeira MG. Inflammatory bowel diseases. Principles of nutritional therapy. *Rev Hosp Clin.* 2002;57:187–198.

26. Young RJ, Vanderhoof JA. Nutrition in pediatric inflammatory bowel disease. *Nutrition.* 2000;16:78–80.

27. Sax HC. Immunonutrition and upper gastrointestinal surgery: What really matters. *Nutr Clin Pract.* 2005;20:540–543.

28. Nehra V, Swails W, Duerksen D, et al. Indications for total parenteral nutrition in the hospitalized patient: A prospective review of evolving practice. *J Nutr Biochem.* 1999;10:2–7.

29. Gabor S, Renner H, Matzi V, et al. Early enteral feeding compared with parenteral nutrition after oesophageal or oesophagogastric resection and reconstruction. *Br J Nutr.* 2005;93:509–513.

30. Braga M, Gianotti L. Preoperative immunonutrition: Cost-benefit analysis. *JPEN.* 2005;29:57–61.

31. Gianotti L, Braga M, Nespoli L, et al. A randomized controlled trial of preoperative oral supplementation with a specialized diet in patients with gastrointestinal cancer. *Gastroenterology.* 2002;122:1763–1770.

32. Isabel M, Correi TD, Silva RG. The impact of early nutrition on metabolic response and postoperative ileus. *Curr Opinion Clin Nutr Metab Care.* 2004;7:577–583.

33. Jeejeebhoy KN. Permissive underfeeding of the critically ill patient. *Nutr Clin Pract.* 2004; 19:477–480.

34. Yao GX, Wang XR, Jiang ZM, et al. Role of perioperative parenteral nutrition in severely malnourished patients with Crohn's disease. *World J Gastro.* 2005;11:5732–5734.

35. American Gastroenterological Association medical position statement: Parenteral nutrition. *Gastroenterology.* 2001;121:966–969.

36. ASPEN Board of Directors. Standards for specialized nutrition support: Adult hospitalized patients. *Nutr Clin Pract.* 2002;17:384–391.

37. Dray X, Marteau P. The use of enteral nutrition in the management of Crohn's disease in adults. *JPEN*. 2005;29:166–172.

38. Mitsuru S. The role of total parenteral nutrition in the management of patients with acute attacks of inflammatory bowel disease. *J Clin Gastro*. 1999;29:270–275.

39. Kraft MD, Btaiche IF, Sacks GS. Review of the refeeding syndrome. *Nutr Clin Pract*. 2005; 20:625–633.

40. Votik AJ, et al. Experience with elemental diet in the treatment of inflammatory bowel disease. Is this primary therapy? *Arch Surg*. 1973;107:329–333.

41. Griffiths AM. Enteral nutrition in the management of Crohn's disease. *JPEN*. 2005;29:108–116.

42. Yamamoto T, Nakahigashi M, Umegae S, et al. Impact of elemental diet on mucosal inflammation in patients with active Crohn's disease: Cytokine production and endoscopic and histological findings. *Inflamm Bowel Dis*. 2005;11:580–588.

43. Knight C, El-Matary W, Spray C, et al. Long-term outcome of nutritional therapy in pediatric Crohn's disease. *Clin Nutr*. 2005;24:775–779.

44. Ogata H, Hibi T. Does an elemental diet affect operation and/or recurrence rate in Crohn's disease in Japan? *J Gastro*. 2003;38:1019–1021.

45. Verma S, Kirkwood B, Brown S, Giaffer MH. Oral nutritional supplementation is effective in the maintenance of remission in Crohn's disease. *Dig Liver Dis*. 2000;32:769–774.

46. Heuschkel RB, et al. Enteral nutrition and corticosteroids in the treatment of acute Crohn's disease in children. *J Pediatric Gastroenterol Nutr*. 2000;31:8–15.

47. Fell JM, Paintin M, Arnaud-Battandier F, et al. Mucosal healing and a fall in mucosal pro-inflammatory cytokine mRNA induced by a specific oral polymeric diet in paediatric Crohn's disease. *Aliment Pharmacol Ther*. 2000;14:281–290.

48. Sanderson IR, Croft NM. The anti-inflammatory effects of enteral nutrition. *JPEN*. 2005;29: 134–140.

49. Lionetti P, Callegari ML, Ferrari S, et al. Enteral nutrition and microflora in pediatric Crohn's disease. *JPEN*. 2005;29:173–178.

50. U.S. Department of Agriculture. Dietary guidelines for Americans 2005. Available at: www.health.gov/dietaryguidelines/dga2005/document/html/chapter2.htm. Accessed January 16, 2005.

51. Ervin RB, Wright JD, Wang CY, Kennedy-Stephenson J. Dietary intake of fats and fatty acids for the United States population: 1999–2000. Advance data from vital and health statistics; no 348. Hyattsville, Md.: National Center for Health Statistics; 2004.

52. Mills SC, Windsor AC, Knight SC. The potential interactions between polyunsaturated fatty acids and colonic inflammatory processes. *Clin Exp Immunol*. 2005;142:216–228.

53. Simopoulos AP. Omega-3 fatty acids in inflammation and autoimmune diseases. *J Amer Col Nutr*. 2002;21:495–505.

54. Gil A. Polyunsaturated fatty acids and inflammatory diseases. *Biomed Pharmacother*. 2002;56: 388–396.

55. MacLean CH, Mojica WA, Newberry SJ, et al. Systematic review of the effects of n-3 fatty acids in inflammatory bowel disease. *Am J Clin Nutr*. 2005;82:611–619.

56. Belluzzi A. Polyunsaturated fatty acids (n-3 PUFAs) and inflammatory bowel disease (IBD): Pathogenesis and treatment. *Eur Rev Med Pharmacol Sci*. 2004;8:225–229.

57. Sartor RB. Therapeutic manipulation of the enteric microflora in inflammatory bowel diseases: Antibiotics, probiotics and prebiotics. *Gastroenterology*. 2004;126:1620–1633.

58. Penner R, Fedorak RN, Madsen KL. Probiotics and nutraceuticals: Non-medical treatment of gastrointestinal diseases. *Curr Opin Pharmacol*. 2005;5:596–603.

59. Bergonzelli GE, et al. Probiotics as a treatment strategy for gastrointestinal diseases? *Digestion.* 2005;72–68.

60. Jenkins B, Holsten S, Bengmark S, Martindale R. Probiotics: A practical review of their role in specific clinical scenarios. *Nutr Clin Pract.* 2005;20:262–270.

61. Galvez J, Rodriguez-Cabezas M, Zarzuelo A. Effects of dietary fiber on inflammatory bowel disease. *Mol Nutr Food Res.* 2005;49:601–608.

62. Guarner F. Inulin and oligofructose: Impact on intestinal diseases and disorders. *Br J Nutr.* 2005;93S:S61–S65.

63. Bengmark S, Martindale R. Prebiotics and synbiotics in clinical medicine. *JPEN.* 2005;20: 244–261.

64. Wilson A, Reyes E, Ofman J. Prevalence and outcomes of anemia in inflammatory bowel disease: A systematic review of the literature. *Am J Med.* 2004;116S:44S–49S.

65. Gasche C, Lomer M, Cavill I, Weiss G. Iron, anaemia, and inflammatory bowel diseases. *Gut.* 2004;53:1190–1197.

66. Cronin CC, Shanahan F. Anemia in patients with chronic inflammatory bowel disease. *Am J Gastro.* 2001;96:2296–2298.

67. Murphy C, Hahn S, Volmink J. Reduced osmolarity oral rehydration solutions for treating cholera. *Cochrane Database Sys Rev.* 2004;(4):CD003754.

68. Alam NH, Yunus M, Faruque AS, et al. Symptomatic hyponatremia during treatment of hydrating diarrheal disease with reduced osmolariy oral rehydration solution. *JAMA.* 2006;296:567–573.

69. Beyer PB, Caviar EM, McCallum RW. Fructose intake at current levels in the United States may cause gastrointestinal distress in normal adults. *J Am Dietet Assoc.* 2005;105:1559–1566.

70. Thomson AB, Drozdowski L, Iordache C, et al. Small bowel review: Normal physiology, Part 1. *Dig Dis Sci.* 2003;48(8):1546–1564.

71. Beyer PL, Flynn MA. Effects of high- and low- fiber diets on human feces. *J Am Diet Assoc.* 1978;72:271–277.

72. Saltzman JR, Russel RM. Nutritional consequences of intestinal bacterial overgrowth. *Compr Ther.* 1994;20:523–530.

73. Karcher RE, Truding RM, Stawick LE. Using a cutoff of <10ppm for breath hydrogen testing: A review of 5 years' experience. *Ann Clin Lab Sci.* 1999;29:1–8.

74. Teo M, Chung S, Chitti L, et al. Small bowel bacterial overgrowth is a common cause of chronic diarrhea. *J Gastroenterol Hepatol.* 2004;19:904–909.

75. Laine L, Ahnen D, McClain C, et al. Review article: Potential gastrointestinal effects of long-term acid suppression with proton pump inhibitors. *Aliment Pharmacol Ther.* 2000;14:651–658.

76. Reed CA, Nichols DL, Bonnick SL, DiMarco NM. Bone mineral density and dietary intake in patients with Crohn's disease. *J Clin Densitom.* 1998;1:33–40.

77. Bernstein CN, Leslie WD. Review article: Osteoporosis and inflammatory bowel disease. *Aliment Pharmacol Ther.* 2004;19:941–952.

78. Schulte CM. Review article: Bone disease in inflammatory bowel disease. *Aliment Pharmacol Ther.* 2004;4S:43S–49S.

79. Basiotis PP. The healthy eating index 1999–2000. Charting dietary patterns of Americans USDA. Available at: www.cnpp.usda.gov/FENR/FENRV16N1/fenrv16n1p39.pdf. Accessed January 16, 2005.

CHAPTER 12

Acute Pancreatitis

Steve McClave, MD

INTRODUCTION

One of the most rapidly evolving areas of clinical nutrition is the nutritional support of the patient with severe acute pancreatitis. In the past, the overriding precept of management was to put the pancreas to rest, and to this end, provision of parental nutrition (PN) appeared to be ideally suited. As the medical professional knowledge of the role of the gut in critical illness evolved over the past decade, it became apparent that in patients with acute pancreatitis, other issues involving gut integrity unrelated to the pancreas were key factors in ultimate patient outcome. Recent collective clinical experience indicates that enteral nutrition (EN) is safe in pancreatitis, and an increasing number of prospective randomized trials demonstrate improved outcome with use of EN compared to PN (1). Nonetheless, controversy remains with regard to whether the magnitude of benefits from EN therapy justifies its inherent risks.

A study published recently by a sophisticated group of pancreatitis researchers in Glasgow, Scotland, challenged the existing understanding of nutritional therapy in pancreatitis and shed new light on the value of feeding versus risks of exacerbating inflammation within the gland (2). In this study, Eatock randomized patients with severe acute pancreatitis (Acute Physiology and Chronic Health Evaluation [APACHE] II score >6, 25% mortality) to either nasogastric or nasojejunal feeding. EN had to be started within 72 hours of onset of pain. Patients reached goal infusion rate within a mean of 36 hours following initiation of feeds. Study results showed that patients in the two groups behaved indistinguishably. There were no significant differences between the two groups with regard to decreases in C-reactive protein levels, decreasing APACHE II scores, resolving pain scores, overall mortality, days to oral diet, and hospital length of stay. The formula selected was a small-peptide formula with 9% fat (2). Only two patients in the nasogastric group experienced pain. None of the patients in either group developed intolerance to the formula requiring cessation of feeding. The conclusion by these researchers was that nasogastric feeds should now be considered as a therapeutic option in the nutritional management of patients with severe acute pancreatitis (2).

Reactions to this paper were similar to the reactions experienced when the first prospective randomized controlled trial comparing EN and PN in acute pancreatitis was published in 1997 (3). Some clinicians did not believe the study results. Others wondered why this group would bother with nasogastric feeds, that infusing a formula into the stomach of a patient who was really sick with pancreatitis was "playing with dynamite," and could cause some patients to experience a potentially deleterious effect. The lesson learned in this study was that there is wide variation in tolerance; that both level of infusion within the gastrointestinal (GI) tract and content of the formula may be equally important issues as to whether a patient tolerates EN. A surprising number of patients tolerate nasogastric feeds even in the face of severe acute pancreatitis and necrosis within the gland. Finally, that intolerance to feeding may not have as narrow a risk/benefit ratio as previously thought, that a symptomatic flare of disease in response to feeding may not truly endanger the patient.

Certainly this controversial study reinforced the concept that EN in severe acute pancreatitis is a double-edged sword. On one hand, the clinician has the capability of reducing stress with EN by maintaining gut integrity, reducing disease severity, and improving outcome (4,5). On the other hand, some degree of pancreatic stimulation in response to EN could actually increase stress through exacerbation of inflammation and further increases in the systemic inflammatory response syndrome (SIRS). By pushing the concept of EN (to the extent of feeding into the stomach), is the clinician asking for trouble? What is the true benefit of providing EN and how strong is that evidence? What is the risk of stimulating the pancreas? Which patients with acute pancreatitis truly benefit from provision of EN?

CONSEQUENCES OF PROVIDING ENTERAL NUTRITION

Twenty-five years ago, Ranson warned that early advancement to oral diet could actually induce late complications, specifically an increase in the incidence of abdominal abscess in patients with severe acute pancreatitis (6). Prospective randomized trials over the last 10 years would suggest that this is not the case. Instead, the experience from these studies would suggest that three potentially adverse (but for the most part benign) situations result from the provision of EN (see Table 12–1). The first scenario is that of silent stimulation of pancreatic exocrine secretion. In a study involving healthy volunteers and patients with acute pancreatitis, O'Keefe compared the effect of EN versus PN on serum levels of trypsin, amylase, and lipase (7). In both groups (volunteers and patients), provision of EN increased serum levels of trypsin, amylase, and lipase significantly compared to groups receiving PN. Increases were higher in healthy volunteers, but similar effects were seen in the patients with acute pancreatitis. The increases in enzyme levels in the patients with acute pancreatitis were clinically silent and appeared to be tolerated well (7). A second scenario that can occur in response to provision of EN is an uncomplicated exacerbation of symptoms. In a study by McClave, three patients randomized to jejunal feeding showed resolution of symptoms and normalization of amylase over 5

Table 12–1 Potential Adverse Consequences From Use of Enteral Nutrition in Severe Acute Pancreatitis

Event	Clinical Evidence	Incidence
• Silent stimulation of pancreatic secretion	↑ amylase, lipase	100%
• Uncomplicated exacerbation of symptoms	↑ amylase, lipase ↑ abdominal pain ↑ nausea, vomiting	21%
• Exacerbation of disease process	↑ amylase, lipase ↑ symptoms (pain, N/V) ↑ fever, WBC count	4%

Legend: N/V= nausea, vomiting.

days of jejunal feeding (3). When advanced to an oral, clear-liquid diet, all three patients experienced an exacerbation of pain, nausea, vomiting, and a rise in their serum amylase levels. Two of the patients were placed back on jejunal feeds and again experienced resolution of symptoms (and one of these patients required three attempts at an oral, clear-liquid diet before it was finally tolerated). In each patient, the increase in pain quickly resolved by switching back from oral ingestion of clear liquids to the jejunal infusion of a complex formula (3). In a large case series by Levy, a similar, uncomplicated exacerbation of symptoms in response to advancement to oral feeding was experienced in 21% of patients (8). The third scenario of response to EN is a true exacerbation of the disease process. In the study by McClave, one patient randomized to deep jejunal feeding experienced clinical deterioration with an exacerbation of symptoms and an increased pattern of SIRS 1 week after starting EN, the point at which the tip of the feeding tube was displaced from the jejunum back into the stomach (3). Once the tube was placed back into the jejunum, however, the exacerbation of SIRS abated within 24 hours with resolution of the fever and return of the white blood cell count toward normal over the next few days (3). In the case series by Levy, a similar exacerbation of the disease process was seen in 4.3% of patients (8).

This collective experience with EN raises questions as to the ultimate significance of pancreatic rest. Clearly, pancreatic rest as a sole strategy in the management of acute pancreatitis (via use of nasogastric suction, cimetidine, somatostatin, etc.) has been shown to have no effect on clinical outcome (9). Whereas in the past it was thought that pancreatic exocrine secretion had to be reduced to basal unstimulated levels, recent clinical experience would suggest that reducing secretion to subclinical levels of output is enough to allow resolution of inflammation within the gland. Putting the pancreas to rest and utilizing the gut are not incompatible concepts, because both can be achieved simultaneously in the same patient. Fortunately for the clinician, management of the severe pancreatitis patient can be guided by clinical symptoms and does not require measurement of enzyme output at the level of the ampulla. An exacerbation of symptoms of the disease process in response to EN may be ameliorated by subtle changes in the level of infusion or content of formula infused. Such a response does not appear to exert a dangerous deleterious effect for the patient.

BENEFITS OF PROVIDING ENTERAL NUTRITION

Some of the strongest data in the literature supporting a benefit from providing EN have been documented in the setting of acute pancreatitis (Table 12–2) (1). In general, the provision of EN maintains gut integrity, resulting in less bacterial challenge to the immune system, and less systemic endotoxemia (10,11). Feeding into the gut helps set the tone for systemic immunity by influencing lymphocyte subset cellular proliferation (12). EN attenuates the stress response and as a result, appears to reduce overall disease severity (4). Patients experience faster resolution of the disease process, as evidenced by shorter duration of SIRS, decreased duration of nutritional therapy, and reduced hospital length of stay (4,13,14). Patients receiving EN experience fewer complications with regard to infection and need for surgical intervention when compared to those patients in whom the gut is not utilized (15). Although animal models have helped elucidate the fine details of the mechanism of these principles, the vast majority of outcome data is well documented in clinical studies involving patients with pancreatitis (1).

Table 12–2 Benefits of Enteral Nutrition in Severe Acute Pancreatitis (compared to parenteral nutrition)

- Maintenance of gut integrity
  Less bacterial challenge to immune system
  Less systemic endotoxemia
- Setting the tone for systemic immunity via lymphocyte subset populations
- Attenuation of the stress response, reduction in disease severity
- Faster resolution of the disease process
  Shorter duration of SIRS
  Decreased duration of nutritional therapy
  Reduced hospital length of stay
- Fewer complications
  Reduced infectious morbidity
  Less need for surgical intervention
  Possibly less organ failure

Legend: SIRS = systemic inflamatory response syndrome.

At the heart of this discussion is the paradigm shift in our perspective of the role of the gut in critical illness. In the past, the gut was thought to be a passive organ that did not need to be utilized at a time when the patient was severely ill. Concern about dysfunction of the gut centered around stress gastropathy, bleeding, and whether ileus was severe enough to require PN. In general, the gut was thought to be an organ of inconvenience. Critical care intensivists now realize that the gut is a dynamic organ in critical illness. Failure to utilize the gut may contribute to an exacerbation of the disease process. Concern about gut dysfunction now focuses on the consequent increases in permeability, bacterial challenge to the immune system, flaring of SIRS, and an up-regulation of the overall immune response (10,12). Through these mechanisms, the gut becomes a proinflammatory organ when not utilized in critical illness. In the past, the concept of gut failure centered on the "vital organs" such as the heart, lungs, and kidneys. It is now important for the clinician to realize that the gut may be a key organ involved in multiple organ failure syndrome; that failure of the gut may lead to failure of other organs (16).

A severe injury generates a dynamic process that causes these paracellular channels to open, resulting in increased permeability and bacterial translocation. By maintaining gut integrity, enteral feeding helps keep the channels between the epithelial cells closed (10–12) (Table 12–3). Feeding stimulates the release of secretory IgA and bile salts, which help to coat bacteria and prevent their adherence to the intestinal epithelium. Peristalsis, stimulated by feeding, helps move bacterial organisms downstream and keeps the overall number of bacteria in check. Feeding also stimulates blood flow to the gut, which prevents ischemia/reperfusion injury (10–12).

Failure to utilize the gut in severe acute pancreatitis results in increases in gut permeability, a phenomenon that is time dependent and which correlates to increases in disease severity (17) (Table 12–3). The consequences of the increase in gut permeability include increased risk of infection and increased risk of organ failure. In a study by Ammori, polyethylene glycol (PEG) was used as a marker for gut permeability (17). This compound is approximately the same size as endotoxin, and should pass through the GI tract unabsorbed unless there are increases in permeability. In a case series of patients with acute pancreatitis, Amori showed that increases in urinary PEG levels (indicating increased permeability and absorption of this marker) correlated significantly with increases in systemic endotoxemia ($p = 0.002$, $R = 0.08$) (17). In a separate study, Windsor measured IgM antibodies to endotoxin and showed that antibody levels increased by 24.8% over a week of nutritional therapy with PN, whereas those patients receiving EN saw a decrease in antibodies by 1.4% ($p < 0.05$) (4). Such increases in permeability would allow the bacteria to engage the immune system.

EN maintains the mass of gut-associated lymphoid tissue (GALT), which in turn contributes to the mass of mucosal-associated lymphoid tissue (MALT) at distant organ sites (Table 12–3). Over 80% of immunoglobulin produced in the body is generated at the level of the gut (18,19). Proliferating lines of B-cells and plasma cells generated at the gut by antigen presentation go out to distant sites to form

Table 12–3 Differential Effects of Feeding Versus Starvation in Severe Acute Pancreatitis and Critical Illness

Parameter	Feeding	Starvation
• **Gut integrity**		
Permeability	Contained, minimized	Increased
Peristalsis	Increased	Decreased, ileus
Splanchnic blood flow	Increased	Decreased
• **Bacterial gut flora**		
Type	Commensal	Pathogenic
Number	Normal	Overgrowth
Phase	Normal	Virulence, adherence
• **Effect on lymphoid tissue**		
GALT	Mass sustained	Up to 50% loss of mass
MALT at distant sites	Sustained delivery from gut	Reduced delivery from gut
• **Effect on systemic immunity**		
Innate response (macrophages, neutrophils)	$\downarrow$ activation Th2 subset proliferation	$\uparrow$ activation Th1 subset proliferation
Acquired response (CD_4 helper lymphocytes)	$\downarrow$ oxidative stress $\downarrow$ disease severity	$\uparrow$ oxidative stress $\uparrow$ inflammation, SIRS
Clinical effect		$\uparrow$ disease severity

Legend: GALT = gut-associated lymphoid tissue; MALT = mucosal-associated lymphoid tissue; SIRS = systemic inflammatory response syndrome.

MALT tissue at distant organs, described as BALT, TALT, and NALT for such tissues localized to the bronchi, tonsils, and nasal passages, respectively (10,11, 20,21). Patient studies involving children with dysfunctional colostomies and infants placed on PN show that starvation can result in a drop by as much as 50% in the mass of secretory IgA-producing immunocytes at the level of the gut (12,19,22). In animal models, starvation following injury reduces the level of secretory IgA produced in the lungs and increases susceptibility to viral infection. Reinstating EN at the level of the gut restores immunity at this distant organ site and promotes eradication of the virus (22). Although such studies have not yet been documented in pancreatis, one of the most common infections reduced by use of EN in pancreatitis is pneumonia (1).

Enteral feeding supports the role of commensal bacteria (Table 12–3). When a child is born, the gut is sterile and becomes colonized over the first month of life. GALT develops over the first 6 months of life. As a result of these processes developing simultaneously, the immune system demonstrates tolerance for the commensal bacteria (10,12). A protective effect is exerted by the commensal bacteria indirectly through prevention of colonization of pathogenic bacteria such as pseudomonas. Direct protection by commensal bacteria is provided through the release of disaccharidase enzymes, which break down the toxin produced by pathogenic bacteria. Studies by Alverdy have shown that bacteria can sense stress through decreases in gut lumenal pH or oxygen levels and switch on virulence genes (23). Once the genes are expressed, contact-dependent activation of intestinal epithelial cells occurs through adherence of the bacteria to the gut epithelium (10). This process increases permeability (by loosening tight junctions), activates release of cytokines, promotes cell apoptosis, and leads to activation of neutrophils flowing through the circulation of the gut (10,23). In such animal models, Alverdy has shown that the bacterial colonization of the gut at the time of injury or shock is a factor in the degree of inflammatory response generated by the gut (23). Colonization by normal commensal bacteria results in the release of the lowest level of inflammatory mediators (tumor necrosis factor and IL-6). In the setting of gut disuse, bacterial overgrowth of normal organisms results in the release of higher levels of mediators in response to shock, with the greatest level of response seen in a setting of bacterial overgrowth by pathogenic organisms (23).

The protective effect of commensal bacteria has been demonstrated in acute pancreatitis through the role of probiotic therapy. In a study by Olah, patients with severe acute pancreatitis were randomized to receive enteral feeding with a live *lactobacillus* organism (24). Control subjects received the same formula with the same bacteria, but the organisms were heat killed prior to infusion. Results of the study showed a highly significant reduction in infected pancreatic necrosis and abdominal abscess from 30.4% (in control subjects) down to 4.5% in the study patients receiving the live *lactobacillus* (p = 0.02) (24). Hospital length of stay was reduced from 21.4 days in control patients to 13.7 days in the study patients, although this difference did not reach statistical significance (24).

Gut disuse stimulates the innate immune response in patients with acute pancreatitis (Table 12–3). The gut serves as a priming bed for macrophages and neutrophils and thus becomes a proinflammatory organ capable of exacerbating oxidative stress (12). In a setting of gut disuse, macrophages at the level of the gut become activated, presumably by either ischemia/reperfusion injury or by bacterial challenge from increased permeability (25–28). Once macrophages are activated, neutrophils flowing through the splanchnic circulation can become primed. These neutrophils then pass out to a distant site such as the lungs, the liver, or the kidneys. A second insult from hypoxemia or hypotension activates the neutrophils, allowing them to move out of the vascular space, enter the organ, and generate an oxidative burst. The activated neutrophils and the increase in free oxygen radical species at these distant sites contribute to the development of organ failure and infection (25,27).

EN helps set the tone for the acquired immune response (12) (Table 12–3). A dendritic macrophage is a professional antigen-presenting cell located in the intestinal epithelium. With long fimbriae, this cell samples lumenal contents of the gut. In a setting of enteral feeding, this macrophage senses a normal number of organisms, comprised primarily of commensal bacteria. The macrophage also senses antigen from the protein of the food infused into the gut. As a result, this cell releases IL-4 (12). In contrast, in the setting of gut disuse, the same cell senses bacterial overgrowth, which may be comprised of pathogenic bacteria. No food antigen is detected. As a result, the cell releases IL-12 (12). The specific cytokine released by this cell has a profound effect on the proliferation of CD_4 helper T-cell lymphocytes located immediately underneath within the lamina propria of the gut. With gut disuse and the release of IL-12, these naïve CD_4 helper lymphocytes proliferate along a Th1 line of cells, which further generates interferon and tumor necrosis factor (12). This proinflammatory pathway of cells spills out into the systemic circulation. In contrast, in a setting of gut use and enteral feeding, the release of IL-4 causes the same naïve lymphocytes to proceed down a Th2 pathway, which contributes further increases in IL-4 and IL-10, which directly oppose the proinflammatory Th1 pathway (12). The Th2 pathway has a clinical effect of down-regulating inflammation at the level of the gut, which in turn spills over into the systemic circulation. In addition, IL-4 stimulates the Th1 and Th3 pathways associated with oral tolerance that go on to produce increased levels of transforming growth factor–beta (TGF-β) (12). The proliferation of these cell lines and their respective cytokines have a down-regulatory effect and contribute to further reductions in inflammation at the level of the gut.

Multiple studies in patients with acute pancreatitis have now shown this differential effect on oxidative stress and overall disease severity in response to the route of feeding and whether the gut is utilized for provision of nutrition support (3,4,13) (Table 12–3). Evidence of greater oxidative stress was shown in a study by McClave, in which patients with acute pancreatitis randomized to PN demonstrated a statistically significant increase in stress-induced hyperglycemia over the first 6 days of nutritional therapy, an increase that was not seen in those patients randomized to EN (3). In the Windsor study, patients randomized to PN saw a decrease in antioxidant capacity by 27.7% over the first week of nutrition therapy, whereas patients randomized to EN saw an increase by 32.6% (4). C-reactive protein levels, a poor man's marker for the stress response, decreased significantly from 156 down to 84 over a week of EN, but remained unchanged in the group receiving PN (125 decreasing to 124) (4). Whereas both groups had a similar number of patients with SIRS upon entering the study, nearly all of the patients in the enteral group resolved their SIRS over a week of nutritional therapy (9 out of 11), which was significantly greater than the 2 out of 12 patients who resolved SIRs in the parenteral group (4). In a different study by Abou-Assi, time to resolution of the disease process was defined by resolution of abdominal pain, near normalization of amylase, and successful advancement to a clear-liquid diet (13). This time duration to resolution was significantly shorter in the EN group at 6.2 days than the PN group at 11.8 days (p <0.05) (13).

The profound physiologic benefits from EN over PN demonstrated in these studies do correlate to improved outcome. In a recent meta-analysis, McClave aggregated data from seven prospective randomized trials involving 291 patients and showed that use of EN reduced infection by 54% (RR = 0.46, 95% CI 0.29–0.74) compared to PN (1). Aggregating data from four of these studies involving 202 patients showed that use of enteral feeding reduced hospital length of stay by nearly 4 full days (weighted mean difference –3.94, 95% CI –5.86, –2.02) (1). In the same study, use of enteral feeding showed a trend toward reduced organ failure by as much as 41% (RR = 0.59, 95% CI 0.28, 1.27, p = 0.18) (1). In a separate meta-analysis, Marik aggregated data from four studies (214 patients) and showed that the need for surgical intervention due to complications of pancreatitis was reduced by 52% with use of EN compared to PN (RR = 0.48; 95% CI 0.23, 0.99; p <0.05) (15).

WHO NEEDS NUTRITIONAL THERAPY?

In general, the greater the severity of acute pancreatitis, the more important the need for maintaining gut integrity and the more likely that provision of EN will alter patient outcome (see Table 12–4). In the study by Ammori using PEG as a marker for intestinal permeability, patients with mild pancreatitis showed no increases in permeability, with urinary PEG levels that were not significantly different from control subjects with no pancreatitis (17). Patients who had severe, uncomplicated pancreatitis had a fourfold increase in permeability, and those with severe pan-

Table 12–4 Need for Specialized Nutrition Support as Related to Disease Severity

Disease Severity	Mild-Moderate	Severe
• **Objective scores**		
Ranson criteria	≤2	≥3
APACHE II	≤9	≥10
Δ APACHE II over 3 d	↓ by 1	↑ by 3
• **Morbidity, mortality**		
Pancreatic necrosis	No	Yes
Complications	6%	38%
Mortality	0%	19%
• **Nutrition support**		
Advance to PO diet (7 d)	81%	0%
EN changes outcome	No	Yes
Specialized support needed	No	Yes
PN utilized	No	Yes (EN intolerant)

Legend: APACHE = acute physiology and chronic health evaluation; EN = enteral nutrition; PN = parenteral nutrition; PO = per os.

creatitis complicated by multiple organ failure had another fourfold increase above that (17). Comparing the first four prospective randomized trials of EN versus PN feeding in acute pancreatitis, the greater the percentage of patients with severe pancreatitis, the more likely the route of feeding impacted patient outcome (3–5,13). In the study by McClave, only 19% of the patients had severe pancreatitis and no outcome parameters were different between the two groups (3). In the studies by Abou-Assi and Windsor, 35%–38% of patients had severe pancreatitis, and use of EN was shown to result in faster resolution of SIRS and shorter duration of time to resolution of the disease process (4,13). In the Greek study by Kalferentzos, where 100% of patients had severe pancreatitis, significant reductions were seen in overall complications from 75% in the PN group to 44% in the EN group (p <0.05), and septic complications were decreased by half (from 50% to 28%, comparing the PN to EN groups, respectively, p <0.05) (5).

On admission, patients with severe acute pancreatitis may be identified as having an APACHE II score ≥10, with ≥3 Ranson criteria (29–33) (Table 12–4). These patients should have necrosis on computerized tomography (CT) scan, have a complication rate close to 38%, and a mortality rate of 19% (30,33). Their chance of advancing to oral diet successfully within 7 days is close to 0% (32). EN is most likely to change the clinical outcome of this group of patients. In contrast, patients with ″2 Ranson criteria or APACHE II scores ″9 demonstrate mild to moderate pancreatitis, will tend not to have necrosis on CT scan, have a low complication rate of 6%, and a near 0% mortality rate (29,30,33). Over 80% of these patients should advance successfully to oral diet within 7 days (32). Their management is supported with fluid resuscitation and intravenous analgesia and no nutritional therapy is required. Presence of necrosis on CT scan or the development of complications such as pseudocysts, ascites, or need for surgical intervention do not obviate the need for EN (34–37). PN should be reserved only for those patients with severe pancreatitis who require nutrition support but have demonstrated intolerance to EN.

These objective scoring systems have greater sensitivity for identifying the patient with severe pancreatitis than bedside clinical judgment. On admission, the sensitivity of clinical assessment for identifying patients with severe pancreatitis is only 34%–44%, while the APACHE II score has a sensitivity of 63% (30,33). At 48–72 hours, the sensitivity of clinical assessment increases only to 44%–66%, while that of the APACHE II score and Ranson criteria range between 75% and 82% (30,33). Thus on admission, if the patient looks good clinically, but these objective scores suggest severe pancreatitis, the objective scoring systems are more reliable than clinical assessment at identifying those patients who will benefit from placement of a feeding tube and initiation of EN therapy.

WHAT FACTORS AFFECT TOLERANCE?

The biggest roadblock to provision of EN in acute pancreatitis involves issues related to tolerance. Increasing experience with EN in acute pancreatitis has led to the identification of a number of factors that affect tolerance (Table 12–5). These

Table 12–5 Factors Affecting Tolerance of Enteral Nutrition in Severe Acute Pancreatitis

- Level of infusion within the gastrointestinal tract
- Content of infused formula
- Duration of ileus prior to feeding
- Institutional variability in experience, expertise
- Individual patient variability

---

factors include level of infusion, content of the formula, duration of ileus, institutional experience, and individual variation in response.

Tolerance to enteral feeding has been previously defined as "provision of nutritional therapy without ill effect" (38); thus, the concept of tolerance in patients with acute pancreatitis is tightly linked to safety. Documenting the safety of EN in acute pancreatitis was the primary endpoint of the first prospective randomized trial by McClave (3). Safety of EN compared to PN was confirmed in this study, because both groups behaved indistinguishably with regard to days at normalization of amylase, days to advancement to oral diet, overall length of hospitalization, length of stay in the intensive care unit, incidence of nosocomial infection, and mortality (3).

A key factor in tolerance to EN in acute pancreatitis relates to the level of infusion of formula within the GI tract. Multiple levels of stimulation of pancreatic exocrine secretion exist and are organized into a cephalic, gastric, and intestinal phase (39). Multiple factors are involved at each level, and include vagal, mechanical, chemical, and hormonal stimuli. Presumably, the lower the level of infusion of formula within the GI tract, the fewer the number of stimulatory factors that are invoked. When the feeding is low enough in the GI tract, the number of inhibitory factors that may be elicited (such as pancreatic inhibitory polypeptide, pancreatic polypeptide YY, and bile salts) may offset what few stimulatory factors are being invoked (39). This effect of level of infusion on stimulation of the pancreas has been documented in studies in which patients served as their own controls for different levels of infusion of formula within the GI tract. In a study by McClave, patients who were tolerant of an infusion of an intact polymeric formula into the jejunum demonstrated a flare of symptoms when advanced to oral clear liquids (3). Similarly, a patient who appeared to be tolerant of infusion of a polymeric formula into the jejunum had a flare with an exacerbation of SIRS when the same formula was infused into the stomach (3).

Content of formula infused in the gut is also a factor in tolerance and the degree to which the pancreas is stimulated. Formulas with higher osmolarity have greater stimulation that those with lower osmolarity (34). Formulas comprised of intact protein or individual amino acids appear to have greater stimulation than formulas comprised of oligopeptides (34,39). Fat is probably the greatest stimulant of pancreatic exocrine secretion, and the longer the chain fat, the greater the degree of stimulation (34,39). Thus, formulas comprised of medium-chain triglyceride (MCT) oil may have less stimulation. In a study by Grant, EN formulas were infused through a jejunostomy tube, while pancreatic enzyme secretions were collected through a tube positioned in the duodenum opposite the ampulla (40). Changing from fat-free elemental formulas (Vivonex or Criticare) to a formula containing long-chain fat (Osmolite), resulted in a statistically significant increase in lipase output from the pancreas (40). In a case series involving patients languishing in the hospital with acute pancreatitis, Parekh showed that oral ingestion of an elemental, fat-free formula (Precision LR) resulted in resolution of pain and normalization of serum amylase levels (34). Advancement to a full ward regular diet resulted in return of pain and an increase in amylase levels above normal. Placing patients back on oral Precision LR resolved symptoms again and normalized the amylase levels (34). These studies suggest that tolerance is a graded scale determined by the degree of necrosis within the gland. With greater degrees of necrosis and disease severity, the level of infusion of formula may need to be displaced further down into the GI tract, and content of the formula may need to be modified to reduce fat, decrease osmolarity, and modify protein to small peptides.

Institutional variation is a factor in tolerance. The success with which a program establishes enteral access and maintains deep jejunal feeding may be an issue in the degree to which their patients tolerate EN (4). In a study by Windsor, problems with ileus occurred in only 5 out of 16 patients randomized to EN (4). The rate of infusion had to be decreased in these five patients briefly for 2 to 4 days, before resuming full goal rate of infusion. In contrast, in a study by Schneider from the same country, only 50% of patients in whom EN was attempted actually tolerated the feeding (41). The other 50% of patients received either PN alone or no nutritional support. Having local expertise for achieving enteral access and having protocols in place to facilitate delivery of EN may enhance the degree to which it is tolerated.

Duration of ileus and the rapidity with which enteral access is achieved may be a factor in tolerance. In a study by Cravo, no patients in whom the duration of ileus lasted ≥6 days tolerated EN, and instead had to be placed on PN (42). If the duration of ileus was " 5 days, then 50% of those patients tolerated EN. Only by limiting the duration of ileus to " 2 days was EN tolerated in 92% of patients (42).

Recent studies suggest that there is tremendous individual variation in tolerance to the same level of infusion and content of formula. The Eatock study from Glasgow, Scotland, demonstrated that in a large number of patients with severe pancreatitis, nasogastric feeds could be tolerated just as well as nasojejunal feeds (2). In contrast to that experience, a patient described by O'Keefe in whom the tube was positioned well below the Ligament of Treitz showed intolerance to nasojejunal feeds at very low rates of infusion with exacerbation of pain and increases in serum amylase (7). The patient had to be switched to PN for a short duration before reattempting EN at a later time.

OPTIONS FOR NUTRITIONAL SUPPORT

When evaluating patients with acute pancreatitis for the need for nutritional support, three options are actually available: provision of EN, provision of PN, or standard therapy (STD) in which no artificial nutritional support is provided and patients are on their own to advance over time to an oral diet. The choice or option in the individual patient is based on disease severity, timing, and tolerance (Table 12–6). As implied earlier in this discussion, disease severity is the primary determinant of whether specialized nutrition support by either enteral or parenteral route is indicated. In patients with mild to moderate acute pancreatitis, STD with no artificial nutritional support is indicated. Patients may be managed with intravenous fluid resuscitation alone or with narcotic analgesia. Only if a complication develops or the patient fails to advance to oral diet after 1 week of hospitalization should specialized nutritional support be considered.

Although the studies already described indicate a greater benefit on outcome with use of EN compared to PN (1), the benefit of EN over STD is not as well documented in the population of patients with acute pancreatitis. In one study of patients

Table 12–6 Prioritization of Specialized Nutritional Therapy Over the Course of Hospitalization

- Severe acute pancreatitis

AFTER FIRST 5 DAYS		FIRST 5 DAYS OF HOSPITALIZATION
	1st Choice	
Enteral nutrition		Enteral nutrition
	2nd Choice	
Parenteral nutrition		Standard therapy
	3rd Choice	
Standard therapy		Parenteral nutrition

- Mild to moderate acute pancreatitis

AFTER FIRST WEEK		FIRST WEEK OF HOSPITALIZATION
	1st Choice	
Enteral nutrition		Standard therapy
	2nd Choice	
Parenteral nutrition		Enteral nutrition
	3rd Choice	
Standard therapy		Parenteral nutrition

Legend: Standard therapy = no specialized nutrition support.

admitted for severe acute pancreatitis, Powell randomized patients to receive either EN or STD (43). The study was limited in that it was only 4 days in duration and only 27 patients were enrolled. Results suggested less oxidative stress in the group receiving EN, as suggested by lower serum levels of tumor necrosis factor, IL-6 and C-reactive protein in those patients receiving EN compared to those randomized to STD, but differences did not reach statistical significance (43). There was no difference in outcome between the two groups. However, in patients undergoing surgical intervention for complications of pancreatitis, a recent meta-analysis suggested a reduction in mortality from use of EN (1). Aggregating the data from two studies involving 71 patients, use of EN showed a trend toward a reduction in mortality by as much as 74% compared to use of STD (RR = 0.26; 95% CI 0.06, 1.09; p = 0.06) (1).

The role of PN in acute pancreatitis is therefore becoming increasingly controversial and the specific timing of initiation of PN may be the biggest determinant in whether benefit is seen from this mode of nutritional therapy. In an early prospective randomized trial of 54 patients with mild acute pancreatitis, PN initiated within the first 24 hours of admission resulted in a length of hospitalization that was 1 week longer, and a rate of catheter sepsis that was tenfold greater than controls who were randomized to STD (32). PN provided too early in the course of disease at the height of the inflammatory response may be a greater liability than benefit to patients with acute pancreatitis. Early on in the first 72 hours of admission to the hospital, the priorities of nutritional support are to modulate the immune response and attenuate oxidative stress. Difficulties in maintaining gut integrity and the likelihood for exacerbating hyperglycemia dictate the liability of PN. Meeting calorie and protein requirements early after admission may not be as important as it is later in the hospital course toward the end of the first week, where inadequacies of nutritional therapy begin to affect overall nutritional status.

Clinical experience has shown, however, that a significant number of patients with severe acute pancreatitis at various institutions do not tolerate EN and are relegated instead to consideration for PN. The timing of initiation of PN and allowing for some delay in the start of parenteral therapy may improve chances for a beneficial effect on outcome. In a recent Chinese study, Xian-Li randomized patients with severe acute pancreatitis to STD, PN, or PN supplemented with parenteral glutamine (44). Patients were entered in the study only after full fluid resuscitation, and feeds had to be started within 48 hours of randomization. As a result, patients receiving PN in this study may have done so further along in the course of hospitalization than those patients in the Sax study. Provision of PN was shown to significantly reduce mortality (from 43.5% in the STD group to 14.3% in the PN group, p <0.05) (44). Overall, complications were reduced significantly from 21% to 11%, and hospital length of stay was reduced significantly from 39.1 days down to 28.6 days, comparing the STD group to the PN group, respectively (all differences p <0.05) (44). Supplementation of PN with parenteral glutamine resulted in further improvement in complications and pancreatic infection compared to the group receiving PN alone.

These studies would suggest that in those patients with severe pancreatitis in whom nutritional support is indicated, EN is clearly the optimum choice and first line of therapy. If there is intolerance to EN or enteral feeding is not feasible, PN should be considered, but should be initiated probably after the first 5 days of hospitalization, to begin after the peak of the inflammatory response.

CONCLUSION

The clinical experience of providing nutritional support to patients with severe pancreatitis has seen revolutionary changes over the past 10 years. Although pancreatic rest may be an issue in tolerance to EN, the benefit of maintaining gut integrity and reducing oxidative stress is a much greater factor in influencing patient outcome. Exacerbation of symptoms and even the disease process in response to EN may not be as dangerous as previously thought and usually subtle changes in the content or level of infusion of formula are successful in improving tolerance. Disease severity dictates whether specialized nutrition support is provided at all and tolerance and timing dictate the manner in which PN is utilized. The clinical experience of providing EN to patients with pancreatitis demonstrates the degree to which events at the level of the gut influence overall systemic immunity, oxidative stress, and the inflammatory response. Although the strategies involved in providing PN may be modified in the future to enhance its efficacy, EN at the present time is clearly the gold standard of therapy for nutritional support.

REFERENCES

1. McClave SA, Chang WK, Dhaliqal R, Heyland DK. Nurition support in acute pancreatitis: A systematic review of the literature. *JPEN J Parenter External Nutr.* 2006; 30:143–156.

2. Eatock FC, Chong P, Menezes N, et al. A randomized study of early nasogastric versus nasojejunal feeding in severe acute pancreatitis. *Am J Gastroenterol.* 2005;100:432–439.

3. McClave SA, Greene LM, Snider HL, et al. Comparison of the safety of early enteral vs parenteral nutrition in mild acute pancreatitis. *JPEN.* 1997;21:14–20.

4. Windsor AC, Kanwar S, Li AG, et al. Compared with parenteral nutrition, enteral feeding attenuates the acute phase response and improves disease severity in acute pancreatitis. *Gut.* 1998;42:431–435.

5. Kalfarentzos F, Kehagias J, Mead N, Kokkinis K, Gogos CA. Enteral nutrition is superior to parenteral nutrition in severe acute pancreatitis: Results of a randomized prospective trial. *Br J Surg.* 1997;84:1665–1669.

6. Ranson JH, Spencer FC. Prevention, diagnosis, and treatment of pancreatic abscess. *Surgery.* 1977;82:99–106.

7. O'Keefe SJ, Broderick T, Turner M, Stevens S, O'Keefe JS. Nutrition in the management of necrotizing pancreatitis. *Clin Gastroenterol Hepatol.* 2003;1:315–321.

8. Levy P, Heresbach D, Pariente EA, et al. Frequency and risk factors of recurrent pain during refeeding in patients with acute pancreatitis: A multivariate multicentre prospective study of 116 patients. *Gut.* 1997;40:262–266.

9. Helton WS. Intravenous nutrition in patients with acute pancreatitis. In: Rombeau JL, ed. *Clinical Nutrition. Parenteral Nutrition.* Philadelphia, Pa.: WB Saunders. 1990:442–461.

10. DeWitt RC, Kudsk KA. The gut's role in metabolism, mucosal barrier function, and gut immunology. *Infect Dis Clin North Am*. 1999;13:465–481.

11. Kagnoff MF. Immunology of the intestinal tract. *Gastroenterology*. 1993;105:1275–1280.

12. Jabbar A, Chang WK, Dryden GW, McClave SA. Gut immunology and the differential response to feeding and starvation. *Nutr Clin Pract*. 2003;18:461–482.

13. Abou-Assi S, Craig K, O'Keefe SJ. Hypocaloric jejunal feeding is better than total parenteral nutrition in acute pancreatitis: Results of a randomized comparative study. *Am J Gastroenterol*. 2002;97:2255–2262.

14. Gupta R, Patel K, Calder PC, Yaqoob P, Primrose JN, Johnson CD. A randomised clinical trial to assess the effect of total enteral and total parenteral nutritional support on metabolic, inflammatory and oxidative markers in patients with predicted severe acute pancreatitis (APACHE II > or = 6). *Pancreatology*. 2003;3:406–413.

15. Marik PE, Zaloga GP. Meta-analysis of parenteral nutrition versus enteral nutrition in patients with acute pancreatitis. *BMJ*. 2004;12(328):1407.

16. Doig CJ, Sutherland LR, Sandham JD, Fick GH, Verhoef M, Meddings JB. Increased intestinal permeability is associated with the development of multiple organ dysfunction syndrome in critically ill ICU patients. *Am J Respir Crit Care Med*. 1998;158:444–451.

17. Ammori BJ, Leeder PC, King RF, et al. Early increase in intestinal permeability in patients with severe acute pancreatitis: Correlation with endotoxemia, organ failure, and mortality. *J Gastrointest Surg*. 1999;3:252–262.

18. Bengmark S. Gut microenvironment and immune function. *Curr Opinion Clin Nutrit Metab Care*. 1999;2:1–3.

19. Brandtzaeg P, Halstensen TS, Kett K, et al. Immunobiology and immunopathology of human gut mucosa: Humoral immunity and intraepithelial lymphocytes. *Gastroenterology*. 1989;97:1562–1584.

20. Targan SR, Kagnoff MF, Brogan MD, Shanahan F. Immunologic mechanisms in intestinal diseases. *Ann Intern Med*. 1987;106:853–870.

21. Dobbins WO. Gut immunophysiology: A gastroenterologist's view with emphasis on pathophysiology. *Am J Physiol*. 1982;242:G1–G8.

22. Kudsk KA. Importance of enteral feeding in maintaining gut integrity. *Tech Gastro Endosc*. 2001;3:2–8.

23. Alverdy JC, Laughlin RS, Wu L. Influence of the critically ill state on host-pathogen interactions within the intestine: Gut-derived sepsis redefined. *Crit Care Med*. 2003;31:598–607.

24. Olah A, Belagyi T, Issekutz A, Gamal ME, Bengmark S. Randomized clinical trial of specific lactobacillus and fibre supplement to early enteral nutrition in patients with acute pancreatitis. *Br J Surg*. 2002;89:1103–1107.

25. Fink MP. Why the GI tract is pivotal in trauma, sepsis, and MOF. *J Crit Illness*. 1991;6:253–269.

26. Moore FA, Feliciano DV, Andrassy RJ, et al. Early enteral feeding, compared with parenteral, reduces postoperative septic complications. The results of a meta-analysis. *Ann Surg*. 1992;216:172–183.

27. Moore EE, Moore FA. The role of the gut in provoking the systemic inflammatory response. *J Crit Care Nutr*.1994;2:9–15.

28. Frost P, Bihari D. The route of nutritional support in the critically ill: Physiological and economical considerations. *Nutrition*. 1997;13(9 suppl):58S–63S.

29. Banks PA. Pancreatitis for the endoscopist. ASGE Postgraduate Course, Digestive Disease Week, San Francisco, Calif. May 23–24, 1996.

30. Larvin M, McMahon MJ. APACHE-II score for assessment and monitoring of acute pancreatitis. *Lancet*. 1989;22;2:201–205

31. Corfield AP, Cooper MJ, Williamson RC, et al. Prediction of severity in acute pancreatitis: Prospective comparison of three prognostic indices. *Lancet.* 1985;24;2:403–407.

32. Sax HC, Warner BW, Talamini MA, et al. Early total parenteral nutrition in acute pancreatitis: Lack of beneficial effects. *Am J Surg.* 1987;153:117–124.

33. Wilson C, Heath DI, Imrie CW. Prediction of outcome in acute pancreatitis: A comparative study of APACHE II, clinical assessment and multiple factor scoring systems. *Br J Surg.* 1990;77: 1260–1264.

34. Parekh D, Lawson HH, Segal I. The role of total enteral nutrition in pancreatic disease. *S Afr J Surg.* 1993;31:57–61.

35. Pupelis G, Austrums E, Jansone A, Sprucs R, Wehbi H. Randomised trial of safety and efficacy of postoperative enteral feeding in patients with severe pancreatitis: Preliminary report. *Eur J Surg.* 2000;166:383–387.

36. Voitk A, Brown RA, Echave V, McArdle AH, Gurd FN, Thompson AG. Use of an elemental diet in the treatment of complicated pancreatitis. *Am J Surg.* 1973;125:223–227.

37. Bury KD, Stephens RV, Randall HT. Use of a chemically defined, liquid, elemental diet for nutritional management of fistulas of the alimentary tract. *Am J Surg.* 1971;121:174–183.

38. Mallampalli A, McClave SA, Snider HL. Defining tolerance to enteral feeding in the intensive care unit. *Clin Nutr.* 2000;19:213–215.

39. Corcoy R, Ma Sanchez J, Domingo P, Net A. Nutrition in the patient with severe acute pancreatitis. *Nutrition.* 1998;4:269–275.

40. Grant JP, Davey-McCrae J, Snyder PJ. Effect of enteral nutrition on human pancreatic secretions. *JPEN J Parenter External Nutr.* 1987;11:302–304.

41. Schneider H, Boyle N, McCluckie A, Beal R, Atkinson S. Acute severe pancreatitis and multiple organ failure: Total parenteral nutrition is still required in a proportion of patients. *Br J Surg.* 2000;87:362–373.

42. Cravo M, Camilo ME, Marques A, Pinto Correia J. Early tube feeding in acute pancreatitis. A prospective study. *Clin Nutrit.* 1989;8(suppl):14.

43. Powell JJ, Murchison JT, Fearon KC, Ross JA, Siriwardena AK. Randomized controlled trial of the effect of early enteral nutrition on markers of the inflammatory response in predicted severe acute pancreatitis. *Br J Surg.* 2000;87:1375–1381.

44. Xian-Li H, Qing-Jiu M, Jian-Guo L, Yan-Kui C, Xi-Lin D. Effect of total parenteral nutrition (TPN) with and without glutamine dipeptide supplementation on outcome in severe acute pancreatitis (SAP). *Clin Nutrit Suppl.* 2004;1:43–47.

CHAPTER 13

Nutritional Management of Short Bowel Syndrome

Charlene Compher, PhD, RD, FADA, CNSD;
Marion Winkler, MS, RD, CNSD;
and Joseph I. Boullata, PharmD, RPh, BCNSP

INTRODUCTION

The purpose of this chapter is to address the clinical management of patients with short bowel syndrome, focusing on expected nutrition support outcomes, dietary and pharmacologic management, complications, and quality of life. In addition, a brief update on intestinal transplantation is provided. This review is focused primarily on adult patients.

SHORT BOWEL SYNDROME

Short bowel syndrome (SBS) is defined as the loss of absorptive capacity of the small bowel due to surgical resection for thrombosis or disease. The condition develops when gastrointestinal function is inadequate to maintain the nutrition and hydration of the individual without orally or intravenously administered nutrients and may occur with or without concurrent gastric and pancreatic insufficiency (1). In adults, SBS typically results from multiple intestinal resections due to inflammatory bowel disease including Crohn's disease or mesenteric ischemia from thrombosis or volvulus.

Absorption may vary in patients with SBS depending on the residual small bowel length, the presence or absence of the colon and ileocecal valve, and the health of the remaining intestine. Normal lengths of the small intestine and colon are 365–600 cm and 150 cm, respectively. SBS is generally defined as less than 150 cm of jejunum and/or ileum in the absence of a colon, or 60–90 cm of jejunum or ileum with an intact colon in continuity (2). The greatest likelihood of prolonged parenteral nutrition (PN) dependence has been defined as jejunoileal anastomosis with <35 cm residual small bowel (SB); jejunocolic or ileocolic anastomosis with <60 cm residual small bowel, or end jejunostomy with <115 cm residual SB (3). Thompson and Langnas summarized data from their work and from a number of investigators to differentiate severity of SBS and the degree of PN dependence (see Table 13–1) (4).

SBS is characterized by severe diarrhea, malabsorption, dehydration, electrolyte abnormalities, and weight loss. The pathophysiology leading to these symptoms includes alteration in motility, bacterial overgrowth, gastric hypersecretion resulting in deconjugation and dehydroxylation of bile acids, and impaired micellar solubilization as well as secondary pancreatic insufficiency. Patients with severe SBS are dependent on PN for hydration and nutrient provision, not only from lost surface area, but also accelerated transit time such that nutrient digestion and absorption are impaired. In eight patients with jejunostomy or short ileostomy (5), total mouth-to-anus transit time was <3 hours and <10 hours in 43 patients with SBS of variable anatomy (6). By scintigraphy, mouth-to-ostomy transit was <5 minutes for liquids and approximately 60 minutes for solids (normal = 18 minutes and 103 minutes, respectively) (7).

Anatomically, the presence of the ileocecal valve, acting as an intestinal brake, influences success in achieving nutritional autonomy. Having an ileocecal valve prolongs transit time and prevents colonic bacteria from migrating back into the SB, resulting in bacterial overgrowth.

Clinicians caring for patients with SBS must have a clear understanding of the gastrointestinal anatomy to both help guide the therapeutic approach and to anticipate the need for PN or intravenous fluids. This is also critical for documentation of medical necessity for insurance coverage and reimbursement. Ideally, the residual bowel is measured intraoperatively, both the amount of intestine resected and the remaining SB. Radiographical studies may be used to estimate residual bowel and to document transit time. It is also important to evaluate a patient's adherence with diet and the role this factor plays on PN dependency.

Table 13–1 PN Dependence and the Severity of SBS

- PN unlikely in patients with >180 cm residual SB
- Less than 6 months duration with 90–120 cm residual SB and colon
- About 6 to 12 months duration with 60–90 cm residual SB with or without the colon in continuity
- Permanent with <60 cm residual SB

NUTRITIONAL GOALS

The goals for patients with SBS are (8):

1. to provide adequate nutrition to replete or prevent protein-energy malnutrition, micronutrient deficiencies, and dehydration
2. to correct and prevent acid-base disturbances
3. to control disabling diarrhea
4. to maintain urine output greater than 1 L and urinary sodium greater than 20 mEq/L
5. to improve quality of life

A number of therapeutic options exist for the management of patients with SBS based in part on the phase of disease and their clinical presentation.

POSTOPERATIVE PERIOD

In those patients with SBS due to surgical resection, PN is often required in the immediate postoperative phase. It is important to maintain detailed, accurate intake and output records during this time. The plan should be established according to baseline fluid maintenance requirements, any ongoing abnormal losses (from stomal output or diarrhea), and any previous deficits. Nutrient goals should be determined on the basis of preoperative nutritional status. There should be careful management of serum electrolytes, including magnesium, and acid-base balance. Gastric hypersecretion and subsequent volume losses occur in the postoperative period and for up to 6 months following massive small bowel resection and may lead to metabolic alkalosis, hypokalemia, and dehydration (9). Patients should receive standard multivitamin, mineral, and trace element supplementation via PN with additional zinc to make up for losses via stomal output or stool (10). In the postoperative period, an oral diet should be introduced; usually with clear liquids, then a rapid transition to simply prepared solid foods. Food and fluid intake as well as urine, stool, or stomal output should be meticulously monitored. Serum chemistries including all of the electrolytes, as well as urine sodium concentration to assess hydration status should be monitored. The monitoring of body weight is essential.

"An aggressive attempt to wean PN should be undertaken in all patients with SBS, regardless of bowel anatomy" (11). The ability to wean a patient from PN requires an intense level of monitoring along with good clinical judgment. Some patients will be able to achieve nutritional adequacy with oral and/or enteral feeding, while others may remain partially or totally dependent on PN due to an inability to maintain weight, strength, hydration, or nutritional status via oral and/or enteral nutrition support (12). If home PN is required, cycled or overnight infusions are typically introduced during the hospital stay in preparation for discharge to home. The length of infusion should be based on the patient's fluid needs, glycemic control (patients with diabetes may need longer infusion to attain adequate glycemic control), frequency of urination during infusion (especially at night), the need for other intravenous therapies including antibiotics, and caregiver or home health care provider availability.

DIETARY MANAGEMENT

The cornerstone of dietary management for patients with SBS is to encourage an oral diet. Early after SBS, absorption of oral nutrients may be very limited, so that provision of complete nutrient needs by PN is advised. Over time, however, in response to oral food intake, the remaining segment of small bowel hypertrophies and nutrient absorption is improved, a process referred to as *gut adaptation*. The progress with and prognosis for adaptation is dependent on the extent of resection, the segments remaining, and the integrity of the bowel that is left (e.g., active Crohn's disease, radiation enteritis, etc.). Maximal adaptation is generally achieved by 2 years, and patients may discontinue their PN or be reduced to several days per week for their remaining lifetime.

Patients' gradual improvement in their ability to absorb oral nutrients through gut adaptation will result in steady weight gain (if this is the goal) or maintenance while PN is tapered. This provides a signal to reduce calories provided in the PN. Food diaries are important not only to quantify food and fluid intake, but also to monitor what is eaten, patterns between time of eating, and stool or ostomy output or gastrointestinal symptoms during periods of weaning from PN. Weight change and records of urine and stomal or stool output are essential to monitor as well as physical assessment of hydration status. Among the most important nutritional outcomes for this patient population are strength, stamina, endurance, sense of well-being, and quality of life. Unless patients are able to absorb >84% of basal energy requirements and >1.4 L of fluid daily (which may actually require an intake of up to 400% of energy needs and 7 L of fluid daily), it is unlikely they will become independent of PN (7). This requires a grazing food pattern with many small frequent meals during waking hours. Adaptive hyperphagia has been described as spontaneous oral intake of 46–48 kcal/kg/d and protein as 20% of energy intake with significant increases over time after SBS (13).

General dietary guidelines for SBS are summarized in Table 13–2. Complex carbohydrates, in addition to being most easily digested and absorbed, can be scavenged by colonic bacteria for production of short-chain fatty acids, which, in turn, provide an additional 200–1000 kcal daily in those patients with a colonic segment intact (14). By contrast, ingestion of simple sugars causes secretion of fluid into the intestinal lumen, thus worsening effluent output or diarrhea.

Foods containing proteins of high biological value should be a staple of the diet in patients with SBS. Because most of these patients have low-serum cholesterol (total and low-density lipoprotein), there is no need to restrict cholesterol-containing foods. In addition, eggs and peanut butter provide dietary choline, a

Table 13–2 Dietary Guidelines for Patients With SBS

	Jejunostomy or Ileostomy	*Colon in Continuity*
Challenges to absorption	Fluid	Chronic diarrhea
	Magnesium, calcium	Oxalate absorption increases risk of nephrolithiasis
	Calories	Bacterial overgrowth
	No vitamin B_{12} absorption	

Strategies to Maximize Intestinal Adaptation

Meal size	Grazing pattern with many small meals and snacks	
Carbohydrate	Enjoy complex carbohydrates; avoid simple sugars	
Protein	High biological value protein foods at most meals	
Fat	High fat to increase calorie absorption	Low fat to limit steatorrhea, calcium loss
	Avoid MCT supplements	Use MCT supplements
Fluids	Drink salty fluids for rehydration, avoid sugary fluids	
	Drink fluids 30–45 minutes after a solid foods meal	
Fiber	Soluble fiber to thicken ostomy effluent	Soluble fiber and resistant starch to increase kcal absorption
Supplements	Vitamin B_{12} injections	Vitamin B_{12} injections
	Multiple vitamin on noninfusion days	Oral calcium to bind fatty acids and oxalate

nutrient not available in PN regimens and deficiency of which has been associated with hepatic steatosis. Legumes, if individual patients tolerate them, may also enhance adaptation by their fermentation to short-chain fatty acids.

Dietary fat absorption is generally less efficient than that of protein and carbohydrates. Carbohydrate is absorbed at 61%–79% and protein at 61%–81% but fat at only 52%–54% of that ingested (10,15). The presence of both medium-chain and long-chain triglycerides increases the intestinal absorption of fat and total calories but reduces carbohydrate and protein absorption significantly in patients with no colon. As a result, medium chain triglyceride (MCT) supplements are only advised for patients with an intact colon (16). In addition, patients who have a colon in continuity risk development of calcium-oxalate renal stones when they ingest a high-fat diet. The excess unabsorbed fatty acids bind with dietary calcium, which would otherwise bind to dietary oxalate, preventing absorption in the colon. With less calcium available, more of this oxalate is absorbed.

Fruits that provide either resistant starch (fairly green bananas) or pectin (oranges, grapefruits, apples) are generally well tolerated and may slow transit or thicken stool (17). By contrast, fruit juices produce diarrhea due to the concentrated fructose content. Fruits that are sweet and semiliquid, such as watermelon, also produce diarrhea.

In the first 6 months after initial bowel resection, a limitation in oral fluid intake to 500–1000 mL daily in addition to use of proton pump inhibitors or histamine 2 antagonists may be needed to control intestinal fluid losses that are due to gastric hypersecretion (9). While a sense of thirst serves as the driving force for fluid intake in patients prior to SBS, limiting oral fluid intake and depending on intravenous fluid support is the most effective strategy after SBS. In addition, fluids taken orally are best absorbed when they contain salt (e.g., soup broth, rehydration fluids). The use of oral rehydration solution may be considered to defray fluid losses in SBS (18). Certainly, avoidance of hypotonic and hypertonic fluids is indicated (9). The fact that transit time is shorter with liquids than solids is the basis for holding fluid intake for 30–45 minutes after a meal in order to prevent wash through of solid foods, preventing digestion and absorption of nutrients. For patients who are able to eat an oral diet, but who have difficulty maintaining adequate urine output and are unable to consume oral rehydration solutions, nocturnal enteral rehydration may facilitate weaning from PN (12). Still others may be able to achieve adequate hydration by limiting total fluid intake, restricting both hypotonic and hypertonic fluids, while sipping isotonic oral rehydration solutions throughout the day and adding salt to the diet or to commercial sports drinks.

PHARMACOLOGIC MANAGEMENT

Pharmacologic management of the patient with SBS is complex. First, patients with SBS are just as likely to receive medication *not* directly related to their intestinal dysfunction as any other patient. The difference with these patients is that the limited surface area available may compromise the rate and/or extent of oral drug absorption. Second, there are specific medications administered to patients with SBS to minimize gastrointestinal symptoms. These include antisecretory and antimotility agents, resulting in enhanced nutrient absorption, as well as drugs whose goal is to promote gut adaptation. General guidelines for drug dosing in SBS have been reviewed elsewhere (19), but generally are best administered before meals. What follows is a review of medications specifically used in the management of patients with SBS.

Patients with SBS often present with hypergastrinemia and increased gastric and pancreatic secretions that further aggravate their fluid and electrolyte losses. Aside from volume loss, the risk for mucosal damage and ulceration also increases in this situation. These increased secretions are expected to decrease with time following a resection, however antisecretory medications are warranted. Several classes of drugs are available for use: histamine type-2 receptor antagonists (H2As) (e.g., famotidine, ranitidine), proton pump inhibitors (PPIs) (e.g., lansoprazole, pantoprazole), or somatostatin analogues (e.g., octreotide).

The H2As and PPIs can decrease gastric acid secretion or hypersecretion, thereby reducing gastric volume output; especially for patients classified as net secretors. Although tolerance to the effects of the H2As over time has been reported, the PPIs can offer a more effective reduction in secretions as they work at the final step of acid secretion. Generally these agents are most effective in patients with the highest outputs (>2.5 L daily). Although H2As and PPIs may be administered orally, intravenous administration is suggested for patients with less than 50 cm of jejunum remaining. The dosing for famotidine is 20–40 mg twice daily (oral), 40 mg daily (via PN), and for ranitidine is 150–300 mg twice daily (oral), 150 mg daily (via PN). The dosing for lansoprazole is 15–30 mg daily (oral), and for pantoprazole 40 mg daily (oral or intravenously but not via PN) (20). Any improvement of fat, carbohydrate, or nitrogen absorption as a consequence of using H2As or PPIs is not expected to be significant. Long-term suppression of gastric secretion can increase the risk for bacterial overgrowth with its own contribution to malabsorption, malabsorption of dietary vitamin B_{12}, and rarely D-lactic acidosis.

Octreotide may decrease output by as much as 30% by reducing stimulated gastric, biliary, and pancreatic secretions without significant impact on fat absorption (21). Initial dosing of octreotide is 50 µg two to three times daily by subcutaneous injection. Allowing the drug to warm to room temperature before administration may reduce the acute pain of the injection. Octreotide may best be reserved for patients with significant losses (>3–4 L daily), for a short-term trial at reducing output. Risks to the use of octreotide include gallstone formation, hyperglycemia or hypoglycemia, and potential interference with gut adaptation by suppressing secretion of needed growth factors.

The rapid transit of material through the intestinal lumen of patients with SBS is an indication for medication to reduce motility and enhance absorption. Opioid-like agents (e.g., loperamide) remain a cornerstone for managing rapid gastrointestinal transit in patients with SBS. Loperamide at a dose of 2–8 mg administered orally 15–45 minutes before a meal not only reduces motility, but may also reduce pancreaticobiliary secretions. The prolonged transit time allows for a 20%–30% decrease in volume loss. Because loperamide normally undergoes enterohepatic recirculation, any interruption of that process due to the combination of rapid transit with diminished absorptive surface area can require larger doses than used in patients without SBS. This drug infrequently exhibits systemic effects such as drowsiness and dry mouth. Less commonly used are opioid-agonists due to sedation and tolerance, and diphenoxylate with atropine due to adverse central nervous system CNS effects.

For some patients, the use of pancreatic enzymes may improve tolerance to oral intake. The enzymes should be taken before, during, and after meals at doses approximating 20,000–30,000 units of lipase from a nonenteric-coated formulation per meal. The enteric-coated products, which would normally allow for the enzymes to be protected at gastric pH and released in the higher pH of the small intestinal lumen, are more expensive than the immediate release products. Furthermore, with concurrent use of PPIs, the gastric pH would be elevated and in part defeat the value of using enteric-coated products. The use of cholestyramine to reduce bile acid–induced diarrhea is rarely well tolerated by patients with SBS and runs the risk of binding other medications and fat-soluble vitamins, although it remains of value in patients experiencing cholerrhea.

Beyond the symptomatic control of gastrointestinal complaints is the potential to enhance, structurally and functionally, intestinal adaptation through drug therapy. Although a number of growth factors have been studied in animal models, only growth hormone and glucagon-like peptide-2 have been evaluated in humans.

Growth hormone (GH), an anabolic and anticatabolic factor that supports total body protein synthesis, is one of several factors involved in the regulation of bowel proliferation (22). Its mechanism of action involves direct binding to specific tissue receptors as well as an indirect effect through increased production of insulin-like growth factors (i.e., IGF-1). These factors, in conjunction with their respective binding proteins, then interact with IGF receptors to initiate a cascade of events. Receptors for GH and IGF-1 can be found in a variety of tissues including the intestinal and colonic mucosa. The development of purified preparations of human GH by recombinant DNA technology for subcutaneous administration has allowed testing of this growth factor for various clinical applications. The evaluation of GH in patients with SBS has been surrounded by debate regarding the issues of combination therapy, patient selection, and dosing regimen.

As part of a rehabilitation program for patients with SBS requiring PN, GH in a regimen that included glutamine and dietary modification was associated with select improvements in nutrient absorption and reductions in PN requirements with a 14- to 28-day regimen (23–25). These patients had some of or their entire colon in continuity with a mean jejunoileal length of 37 cm (8–90 cm) in one unblinded trial (23) and a mean jejunoileal length of 23 cm (0–50 cm) in a case series (25). This is in contrast to most patients with no colon in continuity with a mean jejuno-ileal length of 71 cm (55–120 cm) in the randomized, double-blind, controlled trial (24). The results indicating improved sodium and potassium absorption in the latter trial occurred in the absence of any significant documented changes in mucosal morphology.

A trial examining the effect of GH (120 µg/kg/d) and glutamine in the absence of dietary modification in a small group of patients with SBS, half without colon in continuity, for a 28-day regimen revealed no benefit on nutrient absorption when evaluated a few days after discontinuing the regimen (26). This suggested that GH did not contribute significantly to the adaptation noted clinically in the previous studies or that any effects were only transient. Given the use of high doses in those trials (120–140 µg/kg/d) and their associated adverse effects, lower doses of GH were evaluated.

A small trial administered GH 24 µg/kg/d for 8 weeks, revealing increases in body weight and lean body mass, in parallel with increases in IGF levels, but no changes in absorptive capacity (27). The improvements in body composition dissipated after withdrawal of treatment. At a GH dose of 50 μg/kg/d administered subcutaneously for 21 days, benefits were observed in nutrient absorption, body weight, and lean body mass in a group of patients with SBS, 75% with residual colon and mean small bowel length of 48 cm (28). Of interest in this latter study, patients' spontaneous oral intake exceeded by ~20%–50% that in the studies mentioned previously.

Armed with these data and some unpublished information, the FDA approved a specific GH product for a 4-week regimen at a dose of 100 μg/kg/d administered subcutaneously (to a maximum of 8 mg daily) for use in PN-dependent adult patients with SBS as a means of reducing PN volume and caloric requirements (29). Trials of GH have typically excluded patients with cancer, diabetes, chronic renal impairment, and hepatic dysfunction. The drug is degraded renally with some hepatic metabolism as well. For clinical trials documenting increases in body weight and lean body mass, mechanisms other than enhanced nutrient absorption need to be clarified.

Aside from the questionable benefit on adaptation in several clinical reports, adverse effects of GH were evident. Virtually all patients receiving high-dose GH treatment (>50 μg/kg/d) experience some adverse event, although not all may be attributable to drug therapy (30). Adverse consequences of GH use that may respond to dose reduction include peripheral and facial edema and arthralgia with some patients requiring diuretics and analgesics, respectively (23–26). Less frequently reported are hyperglycemia, nausea, vomiting, rhinitis, chest pain, and pain at the site of injection. At doses ≥100 μg/kg in critically ill patients receiving adequate nutrition support, GH significantly increased mortality despite improvements in nitrogen balance and growth factor biomarkers (31), thus use of GH during critical illness or septic shock is not advised.

Glucagon-like peptide-2 (GLP-2) is a hormone that regulates food intake, gut motility, and nutrient absorption. This peptide is normally secreted, along with GLP-1, from the L-cells of the distal ileum and colon following a meal. The activity of GLP-2 is mediated through a G-protein–coupled receptor (GLP-2R) found predominantly in the gastrointestinal tract, as well as being found in the central nervous system and lung (32,33). The proliferative (crypt cells) and absorptive (villus) effects of GLP-2 are mediated by as yet unknown enteric neuronal signaling pathways and additionally may be region specific. The effect likely involves reduced gastric emptying and increased synthesis and function of nutrient transporters (e.g., sodium-glucose cotransporter [SGLT-1] and glucose transporters [GLUT-2]) at jejunoileal sites) (34). With the development of peptidase-resistant GLP-2 analogues that have a longer duration of effect than the naturally occurring peptide, utility in clinical trials has become more practical.

Administration of GLP-2 at a dose of 400 μg subcutaneously twice daily for 35 days to stable patients with SBS (no terminal ileum or colon, mean residual jejunal length 94 cm, 30–170 cm) resulted in increases in body weight and lean body mass (35). These changes were associated with significant increases in villus height/crypt depth, increased nutrient absorption, and reduced stomal output. Results of another pilot study suggest that GLP-2 administration also improves bone mineral density (36). A larger, multicenter controlled trial of a GLP-2 analogue, teduglutide, reported safety and tolerance of three doses, as well as significant improvement in intestinal fluid absorption (37).

Exogenous GLP-2 appears to be degraded at the proximal tubules with a hepatic component also possible, thus caution should be exercised in considering GLP-2 administration to patients with renal or hepatic impairment when the drug becomes clinically available (34). Although local erythema and tenderness at the injection site have been reported, no edema has been observed in patients receiving GLP-2 (35). Further data on adverse effects is expected.

The potential effect of growth factors on carcinogenesis needs to be clarified, although it is expected that GLP-2 is much more selective (organ specific) based on receptor distribution than with GH. Long-term safety data on both GH and GLP-2 in patients with SBS will be welcome, even as data on the efficacy of GLP-2, GH, or the combination in subsets of patients with SBS may be explored. Future trials will provide answers to the roles of these and still other growth factors in patients with SBS.

LONG-TERM EFFECTS OF PARENTERAL NUTRITION

The importance of weaning from PN, reducing the amount of PN, or decreasing the frequency of PN infusions cannot be overstated. Any reduction could help minimize the long-term negative effects of PN dependency, including risk of catheter-related infections, venous thrombosis, metabolic bone disease, PN-associated liver disease, and less optimal quality of life.

Catheter-Related Complications

The most common clinical problems associated with home PN are catheter-related complications including infections and thrombosis. Catheter-related bloodstream infections (CRBSI) can be life threatening. With a prevalence of 0.8 infections/1000 catheter days in adult home PN patients (38), CRBSI represent 61% of all PN-related complications (38,39) and may progress to complicated sepsis events and to half of all PN-related deaths (39). Repeated infections have also been correlated with liver disease (40).

Patient-specific risks of CRBSI have been described in a prospective observational study of 827 patients with 988 catheters for outpatient or home infusions over 69,532 catheter days (41). Independent risk factors include use of the catheter for PN (hazard ratio 4.1, 95% CI 2.3–7.2), use of a multilumen catheter (hazard ratio 2.8, 95% CI 1.7–4.7), and previous bloodstream infection (hazard ratio 2.5, 95% CI 1.5–4.2). CRBSI increased from 0.16/1000 catheter days in patients with none of the risk factors just listed to 0.46 with a single risk factor, to 2.22 with two risk factors and 6.77 for those with three or more risk factors (41). Of 42 adult home

PN patients, 50% of patients never had CRBSI over 44 months (2–171 months), while 12% had two, 7% had three, and 2% had eight CRBSI, with the first infection after 60 days (42). Clinical factors related to greater CRBSI included greater colonic resection, but not presence of a stoma (41), and shorter length of small bowel (43). Limiting the frequency of catheter manipulations or drawing blood through the catheter did not predict CRBSI, nor did age of catheter, needleless devices, transparent dressings, chlorhexidine use with dressing changes, antibiotic ointment under the dressing, heparin versus saline flushes, receipt of chemotherapy, diagnosis, age, or educational level of the patient (41).

Three general types of catheters are used commonly for PN infusion: tunneled external catheters, implanted reservoir catheters, and peripherally inserted central venous catheters (PICC). Although the infection risk is greater with multilumen than single-lumen catheters (41), risk is not different with double- than triple-lumen catheters (44). When only single-lumen catheters were used, no difference in CRBSI was observed between tunneled catheters and implanted ports (41,45). Thus, the use of single-lumen catheters may be more important than type of catheter in reducing risk of CRBSI.

Infection can occur due to contamination at the time of catheter insertion, migration of skin organisms along the catheter's surface, contamination of the lumen of the catheter, contaminated infusions, by seeping through the bloodstream from a distant site of infection (46), or by contamination of the catheter hub (47). Essentially all venous catheters develop biofilm on the surface, and longer-use catheters also develop biofilm on the inner lumen, but most are not associated with CRBSI (47). When CRBSI occurs, the infection is related to the number of organisms on the catheter tip. Suggested strategies to control biofilm on catheters include aseptic technique during catheter placement, topical antibiotics, using an in-line filter for intravenous fluids, using a cuffed catheter to create a mechanical barrier, and using catheters coated with antimicrobial agents.

The symptoms associated with CRBSI were fever in 84%, chills in 62%, erythema in 14%, and purulence at the catheter insertion site in 7% (41). In 56%, clinical signs were discrete and resulted in a delay of 6 days between first symptom and diagnosis (42). When patients complain of fever, malaise, chills, erythema, or purulence at the catheter insertion site, blood cultures should be drawn. If the patient is hemodynamically unstable or has a fever of >102°F, presentation to the hospital for evaluation is required, admission is probable, and catheter removal is possible (48). Regular screening for infection using quantitative blood cultures or endoluminal brushing was explored, but had a much lower yield than the more typical response to the appearance of clinical signs of infections (49).

The most common bloodstream infections were gram-positive cocci in 58% (coagulase-negative staphylococci, *Staphylococcus aureus,* enterococci, and corynebacteria); gram-negative rods in 32% (*Klebsiella, Escherichia coli, Acinetobacter,* and *Enterobacter* species); fungi in 10% (most commonly *Candida* species) and polymicrobial infections in 20% (50). Antibiotic therapy is directed against the organism based on its susceptibility. After the antibiotic treatment is completed, a peripheral blood culture should be drawn to assure that the infection is cleared.

Antibiotic locks, which consist of filling the catheter lumen with a concentrated antibiotic solution, have been suggested to treat or prevent infections. The Infectious Disease Society of America, American College of Critical Care Medicine, and Society for Healthcare Epidemiology of America guidelines suggest that with uncomplicated catheter infections with *S. aureus*, coagulase-negative staphylococci, or gram-negative bacilli, an antibiotic lock solution for 2 weeks might be used in addition to standard antibiotic therapy (38). If the patient deteriorates clinically while this therapy is ongoing, the catheter should be removed and antibiotic therapy continued. Most clinicians will remove the catheter for fungal or polymicrobial sepsis.

Venous Thrombosis

Thrombosis is estimated to occur at a rate of 0.03 to 0.04 times/catheter year (38), and superior or inferior vena cava syndromes are diagnosed only rarely. These thromboses occur more frequently in patients with clotting disorders, some malignancies, and mesenteric artery or vein thrombosis. When patients are not able to withdraw blood from the catheter, treatment with thrombolytics may dissolve the fibrin sheath around the catheter (48). Full therapeutic anticoagulation may be needed to prevent both catheter and venous thromboses for high-risk patients. If thromboses cannot be resolved or if superior or inferior vena cava syndrome develops, the catheter may need to be withdrawn and a new one placed at a different site. In a systematic review including five PRCT in 204 home PN patients was used heparin either as flush or as a component of the PN infusion. Thrombosis was not significantly different by heparin use (6% of catheters with heparin and 9% of those without) (51). Although no studies compared low-dose warfarin use in home PN patients, a systematic review of outcomes of this practice with cancer patients who have long-term catheters revealed that 1 mg/d warfarin reduced thromboses but kept prothrombin time within the reference range and heparin flush also reduced the risk. Because of a concern about the risk of bleeding with unmonitored minidose warfarin in cancer patients and the low risk (approximately 3%) of venous thrombosis, the ACCP currently recommends not to use minidose warfarin (52).

Metabolic Bone Disease

A high prevalence of bone disease has been described in patients with home PN dependence, using dual energy X-ray absorptiometry to measure bone mineral density (BMD). Osteopenia prevalence has been reported as 54% to 84% and osteoporosis as 33% to 67% (53–55). Recognition of patients at risk of osteoporosis may enable targeted risk reduction. Risk factors for bone disease in home PN patients are listed in Table 13–3.

Vitamin D deficiency causes a bone mineralization defect that results in increased parathyroid hormone (PTH) secretion, mobilization of calcium from bone and os-

Table 13–3 Risk Factors for Osteoporosis in Home PN Patients

Young age at PN initiation	Weight loss
Female	PN
Steroid use	Nicotine
Excess amino acid intake	Excess alcohol
Long PN duration	Heparin
Inflammatory bowel disease	Warfarin
Physical inactivity	Aluminum contaminants

Sources: (53,56,57)

---

teomalacia, with symptoms of bone and muscle pain and weakness (58). Because vitamin D is needed for calcium absorption, monitoring vitamin D status regularly in this high-risk patient group is important.

Although there is no consensus on optimal serum levels of vitamin D, 25(OH)D levels >30 µg/L (>75 nmol/L) are needed to maximize calcium absorption and vitamin action (59). At levels of 25(OH)D <8 µg/L (<20 nmol/L), osteomalacia has been reported, and values <20 µg/L (<50 nmol/L) have been associated with low BMD, reduced calcium absorption, and a decrease in lower extremity function. In a study of 42 patients with no home PN, the mean 25(OH)D concentration was found to be 13.4 µg/mL (33.5 nmol/L); in 16 (38%) of these patients, it was <8 µg/L (<20 nmol/L) and was associated with elevated PTH and reduced BMD (54).

Attaining adequate vitamin D, calcium, and magnesium intake can be challenging in patients with SBS. Intravenous vitamin D is no longer available as a single entity product. Patients exhibit deficiency in spite of the vitamin D content (5 µg) provided in standard intravenous multivitamin preparations. Although toxicity of vitamin D from oral supplementation is unlikely in patients with SBS, toxicity has been seen in subjects taking more than 250 µg daily. The adequate intake level is 10 µg (400 IU) for adults under 70 years and 15 µg for adults over 70 years (60). The richest food sources of vitamin D are fortified milk and fatty fish.

Absorption of calcium, phosphorus, and magnesium may be limited, even with adequate vitamin D status. Absorption of calcium and magnesium from food in patients with SBS is only 10%–14% and 5%, respectively (61). Both food sources (leafy greens) and oral magnesium supplements exacerbate diarrhea.

Although calcium, phosphorus, and magnesium are added to PN, a disadvantage to adding excess amounts is the risk of incompatibility and aluminum toxicity from contaminants in these products (62), thus, oral calcium carbonate supplements are encouraged.

Regular measurement of vitamin D, PTH with concurrent calcium, magnesium, phosphorus, albumin, and alkaline phosphatase are recommended to adjust nutrient intake. In addition, more frequent monitoring of serum bone minerals is usual practice. A practice guideline for management of bone disease in patients with SBS is in Table 13–4.

Medicare covers the cost of BMD testing every 2 years for estrogen-deficient women, individuals with vertebral abnormalities, those receiving long-term steroid therapy, those with primary hyperparathyroidism, and to monitor the response or efficacy of approved osteoporosis treatment (63). Although guidelines for the home PN patient have not been established, a baseline scan to monitor BMD within the first year of PN support and semiannual scans thereafter is the established practice at many medical centers, including the Hospital of the University of Pennsylvania.

With the recent availability of antiresorptive (bisphosphonates) and bone-forming (teriparatide) agents, treatment of bone disease for patients with SBS holds promise. Adequacy of vitamin D status should be assured prior to initiating antiresorptive therapy, because osteomalacia will not respond to the antiresorptive medication and the treatment will actually worsen osteomalacia. A case report described subclinical osteomalacia due to vitamin D deficiency that resulted in life-threatening hypocalcemia after intravenous bisphosphonate therapy (64).

PN-Associated Liver Disease

The prevalence of PN-associated liver disease in adults (PNALD) is 3% after 5 (65) and 15% after 19 years (66). Death due to PNALD occurred an average of 10.8

Table 13–4 Guidelines for Management of Bone Disease in Home PN Patients

Prevention	Monitoring	Treatment
• Screen for osteoporosis risk • Limit smoking and alcohol use • Ensure adequate Ca, Mg, P, vitamin D intake • Optimize protein intake • Encourage walking, weight lifting • Evaluate vision, hearing, and medication profile for patients with falls	• Obtain regular serum calcium, phosphorus, and magnesium serum; adjust intake as needed • Obtain vitamin D, PTH every 6 months • Obtain baseline BMD • Obtain BMD every 2 years	• Assure normal 25 (OH) D status • Consider intravenous bisphosphonates or teriparatide for patients with osteoporosis

months after the initial bilirubin elevation. Intestinal and/or liver transplantation may soon become a more viable option for many patients (67).

PNALD is multifactorial and can be attributed to the underlying disease process, anatomical changes, and PN-related factors. Repeated septic events and persistent inflammatory states (66), intestinal resections that disrupt enterohepatic circulation, and small bowel bacterial overgrowth due to intestinal stasis (40) have all been associated with PNALD.

Other factors implicated in PNALD development include overfeeding as well as 24-hour infusions that do not allow export of fat from the liver during fasting. In home PN patients, total caloric and glucose supply were correlated with abnormal liver enzymes and inflammatory markers (68). Table 13–5 describes a practice guideline for management of PNALD.

Lipid dose and phytosterol contaminants have been associated with PNALD. Lipid intake of 0.6 g/kg/d was not (68), while lipid >1 g/kg/d was associated with PNALD (69). With severe SBS, essential fatty acid deficiency occurs rapidly with inadequate lipid intake, and symptoms include steatosis, hepatomegaly, and thrombocytopenia (70). Phytosterol contaminants in intravenous lipid infusions accumulate with PNALD (71) and occur in lesser concentration in 20% than in 10% lipid emulsion.

Table 13–5 Guidelines for Management of PN-Associated Liver Disease

Prevention	Monitoring	Treatment
• Prevent catheter sepsis • Avoid overfeeding PN kcal, glucose, lipid • Infuse PN in light-protected conditions • Cycle infusion • Encourage oral choline intake • Avoid manganese or copper toxicity	• Monitor liver enzymes and bilirubin monthly to quarterly • Monitor carnitine status if liver function tests are abnormal or patient c/o myopathy, hypoglycemia • Monitor whole blood manganese, and serum copper q 6 months	• Refer for transplantation evaluation • Consider trial of ursodeoxycholic acid • Minimize lipid dose in PN to 0.6 g/kg/day • Use 20% rather than 10% lipid emulsions • Monitor carnitine status • Monitor manganese and copper levels and remove manganese or copper from PN if elevated, recheck levels quarterly

Deficiencies of choline and carnitine have each been associated with PNALD. Provision of choline in PN to patients with hepatic steatosis significantly improved steatosis after 4 weeks and liver enzymes after 24 weeks (72). Unfortunately, no clinical laboratory assay for choline status or intravenous source of choline is currently available.

Carnitine deficiency is a risk with established PNALD since the final step of carnitine biosynthesis occurs exclusively in the liver (73). Case reports have described cholestasis, muscle weakness, and low-serum carnitine that respond to carnitine supplementation (74). Neurological signs may include encephalopathy, lethargy, somnolence, confusion, stupor, or coma; hypoglycemia is also possible. Intravenous carnitine is available for addition to PN.

Toxicity of manganese (Mn) and copper (Cu) can occur as a result of excess supply or limited biliary excretion due to PNALD. In 24 home PN patients, hypermanganesemia was related to liver enzyme elevation (75). In 12 adult home PN patients, a dose-finding trial suggested that 0.05 mg/d was associated with minimal brain Mn accumulation and lack of deficiency by whole blood Mn (76). Because no available multitrace element preparation meets the recommendation of 0.05 mg/d Mn while providing adequate intake of Cu, zinc, chromium, and selenium for adult patients (77), selection of a 0.1 mg/d preparation with regular monitoring of whole blood Mn concentration is suggested.

In 28 home PN patients undergoing liver biopsies for abnormal liver enzymes, quantitative hepatic Cu was elevated in 89% and correlated with bilirubin and AST, but not serum Cu. However, elimination of Cu during PNALD should not be employed without monitoring Cu status regularly, because copper *deficiency* is associated with pancytopenia (78) and anemia (79). If the whole blood Mn or serum Cu becomes elevated, individual doses of zinc, chromium, and selenium can be added, but the cost and time involved are considerable.

Biochemical measures of liver function are frequently abnormal in home PN patients and do not reflect the degree of liver injury. When biopsy specimens were compared in 51 patients with normal ALT, the entire histologic spectrum of nonalcoholic fatty liver disease, of which PNALD is a subset, was seen and was not different from those with an elevated ALT (80). Thus, liver biopsy should be an early part of the PNALD evaluation. In fact, some clinical groups order liver biopsy when the liver enzymes or bilirubin remain >1.5 times the upper limit of normal for more than 3 months (68,69).

Ursodeoxycholic acid (UDCA), a naturally occurring bile acid, is normally present at approximately 5% concentration in the intestinal lumen and is efficiently taken up by the liver and secreted into bile, increasing bile flow and secretion of bile acids (81). Reducing cholestasis by promoting bile flow and secretion of bile acids may reduce chronic toxicity to hepatic cell membranes, correct abnormal immune responses, and/or reduce stimuli for chronic inflammation, resulting in fibrosis and cirrhosis. In data from four open-label pilot studies using synthetic ursodiol (Actigall) representing 103 patients, most of whom had normal gastrointestinal function, liver enzymes improved after UDCA therapy over 6–12 months; however, improvement in histology was not impressive (79). Because the absorption of synthetic UDCA in patients with SBS is not known, expected therapeutic effects cannot be predicted.

Quality of Life

Published quality of life (QOL) scores of patients receiving home PN are generally lower than healthy individuals, patients with intestinal disease who are not receiving home PN, and renal transplant recipients (82). Physical function resulting in impaired performance status, inability to conduct activities of daily living, and not being able to be meaningfully employed appear to influence overall QOL in home PN patients (82–85). Worsening of QOL is associated with unemployment status, having an external catheter, younger age, having an active complication of the primary disease and a high hospitalization rate, having an intestinal motility disorder, male sex, and number of PN infusions (86). Poor QOL is also associated with length of time on home PN, family coping skills, and financial concerns (87). Better QOL is associated with higher self-esteem, quality relationships, and affiliation with the Oley Foundation (88).

Being dependent on home PN influences lifestyle and activities. While PN-dependent individuals view PN as life-sustaining therapy, still many adaptations and adjustments in their lives must be made. Table 13–6 outlines concerns of patients on home PN.

Clinicians can do many things to support their patients in dealing with lifelong dependency on home PN. A frank discussion of how PN is impacting both physical and psychological health is valuable. Knowledge of the patient's lifestyle, family, and support system should help guide the choice of venous access device and PN administration schedule. Lifestyle concerns should be identified and discussed at each follow-up visit in the clinic, physician's office, or home. Depression should be diagnosed and treated. The benefit of patient support groups should be promoted. The Oley Foundation (*www.oley.org*) is a valuable national support group for home EN and PN consumers that provides up-to-date information, outreach services, conference activities, free educational materials, and emotional support to patients, families, caregivers, and professionals. QOL should be monitored at baseline and periodically reassessed throughout duration of home PN.

INTESTINAL TRANSPLANTATION

Intestinal transplantation is a viable option for patients with severe SBS who have severe PN-related complications. Recurrent catheter sepsis, loss of major venous access sites, progressive liver dysfunction, and impaired renal function due to massive GI losses are indications for intestinal transplantation (89). Early referral to a center that specializes in intestinal transplantation is recommended in order to provide optimal management in the pretransplant phase of care.

Table 13–6 Concerns of Patients Dependent on Home PN

Being a burden or dependent on others
Sleep deprivation
Energy level
Feeling alone
Body image
Sexual drive
Missing out on activities due to infusion schedule
Need for further surgery
Worrying about infection
Fear of catheter dislodgement
Worry over pump malfunction or alarms
Being hooked up to the equipment
Weight of the pump and backpack
Fear of liver dysfunction
Running out of access
Losing insurance
Loss of the ability to eat or share meals
Disruption in traveling, leisure activities, and social life

Sources: (87,90–94)

Successful intestinal transplantation has been reported as early as 4–12 months after initial SBS and prior to PNALD (95). The early referral of patients with extreme SBS (<50 cm SB) who are unlikely to wean from PN but are at high risk of PNALD might yield greater success with intestinal transplantation because the patients are not ill and donor livers could be reserved for those with isolated liver disease (96). In more typical practice, patients are referred for liver and small bowel transplant evaluation when PNALD is progressive (sustained elevations in liver enzymes; histologic fibrosis or cirrhosis; and hepatomegaly). The transplant surgeon must decide whether an isolated intestine graft will permit the patient's native liver to recover function or combined liver and small bowel grafts are needed. Thus thorough evaluation of degree of liver injury and referral once the pattern is clear is a very important practice.

SBS was the most common indication for transplantation in a recent summary of what is believed to be all intestinal transplants worldwide between April 1985 and May 2003 (67). Patient and graft survival rates have improved significantly since 1998, with current levels of 65%–77% small intestine alone versus 60% with small bowel and liver (67). Of the patients surviving more than 6 months at the point of data collection, 81% (328) remained off PN, 3.9% required intravenous fluids, and 6.4% required partial PN (67). Intestinal transplantation is associated with improved Karnofsky performance scores (97) and allows a patient to resume a more normal lifestyle and to experience improved QOL (92,98). Compared to patients with complicated intestinal failure, QOL as it relates to energy level, emotional status, and physical function was significantly better following small bowel transplantation (82). Quality of life alone is not a current indication for intestinal transplantation; however; it is expected to become more common as transplantation risks are minimized and results improve.

CONCLUSION

Management of the complexities of SBS can be challenging because of the underlying disease, metabolic sequelae, and lifelong dependency on home PN. A holistic approach that considers physiological factors, the patient's ability to adhere to dietary and medical treatments, potential complications, and QOL will provide the most satisfying outcomes for the patient and the clinical staff.

REFERENCES

1. Grant JP. Anatomy and physiology of the gastrointestinal tract. In: Matarese LE, Steiger E, Seidner DL, eds. *Intestinal Failure and Rehabilitation—A Clinical Guide.* Boca Raton, Fla.: CRC Press; 2005.

2. Cleveland Clinic Foundation. Short bowel syndrome: Etiology, pathophysiology and management; 2003.

3. Buchman AL, Scolapio J, Fryer J. AGA technical review on short bowel syndrome and intestinal transplantation. *Gastroenterology.* 2003;124:1111–1134.

4. Thompson JS, Langnas AN. Small intestinal insufficiency and the short bowel syndrome. In: Zuidema GD, Yeo CJ, eds. *Shackelford's Surgery of the Alimentary Tract.* 5th ed. Toronto, Canada: W.B. Saunders Company; 2002.

5. Woolf GM, Miller C, Kurian R, Jeejeebhoy KN. Diet for patients with a short bowel syndrome: Evaluation of fluid, calorie, and divalent cation requirements. *Dig Dis Sci.* 1983;32:8–15.

6. Jeppesen PB, Mortensen PB. Intestinal failure defined by measurements of intestinal energy and wet weight absorption. *Gut.* 2000;46:701–706.

7. Nightingale JM, Lennard-Jones JE, Gertner DJ, Wood SR, Bartram CI. Colonic preservation reduces need for parenteral therapy, increases incidence of renal stones, but does not change high prevalence of gall stones in patients with a short bowel. *Gut.* 1992;33:1493–1497.

8. Merritt RJ. *The ASPEN Nutrition Support Practice Manual.* Silver Spring, Md: American Society for Parenteral and Enteral Nutrition; 1998.

9. Buchman AL. The clinical management of short bowel syndrome: Steps to avoid parenteral nutrition. *Nutrition.* 1997;13:907–913.

10. Woolf GM, Miller C, Kurian R, Jeejeebhoy KN. Nutritional absorption in short bowel syndrome evaluation of fluid, calorie, and divalent cation requirements. *Dig Dis Sci.* 1987;32:8–15.

11. DiBaise JK, Young RJ, Vanderhoof JA. Intestinal rehabilitation and the short bowel syndrome. Part 2. *Am J Gastroenterol.* 2004;99:1823–1832.

12. ASPEN Board of Directors, Force. CGT. Guidelines for the use of parenteral and enteral nutrition in adult and pediatric patients. *JPEN.* 2002;26(1 suppl):1SA–138SA.

13. Crenn P, Morin MC, Joly F, Penven S, Thuillier F, Messing B. Net digestive absorption and adaptive hyperphagia in adult short bowel patients. *Gut.* 2005;53:1279–1286.

14. Nordgard I, Hansen BS, Mortensen PB. Importance of colonic support for energy absorption as small-bowel failure proceeds. *Am J Clin Nutr.* 1996;64:222–231.

15. Messing B, Pigot F, Rongier M, Morin MC, Neindoum U, Rambaud JC. Intestinal absorption of free oral hyperalimentation in the very short bowel syndrome. *Gastroenterol.* 1991;100:1502–1508.

16. Jeppesen PB, Mortensen PB. The influence of a preserved colon on the absorption of medium chain fat in patients with small bowel resection. *Gut.* 1998;43:478–483.

17. Rabbani GH, Teka T, Saha SK, et al. Green banana and pectin improve small intestinal permeability and reduce fluid loss in Bangladeshi children with persistent diarrhea. *Dig Dis Sci.* 2004; 49:475–484.

18. MacMahon RL. The use of the World Health Organization's oral rehydration solution in home parenteral nutrition patients. *JPEN.* 1984;8:720–731.

19. Speerhas RA BA, Wagner S. Medication delivery in intestinal failure. In: Matarese LE SE, Seidner DL, eds. *Intestinal Failure and Rehabilitation: A Clinical Guide.* Boca Raton, Fla.: CRC Press; 2005:321–332.

20. *AHFS Drug Information Essentials.* Bethesda, Md.:American Society of Health-System Pharmacists, 2006.

21. Huan-Long Q, Zhen-Dong S, Yang Z, You-Ben F. Effect of parenteral and enteral nutrition combined with octreotide on pancreatic exocrine secretion of patients with pancreatic fistula. *World J Gastroenterol.* 2004;10(16):2419–2422.

22. Ulshen MH, Dowling RH, Fuller CR, et al. Enhanced growth of small-bowel in transgenic mice overexpressing bovine growth hormone. *Gastroenterology.* 1993;104:973–980.

23. Byrne TA, Morrissey TB, Nattakom TV, Ziegler TR, Wilmore DW. Growth hormone, glutamine, and a modified diet enhance nutrient absorption in patients with severe short bowel syndrome. *JPEN.* 1995;19:296–602.

24. Scolapio JS, Camilleri M, Fleming CR, et al. Effect of growth hormone, glutamine and diet on adaptation in short-bowel syndrome: A randomized controlled study. *Gastroenterology.* 1997;113:1074–1081.

25. Wilmore DW, Lacey JM, Soultanakis RP, et al. Factors predicting a successful outcome after pharmacologic bowel compensation. *Ann Surg.* 1997;226:288–293.

26. Skudlarek J, Jeppesen PB, Mortensen PB. Effect of high dose growth hormone with glutamine and no change in diet on intestinal absorption in short bowel patients: A randomized, double blind, crossover, placebo controlled study. *Gut.* 2000;47:199–205.

27. Ellegard L, Bosaeus I, Nordgren S, Bengtsson BA. Low-dose recombinant human growth hormone increases body weight and lean body mass in patients with short bowel syndrome. *Ann Surg.* 1997;225:88–96.

28. Seguy D, Vahedi K, Kapel N, et al. Low-dose growth hormone in adult home parenteral nutrition-dependent short bowel syndrome patients: A positive study. *Gastroenterol.* 2003;124:293–302.

29. Serono, Inc. Somatropin (rDNA origin) for injection (Zorbtive). Full prescribing information; 2003. Available at: www.fda.gov/cder/foi/label/2003/20604s026_zorbtive_lbl.pdf. Accessed October 1, 2005.

30. Keating GM, Wellington K. Somatropin (Zorbtive) in short bowel syndrome. *Drugs.* 2004;64: 1375–1381.

31. Ruokonen E, Takala J. Dangers of growth hormone therapy in critically ill patients. *Curr Opin Clin Nutr Metab Care.* 2002;5:199–209.

32. Baggio LL, Drucker DJ. Glucagon-like peptide-1 and glucagon-like peptide-2. *Best Pract Res Clin Endocrinol Metab.* 2004;18:531–554.

33. Mayo KE, Miller LJ, Bataille D, et al. International union of pharmacology, XXXV: The glucagon receptor family. *Pharmacol Rev.* 2003;55:167–194.

34. Thulesen J. Glucagon-like peptide 2 (GLP-2), an intestinotrophic mediator. *Curr Protein Peptide Sci.* 2004;5:51–65.

35. Jeppesen PB HB, Thulesen J, et al. Glucagon-like peptide 2 improves nutrient absorption and nutritional status in short-bowel patents with no colon. *Gastroenterology.* 2001;120:806–815.

36. Haderslev KV, Jeppesen PB, Hartmann B, et al. Short-term administration of glucagons-like peptide-2: Effects on bone mineral density and markers of bone turnover in short-bowel patients with no colon. *Scand J Gastroenterol.* 2002;37:392–398.

37. Jeppesen PB, Sanguinetti EL, Buchman AL, et al. Teduglutide (ALX-600), a dipeptidyl peptidase IV resistant glucagon-like peptide 2 analogue, improves intestinal function in short bowel syndrome. *Gut.* 2005;54:1224–1231.

38. Buchman AL. Complications of long-term home total parenteral nutrition: Their identification, prevention and treatment. *Dig Dis Sci.* 2001;46:1–18.

39. Van Gossum A, Vahedi K, Abdel M, et al. Clinical, social and rehabilitation status of long-term home parenteral nutrition patients: Results of a European multicentre survey. *Clin Nutr.* 2001; 20:205–210.

40. Kaufman SS, Gondolesi GE, Fishbein TM. Parenteral nutrition associated liver disease. *Sem Neonatol.* 2003;8:375–381.

41. Tokars JI, Cookson ST, McArthur MA, Boyer CL, McGeer AJ, Jarvis WR. Prospective evaluation of risk factors for bloodstream infection in patients receiving home infusion therapy. *Ann Intern Med.* 1999;131:340–347.

42. Reimund J, Duclos B, Cuby C, et al. Home parenteral nutrition: Clinical and laboratory analysis of initial experience (1994–1997). Implications for patient management. *Ann Nutr Metab.* 1999; 43:329–338.

43. Terra RM, Plopper C, Waitzberg DL, et al. Remaining small bowel length: Association with catheter sepsis in patients receiving home total parenteral nutrition: Evidence of bacterial translocation. *World J Surg.* 2000;24:1537–1541.

44. Ma TY, Yoshinaka R, Banaag A. Total parenteral nutrition via multilumen catheters does not increase the risk of catheter-related sepsis: A randomized, prospective study. *Clin Infect Dis.* 1998; 27:500–503.

45. Bozzetti F, Mariani L, Boggio Bertinen D, et al. Central venous catheter complications in 447 patients on home parenteral nutrition: An analysis of over 100,000 catheter days. *Clin Nutr.* 2002; 21:475–485.

46. O'Grady MP, Alexander M, Patchen Dellinger E, et al. Guidelines for the prevention of intravascular catheter-related infections. *MMWR.* 2002;51(RR11):1–26.

47. Donlan RM. Biofilm formation: A clinically relevant microbiological process. *Clin Infect Dis.* 2001;33:1387–1392.

48. Grant J. Recognition and treatment of home parenteral nutrition central venous access complications. *JPEN.* 2002;26:S21–S28.

49. Mermel LA, Farr BM, Sherertz RJ, et al. Guidelines for the management of intravascular catheter-related infections. *Clin Infect Dis.* 2001;32:1249–1272.

50. Carratala J. The antibiotic-lock technique for therapy of "highly needed" infected catheters. *Clin Microbiol Infect.* 2002;8:282–289.

51. Klerk CPW, Smorenburg SM, Buller HR. Thrombosis prophylaxis in patient populations with a central venous catheter. *Arch Intern Med.* 2003;163:1913–1921.

52. Geerts MD, Pineo GF, Heit JA, et al. The seventh ACCP conference on antithrombotic and thrombolytic therapy: Evidence-based guidelines. *Chest.* 2004;127:338S–400S.

53. Cohen-Solal M, Baudoin F, Joly K, et al. Osteoporosis in patients on long-term home parenteral nutrition: A longitudinal study. *J Bone Miner Res.* 2003;18:1989–1998.

54. Haderslev K, Jeppesen PB, Sorensen HA, Mortensen PB. Vitamin D status in patients with small intestinal resection. *Gut,* 2003;52:653–658.

55. Pironi L, Moreselli Labate AM, Pertkiewicz M, et al. Prevalence of bone disease in patients on home parenteral nutrition. *Clin Nutr.* 2002;21:289–296.

56. National Osteoporosis Foundation. Osteoporosis: Impact and overview; 2005. Available at: www.NationalOsteoporosisFoundation.org. Accessed September 15, 2005.

57. Iwamoto J, Takeda T, Sato Y. Effects of vitamin K_2 on osteoporosis. *Curr Pharm Des.* 2004;10: 2557–2576.

58. Heaney RP. The vitamin D requirement in health and disease. *J Steroid Biochem Mol Biol* [online]. 2005:1–7.

59. Reginster J-Y. The high prevalence of inadequate serum vitamin D levels and implications for bone health. *Curr Med Res Opin.* 2005;21:579–585.

60. NAS I. *Dietary Reference Intakes for Calcium, Magnesium, Phosphorus, Magnesium, Vitamin D, and Fluoride.* Washington, D.C.: Institute of Medicine; 1997.

61. Haderslev KV, Jeppesen PB, Mortensen PB, Staun M. Absorption of calcium and magnesium in patients with intestinal resections treated with medium chain fatty acids. *Gut.* 2000;46:819–823.

62. Canada T. Aluminum exposure through parenteral nutrition formulations: Mathematical versus clinical relevance. *Am J Health-Syst Pharm.* 2005;62:315–318.

63. DoHHSDCfMMS. Medicare Benefit Policy. CMS Manual System. 2004;Pub 100-02:1–2.

64. Rosen C, Brown S. Severe hypocalcemia after intravenous bisphosphonate therapy in occult vitamin D deficiency. *N Engl J Med.* 2003;348:1503–1514.

65. Jeppesen PB, Staun M, Mortensen PB. Adult patients receiving home parenteral nutrition in Denmark from 1991 to 1996: Who will benefit from intestinal transplantation? *Scand J Gastroenterol.* 1998;338:839–846.

66. Chan S, McCowen KC, Bistrian BR, et al. Incidence, prognosis, and etiology of end-stage liver disease in patients receiving home total parenteral nutrition. *Surgery.* 1999;126:28–34.

67. Grant D, Abu-Elmagd K, Reyes J, et al. 2003 report of the intestine transplant registry. A new era has dawned. *Ann Surg.* 2005;241:607–613.

68. Reimund J-M, Duclos B, Arondel Y, Baumann R. Persistent inflammation and immune activation contribute to cholestasis in patients receiving home parenteral nutrition. *Nutrition.* 2001;17: 300–304.

69. Cavicchi M, Beau P, Crenn P, Degott C, Messing B. Prevalence of liver disease and contributing factors in patients receiving home parenteral nutrition for permanent intestinal failure. *Ann Intern Med.* 2000;132:525–532.

70. Fong DG, Nehra V, Lindor KD, Buchman AL. Metabolic and nutritional considerations in nonalcoholic fatty liver. *Hepatology.* 2000;32:3–11.

71. Iyer KR, Spitz L, Clayton P. BAPS prize lecture: New insight into mechanisms of parenteral nutrition-associated cholestasis: Role of plant sterols. British Association of Paediatric Surgeons. *J Pediatr Surg.* 1998;33(1):1–6.

72. Buchman AL, Ament ME, Sohel M, et al. Choline deficiency causes reversible hepatic abnormalities in patients receiving parenteral nutrition: Proof of a human choline requirement: A placebo-controlled trial. *JPEN.* 2001;25:260–268.

73. Krahenbuhl S. Carnitine metabolism in chronic liver disease. *Life Sci.* 1996;59:1579–1599.

74. Worthley LIG, Fishlock RC, Snoswell AM. Carnitine deficiency with hyperbilirubinemia, generalized skeletal muscle weakness and reactive hypoglycemia in a patient on long-term total parenteral nutrition: Treatment with intravenous $_L$-carnitine. *JPEN.* 1983;7:176–180.

75. Takagi Y, Okada A, Sando K, Masafumi W, Yoshida H, Hirabuki N. On-off study of manganese administration to adult patients undergoing home parenteral nutrition: New indicies in *in vivo* manganese level. *JPEN.* 2001;25:87–92.

76. Takagi Y, Okada A, Sando K, Wasa M, Yoshida H, Hirabuki N. Evaluation of indexes of in vivo manganese status and the optimal intravenous dose for adult patients undergoing home parenteral nutrition. *Am J Clin Nutr.* 2002;75:112–118.

77. Dickerson RN. Manganese intoxication and parenteral nutrition. *Nutrition.* 2001;17:689–693.

78. Fuhrman MP, Hermann V, Masidonski P, Eby C. Pancytopenia after removal of copper from total parenteral nutrition. *JPEN.* 2000;24:361–366.

79. Spiegel JE, Willenbucher RF. Rapid development of severe copper deficiency in a patient with Crohn's disease receiving parenteral nutrition. *JPEN*. 1999;23:169–172.

80. Mofrad P, Contos MJ, Haque M, et al. Clinical and histologic spectrum of nonalcoholic fatty liver disease associated with normal ALT values. *Hepatology*. 2003;37:1286–1292.

81. Angulo P. Use of ursodeoxycholic acid in patients with liver disease. *Curr Gastroenterol Rep*. 2002;4:37–44.

82. Cameron EAB, Binnie JAH, Jamieson NV, Pollard S, Middleton SJ. Quality of life in adults following small bowel transplantation. *Transplant Proc*. 2002;34:965–976.

83. Richards DM, Irving MH. Assessing the quality of life of patients with intestinal failure on home parenteral nutrition. *Gut*. 1997;40:218–222.

84. Jeppesen PB, Langholz E, Mortensen PB. Quality of life in patients receiving home parenteral nutrition. *Gut*. 1999;44:844–852.

85. DeFrancesco A, Boggio BD, Fadda M, Gallenca P, Mlafi G, Palmo A. Long-term parenteral nutrition in adults: Outcomes and quality of life. *Clin Nutr*. 2001;20(S):3–5.

86. Pironi L, Paganelli F, Mosconi P, et al. The SF-36 instrument for the follow-up of health-related quality-of-life assessment of patients undergoing home parenteral nutrition for benign disease. *Transplant Proc*. 2004;3:254–258.

87. Smith CE. Quality of life in long-term total parenteral nutrition patients and their family caregivers. *JPEN*. 1993;17:501–506.

88. Smith CE, Curtas S, Werkowitch M, Leinbeck SVM, Howard L. Home parenteral nutrition: Does affiliation with a national support and educational organization improve patient outcomes? *JPEN*. 2002;26:159–163.

89. Fryer JP. The role of intestinal transplantation in the management of intestinal failure. *Curr Gastroenterol Rep*. 2001;3(4):334–342.

90. Malone M. Longitudinal assessment of outcome, health status, and changes in lifestyle associated with long-term home parenteral and enteral nutrition. *JPEN*. 2002;26:164–168.

91. Ehrenpreis B, Hilf A. Home parenteral nutrition: The consumer's perspective. *Support Line*. 2004;27:21–23.

92. DiMartini A, Rovera GM, Graham TO, et al. Quality of life after small intestinal transplantation and among home parenteral nutrition patients. *JPEN*. 1998;22:357–362.

93. Silver HJ. The lived experience of home total parenteral nutrition: An online qualitative inquiry with adults, children, and mothers. *Nutr Clin Pract*. 2004;19:297–304.

94. Lehoux P, Saint-Arnaud J, Richard L. The use of technology at home: What patient manuals say and sell vs. what patients face and fear. *Soc Health Illness*. 2004;26:617–644.

95. Benedetti E, Testa G, Sankary H, et al. Successful treatment of trauma-induced short bowel syndrome with early living related bowel transplantation. *J Trauma*. 2004;57:164–170.

96. Abu-Elmagd K, Bond G. Gut failure and abdominal visceral transplantation. *Proc Nutr Soc*. 2003;62:727–737.

97. Horslen SM, Sudan D. Long-term outcomes in small bowel transplantation: Survival, nutrition, growth, and quality of life. *Curr Opin Organ Transplantation*. 2003;8:202–208.

98. Rovera GM, Sileri P, Rastellini C, Knight P, Benedetti E, Cicalese L. Quality of life after living related small bowel transplantation. *Transplant Proc*. 2002;34:967–968.

CHAPTER 14

Nutritional Aspects of Wound Healing

Marsha Stieber, MSA, RD, CNSD

INTRODUCTION

The interrelationships between nutrition and wound healing have been a topic of significant interest and debate for centuries, from mothers and wives encouraging their loved ones to eat if they wished to heal, to dietary supplements and medical nutritional product manufacturers developing and promoting their respective products to optimize the rapidity and completeness of the healing of wounds. Interest in and debate over nutrition's role, if any, in wound healing continues to thrive in the 21st century. However, advancements in clearly identifying nutrition's function in the physiologic and anatomic healing or nonhealing of wounds have been slowed by the paucity of random, double-blind, placebo-controlled studies with homogenous components and concise end points; thus, a clearly defined nutritional intervention road map the clinician can safely and confidently follow is unavailable. The use of best clinical judgment remains the wisest course of action.

This chapter will focus on the relationship between nutrition and wound healing in the adult human. To begin, a brief overview of frequently used wound terminology, wound categories, and the integumentary system will be provided to establish a common foundation upon which the discussion of nutrition's role in wound management is constructed. This synopsis is meant to offer guidance in understanding the contents of the chapter and is not intended to eradicate and/or replace currently available knowledge, methods, procedures, or standards.

AN OVERVIEW OF WOUND HEALING

Wound Terminology

A variety of terms frequently are used in discussing wounds and wound care. To clarify the meaning of some of those terms within this chapter, the following definitions are used:

> *Wound* (noun): any physical injury involving a break in the skin, usually caused by an act or accident rather than by a disease; includes a chest, gunshot, or puncture wound
> *Wound* (verb): to cause an injury, especially one that breaks the skin
> *Wound care*: a nursing intervention from the Nursing Interventions Classification (NIC) defined as prevention of wound complications and promotion of wound healing
> *Wound healing*: a process to restore to a state of soundness any injury that results in an interruption in the continuity of external surfaces of the body (1)

Wound Categories

The most well-known and widely accepted categories of wounds are: pressure ulcers, traumatic wounds, surgical wounds, and pathophysiologic wounds. Although there are healing and management commonalities amongst these wound categories, the etiology of each is distinctly different (see Table 14–1).

Integumentary System

Within the practice of nutrition and nutrition science, there is often times an inclination to overlook the physiology and anatomy of the integumentary system as a crucial functional unit of wound management. Instead, there is a tendency to focus on outcome, rather than fully comprehending the minute and delicate intricacies of the wound-healing process, literally from the inside out, beginning from the moment of skin disruption.

The integumentary system is composed of the skin, its appendages, hair, nails, and sweat and sebaceous glands (1). The skin is segmented into three compartments: epidermis (the avascular layer), the dermis, and the subcutaneous layer. The outermost skin compartment, the epidermis, has no vascular structure, but contains five distinct anatomical layers, each having a specific physiologic purpose: stratum corneum, stratum lucidum, stratum granulosum, stratum spinosum, and stratum basale. Together, the total thickness of all five epidermal layers is approximately 0.5–1.1 millimeters (1).

Underneath the epidermis lies the dermis, which is highly vascularized. This skin compartment houses blood and lymphatic vessels, nerves and nerve endings, pressure receptors, sebaceous glands, and hair follicles.

Table 14–1 Wound Categories

Wound Category	Wound Category Definition(s)	Wound Examples
Pressure ulcers (also known as a decubitus ulcer or decubiti [more than one ulcer])	Result from prolonged ischemia-producing external pressure, usually to a soft tissue region overlying a bony prominence (3) Are caused by prolonged pressure and typically occur over bony prominences in bed- or chair-bound individuals (4) Wound characteristics can be used to distinguish pressure ulcers from other types of chronic wounds (4)	Wounds that occur most frequently on the sacrum, elbows, heels, outer ankles, inner knees, hips, shoulder blades, and occipitae bone of high-risk patients, especially those who are obese, elderly, or suffering from chronic diseases, infections, or injuries (1)
Traumatic	Result secondarily to a foreign body or substance disrupting skin integrity	Penetrating injuries, such as knife or gunshot wounds; paper cuts; needle sticks Burn injuries, such as those caused by fire; radiation; frostbite
Surgical	Intentional wounding, as occurs with incisions and excisions	Tracheotomy; gastrostomy; cholecystectomy
Pathophysiologic	Internal and/or external tissue disruption secondary to a pathophysiologic process	Diabetic foot ulcers; collagen diseases; pellagra dermatitis

309

Lastly, the skin's innermost compartment is the subcutaneous layer. The subcutaneous layer is a continuous cover of connective tissue over the entire body between the dermis and the deep fascial investment of the body, such as the muscles. Under normal circumstances, it is composed of an outer fatty layer (adipose tissue) and an inner thin elastic layer (1). The depth and health of the subcutaneous layer is partially dependent on the presence and extent of each individual's adipose tissue component.

Wound Stages

The cellular disruption of any skin compartment (epidermis, dermis, subcutaneous layer) results in anatomical wounding, or, more simply, a wound. The National Pressure Ulcer Advisory Panel (NPUAP), formed in 1987, is an independent, not-for-profit, professional organization dedicated to the prevention and management of pressure ulcers and is composed of leading experts from different health care disciplines (6). In 1989, a wound-staging system was developed by the NPUAP as an outcome of the Consensus Development Conference and is, by far, the most widely cited and used wound-staging system in the United States. The NPUAP wound-staging system has also been employed by health professionals to identify wounds of other etiologies in their respective healing progression and digression stages. The NPUAP staging system consists of four distinct stages. See Table 14–2 for further information on the system.

Phases of Wound Healing

For the healing process to occur (that is, the act or process in which the normal structural and functional characteristics of health are restored to diseased, dysfunctional, or damaged tissues, organs, or systems of the body), distinct and specific physiologic processes must be initiated and permitted to perform their designated actions (1). In wound healing, three fairly characteristic phases have been identified:

1. hemostatic/inflammatory phase
2. proliferative phase
3. remodeling phase

However, it must be noted that these phases may overlap during the healing process and that any part of a wound may digress or progress in the healing process at a different rate from another section of the same wound (see Table 14–3).

Obstacles to Wound Healing

Wounds heal, incompletely heal, or don't heal, due to a multitude of related, interrelated, and nonrelated causal factors. Wound healing can occur quickly or exceedingly slowly, with variable healing times within and among healing phases. The

Table 14–2 NPUAP Wound Staging System

Stages	Definition and Clinical Identifiers
Stage 1	Pressure ulcer is an observable pressure-related alteration of intact skin whose indicators as compared to an adjacent or opposite area on the body may include changes in one or more of the following: skin temperature (warmth or coolness), tissue consistency (firm or boggy feel), and/or sensation (pain, itching). The ulcer appears as a defined area of persistent redness in lightly pigmented skin, whereas in darker skin tones, the ulcer may appear with persistent red, blue, or purple hues.
Stage 2	Partial thickness skin loss involving epidermis, dermis, or both. The ulcer is superficial and presents clinically as an abrasion, blister, or shallow crater.
Stage 3	Full thickness skin loss involving damage to, or necrosis of, subcutaneous tissue that may extend down to, but not through, underlying fascia. The ulcer presents clinically as a deep crater with or without undermining of adjacent tissue.
Stage 4	Full thickness skin loss with extensive destruction, tissue necrosis, or damage to muscle, bone, or supporting structures (e.g., tendon, joint, capsule). Undermining and sinus tracts also may be associated with Stage 4 pressure ulcers.

healing process can progress from one phase to the next and can digress to the prior phase if an insult is inflicted that initiates the digression. Identifiable impediments to wound healing are numerous and may derive from both internal and external causative agents. As a guide to assist the clinician in recalling possible obstacles to wound healing, Stillman created the mnemonic DIDN'T HEAL (3). Although the categories contained within DIDN'T HEAL are not all-encompassing, they are expansive and serve to draw the clinician's attention to potential factors of concern that may be impeding the healing process. Those potential DIDN'T HEAL factors are: *D*iabetes, *I*nfection, *D*rugs, *N*utritional problems, *T*issue necrosis, *H*ypoxia, *E*xcessive tension on wound edges, *A*nother wound, and *L*ow temperature (see Table 14–4).

Other Adverse Influences on Wound Healing

While the anatomy and physiology of wound healing and targeted clinical interventions have received the most attention by both science and health care providers, other aspects of wound healing have been ignored or minimally addressed. Additional adverse influences on wound healing that merit closer attention for each individual are: general medical condition, or systems health; general psychological and

Table 14–3 Phases of Wound Healing

Wound Healing Phase	Duration	Characteristic Processes
Hemostatic/inflammatory	Starts immediately after injury and lasts approximately 2–5 days (3); 3–10 days (7)	• Hemostasis and clot formation • ↑ number of neutrophils → ↑ phagocytosis of bacteria • ↑ number of monocytes → ↑ phagocytosis and release of cytokines TNF, IL-1, IL-6 → angiogenesis and neovascularization of wound bed
Proliferative phase	Follows hemostatic/inflammatory phase and lasts 2 days–weeks (3); generally about 2 weeks (7)	• Granulation: ↑ number of fibroblasts, which create a collagen bed to fill the defect and grow new capillaries (angiogenesis) • Contraction: Myofibroblasts pull the wound edges together to diminish wound size • Epithelialization: Migration of new epithelium occurs from the intact periwound epidermis
Remodeling phase or collagen remodeling	Follows proliferative phase and lasts weeks to years	• Collagen maturation: a gradual replacement of immature, soft, gelatinous collagen with a more organized (mature) collagen (3) • A state of balance between collagen production and degradation (7) • Increased and increasing tensile strength of the healed wound tissue *Note:* The tensile strength of a healed wound is *never* as strong as the original noninjured tissue. Healed wound tissue has about 80% the tensile strength of the original noninjured tissue.

↑ = increased or increasing; → = leads to or results in; TNF= tumor necrosis factor; IL–1 = interleukin-1; IL–6 = interleukin-6

Table 14-4 DIDN'T HEAL: Obstacles to Wound Healing

DIDN'T HEAL Obstacle	Impact on Wound Healing
D = Diabetes	Adverse systemic effects of elevated blood glucose levels on leukocyte function, impairing phagocytosis and potentiating infection
	Long-term disease: restricted blood flow secondary to partial and/or complete sclerosis of either or both micro- and macrovasculature; distal symmetric polyneuropathy may impede pressure, temperature, and/or pain sensation(s), causing new tissue damage to current wound and/or initiating damage at another location
I = Infection	Impairment of collagen formation by stimulating collagen lysis
D = Drugs	Dependent upon type of drug; i.e., corticosteroids have an "antihealing" effect by impeding proliferation of fibroblasts and impairing collagen synthesis
N = Nutritional problems	Macro- and micronutrient insufficiencies/deficiencies and/or energy imbalances can impair tissue healing mechanisms; obesity may disrupt adequate blood flow to wound site
T = Tissue necrosis	Result of local or systemic ischemia caused by inadequate blood flow, and thus oxygen and nutrient delivery to wound site
H = Hypoxia	Caused by vasoconstriction or an interruption in vasculature, resulting in inadequate oxygen perfusion of the wound tissue
E = Excessive tension on wound edges	Can lead to local tissue ischemia and necrosis
A = Another wound	May potentiate competition for oxygen, nutrients, and energy substrates to assist tissue healing and negatively impact both or all injured tissues
L = Low temperature	The relatively low tissue temperature in the distal aspects of the upper and lower extremities is an adjunct to slower tissue healing at these sites; fingers and toes may be 2°–3°F less than normal core body temperature

313

mental health; general medical care; access to care; social health; and financial status and concerns. A discussion of each of these areas is beyond the scope of this chapter. The reader is encouraged to give some or all of these topics consideration in the overall diagnosis or problem identification, treatment, and continuity of care of individuals with wounds.

NUTRITION AND WOUND HEALING: IS THERE A RELATIONSHIP?

If there is a relationship between nutrition and wound healing, what is the depth and extent of the relationship? Many clinicians would readily agree that nutrition and wound healing have close ties; for example, poor nutritional status, however defined, is positively correlated with poor wound healing and/or increased risk for wound occurrence in certain conditions, such as prolonged pressure over bony prominences in decubitis ulcer formation. However, when asked why a wound is mending unsuccessfully in a well-tended, well-nourished individual, the nutrition-healing relationship falters. Given both anecdotal reports and research findings, wounds have been noted to adequately heal in both well-nourished and grossly undernourished conditions, all other known factors considered. Why the dichotomy? The answer remains elusive, although its dimensions are becoming clearer and more distinct.

Part of the difficulty in performing research studies and discussing findings on various aspects of wounds and the healing process is the definition of a healed wound. There is no widely accepted definition amongst health care providers or the research community as to the parameters that define a healed wound—nor is there agreement as to when the healed condition occurs. In other words, has a wound healed when it displays the characteristics defined as healed by the health care provider or is there a more optimal end point of healed that remains to be achieved?

If there is a more optimal end point, what might that be? Is it an end point that can be realistically attained and withstand the rigors of scientific investigation? Studies to date on wound healing, with or without a nutrition component, have been too diverse in hypotheses, methodology, sample size, population composition, treatment regimens, and surrogate markers to provide consistent, concise conclusions as regards healed wounds and fail-safe interventions. The future looks hopeful, however. In the meantime, the clinician must continue to use his or her best judgment in the provision and monitoring of wound care interventions.

The nutritional aspects of wound care interventions are numerous, most of which remain controversial. For example, are there specific nutrients in defined amounts that would facilitate wound healing, such as protein, vitamins A, E, and C, or the minerals selenium and zinc? Does the method by which nutrients are delivered to the human body have an impact, positive or negative, on wound healing (enteral oral, enteral tube, and/or parenteral modes)? Do nutrient forms and/or the timing in which they are conveyed to the human body have an impact on wound healing? Does body weight affect wound healing? To date, there are no definitive, unequivocal answers to these justifiable questions. Each of these aspects will be discussed in greater detail, but again, the clinician must employ his or her own best judgment in deciphering their role in wound care management.

WOUNDS AND NUTRITIONAL RISK

As previously stated, wounds have been noted to heal in the poorly nourished state and not heal in the well-fed state. When identifying individuals at nutritional risk, regardless as to how that is defined and stratified in a given institution or setting, a poorly nourished individual most likely would be classified as having some degree of nutritional risk. If that same individual had one or more wounds, regardless of the cause(s), the degree of nutritional risk would probably be elevated. Conversely, the well-fed individual initially almost certainly would not be deemed to be at nutritional risk. Given the presence of one or more wounds, some degree of nutritional risk likely would be assigned, dependent upon the type and extent of the wound(s). Although nutrition interventions are frequently based on degree of nutritional risk, it would seem inherently reasonable that the greater the number of wounds and/or extent of wounding, the greater the need for nutrition, with nutrition intervention commensurate with degree of nutritional risk and extent of wounding. Those correlations, though, have not withstood scientific scrutiny and may have negative consequences in practice. Therefore, caution should be exercised by the clinician when assessing degree of nutritional risk in an individual with a wound or wounds and in subsequently deciding on particular nutrition interventions. Specific nutrients and nutrition interventions are discussed elsewhere in this chapter.

BODY WEIGHT AS A NUTRITIONAL RISK FACTOR IN WOUND CARE MANAGEMENT

A variety of studies have looked at the relationships amongst body weight, nutritional status, energy and nutrient intake or delivery, and wound healing. In a study by Mathus-Vliegen related to pressure ulcer risk in an elderly, malnourished population, it was determined that, in general, adequate nutritional intake tended to reverse the risk for pressure ulcer *formation*, but its effect on pressure ulcer *healing* was inconclusive (8). A case report by Armstrong on obesity (body mass index ≥ 30) as an intrinsic factor affecting the healing of surgical wounds determined that obesity impaired healing secondary to reduced tissue oxygenation and collagen production at the wound site, regardless of the adequacy of the diet (9). Both these examples highlight the intricate and divergent relationship among body weight, nutritional status, and adequacy of nutritional intake in wound management.

Obesity has long been recognized as an impediment to wound healing due to its effects on the physiology and anatomy of the wounded site. Adipose tissue is poorly vascularized, partly due to its role as a storage depot for excess energy, as compared to the structure and function of the various muscle tissue types, such as cardiac and skeletal muscle. The diminished vascular network in adipose tissue, as compared to muscle tissue, correlates with fewer transportation routes for delivery of oxygen and nutrients necessary for cellular health and function. This situation is partially responsible for some cases of wound dehiscence occurring in obese individuals, although infection remains the primary causative factor (9).

Diminished vascularization of adipose tissue can also precipitate "dead space" in thick, injured layers of tissue, such as injuries that occur secondarily to surgical incisions. It is thought that these areas of dead space may be responsible for reducing the oxygen tension in the affected tissues to less than 15 mm Hg, a condition incongruent with cellular viability. Such conditions have also been noted to impede adequate collagen production and, thus, wound healing (9).

Body weight, at either end of the spectrum, can have detrimental effects on wound healing and may play a role in wound development. Encouraging individuals to attain and/or maintain a sensible weight for height and assisting them in that endeavor appears to be a reasonable course of action for the health care provider to take, for a myriad of reasons.

ENERGY AND WOUND CARE

Wound healing is an energy-requiring process. How much energy (kilocalories) is needed, when it's needed, and the preferred sources remain controversial issues. Energy is compulsory for a host of wound-healing processes, such as collagen formation; leukocyte and erythrocyte formation; cytokine production; angiogenesis; nutrient ingestion, digestion, metabolism, and distribution; and to meet the increased demands placed upon the cardiovascular, lymphatic, respiratory, and integumentary systems. The amount of energy needed for each physiologic process and that needed for integrated systemic processes to support wound healing is largely unknown (10). It may appear intuitive that smaller wounds are less energy demanding than larger wounds, or that multiple wounds greatly increase overall energy needs, but those associations remain to be scientifically proven or dispelled. There has been a tendency among clinicians to positively correlate energy needs with wound size and severity and/or with the total number of wounds. This practice, however, may be more detrimental than advantageous in that it may precipitate excessive intake or exogenous delivery of nutrients (i.e., overfeeding) and may impose unnecessary and undesired physiologic stress on cellular function and organ systems that already may be strained (10–13).

ASSESSMENT OF ENERGY NEEDS

Assessment of energy needs must be made on an individual basis and within the context of the individual's existing physiological and metabolic condition. The most favorable goal is provision of adequate energy (and nutrients) to meet the body's demands at any given point in time, while simultaneously avoiding prolonged occurrences of energy deficits or excesses (11). However, this goal would be extremely difficult to attain, even under the most stringent research conditions. Thus, the clinician must rely on the best scientific evidence to date, integrated with his or her knowledge and skill base, and the existing and projected medical status of the individual patient/client, to determine a reasonable range of energy needs.

Generally speaking, it is recommended a range of 30–35 kcal/kg/day be provided (14,15). If indirect calorimetry is available, its use is suggested to more definitively identify estimated energy needs (11–13). However, 30–35 kcal/kg/day is a recommended range only, and close monitoring of the individual to assess metabolic tolerance and to deter the possible detrimental consequences of overfeeding is encouraged (16,17). Overfeeding, especially during the initial phases of the inflammatory process, should be avoided. Overfeeding can increase the risk of hyperglycemia, as well as precipitate signs of refeeding syndrome (hyperglycemia, hypophosphatemia, hypokalemia, hypoinsulinemia, respiratory distress, and edema), particularly if the individual is already in a malnourished or highly stressed state (16–18). Maintaining tight blood glucose control, in both diabetic and nondiabetic individuals, in stressed or nonstressed states, is encouraged so as to avoid and/ or diminish the deleterious physiologic and anatomic effects of high-serum glucose levels (19–21).

Monitoring for adequacy of energy intake/delivery can be a tedious process for the clinician. One must be aware of all sources of energy substrates and must include their respective energy contributions in calculations of daily total energy intake/delivery. Energy sources from the carbohydrate, protein, and/or fat components of oral feeding, enteral tube feeding, parenteral nutrition (PN) solutions, intravenous hydration solutions, and medication delivery systems must be recognized and tallied. Consistently overlooking or discounting these energy sources can precipitate overfeeding and subsequent adverse outcomes.

ENERGY NEEDS AND BODY WEIGHT

An individual's existing body weight at the time the clinician performs an energy needs assessment is a factor that, correctly or not, plays a role in the subconscious use of predictive equations and energy needs ranges. If at all possible, energy requirements should be based on a dry (absence of edema or ascites) body weight, or a reasonably estimated dry body weight, if direct calculation is not feasible (22). In the undernourished, underfed individual, the initial energy goal should be to retard and/or inhibit additional weight loss, if possible, dependent upon the existing metabolic state. The NPUAP suggests increasing energy intake/delivery to 35–40 kcal/kg/day in these conditions (23). However, good clinical judgment and frequent monitoring must be employed to avoid possible overfeeding and hyperglycemia in this elevated energy range. Energy intake/delivery can be advanced as the clinical condition warrants, but should proceed slowly, with close monitoring, to preclude adverse outcomes.

In the normal-weight individual, the initial energy goal should be to avoid or minimize weight loss; again, dependent upon the existing metabolic condition.

Energy intake/delivery can be advanced as the clinical condition warrants, with close monitoring, to preclude adverse outcomes.

The obese individual, however, presents a more difficult challenge in both estimating and monitoring energy needs. There are no good predictive energy needs equations that apply in all conditions and body weights. The Harris-Benedict equation, the most well-known predictive energy equation, tends to overestimate basal energy expenditure (BEE) in healthy adults by 10% to 15%, but has been shown to accurately predict BEE in obese individuals (body mass index of about 35 to 40) when actual weight was used (24,25). At this time, the Mifflin-St. Jeor equation appears to offer the most accurate estimate of resting energy expenditure in both normal-weight and obese individuals (26,27). As in the underfed and normal-weight individuals, energy intake/delivery can be advanced, if deemed necessary, followed by close monitoring to preclude adverse outcomes.

MACRONUTRIENTS AND WOUND CARE

Macronutrients supply energy (calories) to the body. The percentage of each macronutrient needed by the human body varies with age, gender, body composition, activity level, and any disease or condition that alters metabolism and/or excretion of the nutrient and/or its metabolites. General acceptable macronutrient ranges for the healthy adult human consist of approximately 45%–60% of energy from carbohydrate; 10%–35% of energy from protein; and 20%–35% of energy from fat (28). As regards macronutrient requirements in wound-care management, the exact percentages of carbohydrate, protein, and fat have not been clearly delineated. However, of the three, protein has received the most attention and study, primarily due to its role in collagen formation; angiogenesis; and enzymatic, cytokine, erythrocyte, and leukocyte formation and function.

PROTEIN AND AMINO ACIDS

A variety of studies done on protein requirements in infection, inflammation, and wounds have used positive nitrogen balance as an end point; some have also used wound healing or wound-healing response as a marker (e.g., hydroxyproline content or collagen content) (28,29). Others have looked at *in vivo* protein kinetics of muscle, skin, and wound in injured tissue and protein turnover in skeletal muscle (30,31). However, the use of nitrogen balance as a valid marker of adequate or inadequate protein intake/delivery is fraught with problems, not the least of which is obtaining a legitimate, unadulterated nitrogen collection of all sources of nitrogen excreted from the body, as well as all sources of nitrogen ingested/delivered to the body for a 24-hour period (32). Although "fudge factors," or estimates of smaller nitrogen losses, have been used to account for unmeasured nitrogen components, the outcomes of nitrogen-balance studies outside of the research environment have to be interpreted with great latitude. If a nitrogen-balance study is employed to determine adequacy of protein intake/delivery, the suggested goal is +3 to +5 grams of nitrogen; some resources state +2 to +4 grams of nitrogen. One of the most commonly used equations to determine nitrogen balance is:

Nitrogen balance = Nitrogen intake − Nitrogen output + 2 to 4 grams nitrogen

where the +2 to +4 grams of nitrogen are a "fudge factor" that acts as an estimate of fecal, dermal, miscellaneous, and nonurea nitrogen losses (33).

A significant amount of nitrogen may be lost from draining wounds, and its acquisition for inclusion in nitrogen-balance equations can be difficult. As an alternative, the following guideline can be used to estimate those nitrogen losses:

<10% open wound = 0.02 grams nitrogen per kilogram body weight per day
11% to 30% open wound = 0.05 grams nitrogen per kilogram body weight per day
>31% open wound = 0.12 grams nitrogen per kilogram body weight per day (34)

Interpretation of nitrogen-balance study results and use of that data to adjust or justify alterations in the protein component of the diet or nutrition-support regimen must be done carefully. If it is determined that additional protein is necessary, adequate energy sources are present, and renal and hepatic function are stable, the addition of more protein to the diet or nutrition support regimen can be done. Generally, in wound healing, given adequate renal and hepatic function and reasonable energy sources, 1.0 to 2.0 grams protein per kilogram per day should be sufficient to meet protein demands (8,10,14,23,35,36).

SPECIFIC AMINO ACID SUPPLEMENTATION

In recent years, there has been great interest in the role of specific amino acids in infection, sepsis, and wound healing and prevention. Amino acids drawing the most attention are arginine, glutamine, and a metabolite of leucine, β-hydroxy β-methylbutyrate (HMB).

Arginine

Arginine, a semiessential amino acid, is synthesized endogenously primarily in the proximal renal tubule by conversion of citrulline to arginine (37). In the stressed state, however, arginine may become a conditionally essential amino acid in adults (37,38). Arginine functions in the body as a substrate for protein synthesis, cell proliferation, neurotransmission, vasodilation, calcium release, immunity, and wound healing (39). It is also derived from both endogenous protein breakdown and exogenous protein intake; the jejunum is the principal intestinal site of absorption (37). In the human body, it is metabolized via four known pathways, two of which may indicate a role for arginine in wound healing and immunity (37,39) (see Figures 14–1 and 14–2).

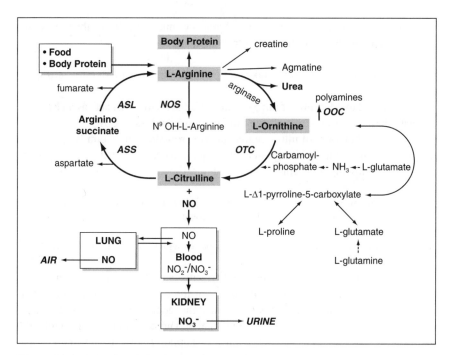

Figure 14–1 Role of Arginine in Acute Wounds

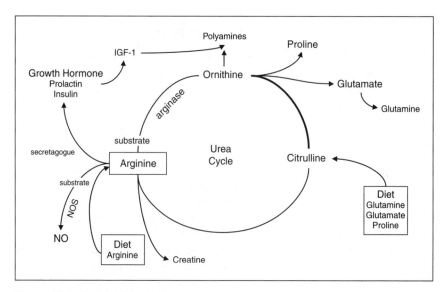

Figure 14–2 Arginine Metabolism

In one of these two pathways, arginine, via the effects of type II arginase, combines with ornithine and urea to create proline and the polyamines. These steps are imperative for cell growth and differentiation and for synthesis of connective tissue (collagen) (37,39). In another pathway, arginine plays an active role in the synthesis of nitric oxide (NO). High levels of NO, synthesized by nitric oxide synthase-2 (NOS-2), also known as inducible NOS or *i*NOS, have been demonstrated to have immunoregulatory functions, such as control or killing of infectious pathogens; modulation of cytokine development; and T-helper cell development (37). Nitric oxide has also been shown to have cytoprotective properties as a free-radical scavenger when stimulated by increased circulating levels of cytokines (TNF-alpha and IL-1, IL-6, IL-8) or microbial products during inflammatory processes (37).

However, caution must be exercised in drawing positive correlations between arginine and the effects of these two metabolic pathways in wound healing. Stechmiller et al. state that arginine has a regulatory role during the course of wound repair and that these two metabolic pathways are sequentially organized in wound healing (39). Cytokines and growth factors stimulate the induction of each pathway, resulting in down-regulation of the opposing pathway (39). Early NOS-2 activity creates an overall cytotoxic wound environment, whereas the type II arginase pathway may promote cell growth proliferation by depleting arginine, the NOS-2 substrate, and by increasing the availability of ornithine, the precursor for the synthesis of collagen (39). The cytotoxic environment created by NOS-2 may be unfavorable if it persists after the initial days of wounding, extending the inflammatory phase of healing. The resultant effect is an interference with cell proliferation, collagen formation, and wound closure (39).

There continues to be great debate amongst the nutrition, medical, and surgical communities as to whether arginine supplementation can positively impact wound healing (10). Research using arginine supplementation has centered mainly on acute surgical wounds, where it has been shown to enhance wound strength and collagen deposition in artificial incisional wounds in rodents and in humans (40,41). Its therapeutic effectiveness in aiding the healing of delayed or chronic wounds remains undefined (10). At this time, it is too early in the advent of arginine and wound-healing research to generally promote routine arginine supplementation for all individuals with all types of wounds.

Arginine Supplementation: Yes or No?

As stated earlier, the findings from research on arginine and wound healing remain controversial and ill defined. Studies have lacked consistency in types of wounds addressed, populations, surrogate markers, presence or lack of comorbidities in the study population, adequacy of nutritional intake/delivery, and the route of arginine supplementation. If arginine supplementation is being considered, the clinician must be aware of the potential risks, especially in the critically ill, secondary to the enhancement of the systemic inflammatory response with high-circulating concentrations of cytokines, which promote greater circulating levels of NOS-2 (42–44).

No definitive amount of arginine has been identified for wound repair in either surgical or chronic wounds, in either the stressed on nonstressed state, nor has a supplemental maximum safe dosage of arginine been established, to date (10).

If, however, a clinical decision is made to provide arginine supplementation, arginine provision from all existing sources should be estimated before additional arginine if any is provided, (see Table 14–5). Additionally, total protein and fluid intake/delivery should also be scrutinized, as well as renal and hepatic function. Arginine, by virtue of being an amino acid, will add to the nitrogen load that must be metabolized by the liver and filtered by the kidneys. If either or both renal and/or hepatic function is impaired, it is suggested arginine supplementation be eliminated from consideration as a wound healing measure.

Glutamine

Glutamine, a nonessential amino acid, is one of the most abundant amino acids in the human body. It performs numerous metabolic functions, some of which play an important role, although not directly, in wound healing. Glutamine is a precursor for nucleotide synthesis; an interorgan nitrogen and carbon transporter; a regulator of protein synthesis and breakdown rates; and an important metabolic fuel source for rapidly replicating cells, to include enterocytes, lymphocytes, fibroblasts, and reticulocytes, amongst other vital functions (45,46). It is probably best known for its role in enterocyte health, bacterial translocation, infection, and immunosuppression in highly catabolic states, such as burns and trauma. All of these conditions can positively or negatively impact the wound-healing process. However, a direct link between glutamine intake/delivery and progression or digression of wound-healing phases has not been established.

Table 14–5 Sources of Arginine

Source	Amount of Arginine (Grams)
Endogenous arginine production	~15–20 grams per day
Dietary protein	1 gram provides 54 mg arginine
Oral diet, dependent upon intake	Generally provides ~3–6 grams per day
Oral liquid supplements	Generally contain ~4.5 grams per 240 mL
Enteral tube feeding formulas: arginine enriched	~12.5–18.7 grams per liter; approximately 2% of total calories
Enteral tube feeding formulas: standard	~1–2 grams per liter
Parenteral amino acid solutions (10%)	~10–12 grams per liter

Currently, the safe maximum supplemental glutamine dosage for adults is 0.57grams/kilogram body weight/day (47). However, research findings on the use of supplemental glutamine as a wound-healing intervention are insufficient to recommend its use, at this time (10,48). If glutamine supplementation is undertaken, monitoring of protein and fluid intake, as well as renal and hepatic status, is suggested.

β-hydroxy β-methylbutyrate

β-hydroxy β-methylbutyrate, also known as HMB, is a metabolite of the amino acid leucine. It regulates muscle proteolysis in animals and in humans and increases collagen deposition in rodents (39). A human study performed using healthy elderly volunteers looked at the effects of an oral supplement containing a combination of HMB, arginine, and glutamine on incisional wound healing (45). While an increase in collagen deposition was noted, the contribution of each supplemented component, individually or synergistically, could not be determined.

Recent research, though, indicates that HMB may have a possible advantageous role in other medical conditions. Positive outcomes have been seen in acquired immunodeficiency virus-associated wasting, cancer-related wasting, and rheumatoid cachexia (49–51). These findings, though, remain to be replicated through additional studies and cannot be extrapolated to infer similar beneficial results in wound healing processes. This is an area for more detailed research in both animals and humans.

OTHER AMINO ACIDS

Other amino acids, not as well researched as arginine and glutamine, may have roles in wound healing. In healing tissue, proline and lysine undergo hydroxylation to hydroxyproline and hydroxylysine before being incorporated into collagen (52). Methionine, which is a precursor for cysteine, is needed for fibroblast proliferation and collagen synthesis (52). Cysteine is most likely used as a cofactor in the enzyme systems involved in collagen synthesis. It also contributes to the proper alignment of the peptide chain of the procollagen helix (52). However, at this time, there is no substantive research in humans to suggest supplementation of these amino acids to promote wound healing (53).

LIPIDS

Lipids, or fats, are a source of energy in the diet, as well as the essential fatty acids (linoleic, alpha-linolenic, and arachidonic acids). They also act as a carrier for the fat-soluble vitamins A, D, E, and K and fat-soluble phytochemicals, such as carotenoids and lycopenes; are incorporated into adipose tissue and perform as energy storage depots to be called upon when energy deficits occur; act as structural (fat) pads to protect vital internal organs and nerves against traumatic injury and shock; are components or precursors of phospholipids and prostaglandins; impart taste and texture to foods; and provide a sense of satiety during eating (38,54). Lipids are energy dense in that they provide more than twice the energy per gram than carbohydrate and protein; that is, approximately 9 kilocalories/gram of fat compared to about 4 kilocalories/gram of carbohydrate and protein.

Lipids have not been as widely studied for their impact on and contribution to the wound-healing process as have carbohydrate and protein (38). General recommendations for energy from fat intake/delivery vary greatly in the literature. Needs are dependent upon gender, age, body size, activity level, and existing medical and/or metabolic conditions or diseases and can range from <20% to 40%. Because of their role as components or precursors of phospholipids and prostaglandins, inadequate intake/delivery of lipid constituents can impair wound healing in both animals and humans (55–57). Impairment is due primarily to the role phospholipids have as constituents of the cellular basement membrane and the participation of prostaglandins in cellular metabolism and inflammation (38).

While, over time, impaired or delayed wound healing may be seen with very low fat intake/delivery or lipid-free PN infusions, there is also concern surrounding the contribution of the various fatty acid types, particularly the omega-6 and omega-3 fatty acids (56–59). While overall insufficient intake/delivery or absence of fat will preclude an adequate supply of all fatty acids types, the supplementation of one fatty-acid type in preference to another may, in effect, impair the healing process (59). This is of primary concern given the anti-inflammatory properties of the omega-3 fatty acids, as compared to the omega-6 fatty acids. Supplementation of omega-3 fatty acids may be detrimental to the wound-healing process by inhibiting the production of eicosanoids, platelet-activating factor, IL-1, and tumor necrosis factor-α, all of which are integral components of the initial, inflammatory phase of wound repair (60,61). A study performed on two groups of rats receiving diets containing 20% lipid in which one group was fed a diet high in omega-3 fatty acids and the other a diet containing omega-6 fatty acids from corn oil showed decreased wound tensile strength after 30 days in the group fed the high omega-3 diet (59). An unexpected finding of this study was that initial wound-healing outcomes at 10 days did not differ between the two groups; the findings at 30 days did (decreased wound tensile strength). Also surprising was that wound collagen content between the two groups was approximately the same. The difference in wound tensile strength was theorized to be due to the impaired quality, cross-linking, or spatial orientation of collagen fibrils in the omega-3 supplemented group (59).

While some clinicians may be inclined to provide omega-3 supplementation to individuals with wounds, caution is suggested. At this time, there is insufficient data to make clinical recommendations as to fatty-acid content, fatty-acid supplementation, and total fat percentage of energy needs in individuals with wounds.

CARBOHYDRATES

The primary sources of energy to drive the metabolic, growth, maintenance, systemic, and physical activity functions of the human body are supplied by adequate intake/delivery of carbohydrate and fat components. Although protein can serve as an energy resource, it is not the preferred fuel source, with the exception of some specialized cells, such as enterocytes, fibroblasts, lymphocytes, and reticulocytes.

The exact amount, source, and structure of carbohydrate needed for wound-healing functions is unknown. The predominant energy preference for most body cells is glucose, a monosaccharide that is dependent on insulin to facilitate its transfer from the bloodstream to cells and muscle fibers. Glucose is the major source of fuel used to generate cellular energy in the form of adenosine triphosphate (ATP), which, in turn, powers the wound-healing process (38). In the setting of inadequate glucose availability and increased demand, gluconeogenesis from amino acid substrates functions to provide the needed glucose. However, this process is an inefficient resource for glucose and can diminish the existing amino acid pool, straining those physiologic systems, such as collagen production, that are reliant upon a sufficient and appropriate amino acid reserve to perform optimally. Additionally, gluconeogenesis can result in the production of surplus amounts of glucose, which may complicate various wound-healing processes, especially in diabetic individuals with poor glycemic control (38).

Although delayed or poor wound healing is often noted in diabetic individuals, the exact etiologies vary from person to person, both as single causative agents and as intertwined mechanisms. Hyperglycemia, peripheral and autonomic neuropathies, and microvascular sclerosis all singly can have a detrimental effect on wound healing; together their negative impact may be greatly magnified. Additionally, in animal studies, diabetes appeared to exert a negative effect on the early inflammatory response and directly inhibited fibroblast and endothelial cell activity (62).

In a study by Langouche et al., intensive insulin therapy was shown to protect the endothelium of critically ill patients, both with and without diabetes, prior to the onset of critical illness (63). The vascular endothelium controls vasomotor tone and microvascular flow and regulates trafficking of nutrients and several biologically active molecules (63). Local activation of the endothelium is crucial for infection control, but widespread systemic endothelial activation may lead to deleterious consequences (63). By strictly controlling blood glucose with insulin to maintain normoglycemia (80–110 mg/dl), a protective effect on the endothelium was identified, the etiology of which was direct and/or via inhibition of excessive iNOS-induced nitric oxide release and the resultant proinflammatory effects of high nitric oxide concentrations (63).

The positive impact of tight glycemic control has also been demonstrated in diabetic patients undergoing cardiac surgical procedures. Continuous insulin infusion to maintain blood glucose levels between 150 mg/dL and 200 mg/dL diminished the incidence of deep sternal wound infections by 58% (64). In a study by Van den Berghe et al., in surgical intensive care unit patients, intensive insulin intervention was shown to reduce bloodstream infections, acute renal failure, and critical illness polyneuropathy, but at the cost of a 60% increase in risk of hypoglycemic events in the study group (65,66). Whether the positive effects of tight glycemic control on sequelae in critically ill patients is due to consistently lower blood glucose levels, the anabolic effects of insulin, or other yet-to-be-identified factors, there is some evidence that blood glucose levels may be the primary agent (19,66).

Until more definitive description can be given to the multifactorial consequences of hyperglycemia, regardless of causation, on wound healing, it would appear to be clinically wise to control blood glucose levels to maintain normoglycemia. In this endeavor, the carbohydrate content of the oral diet and/or specialized nutrition support regimens should be considered as an integral, but not sole, part of clinical assessment and intervention.

WATER

Despite the human body being approximately 50%–60% water, this nutrient is often overlooked as an essential nutrient. Water is vital to health and wound healing because it comprises a significant portion of the blood, and consequently, blood pressure (67). Adequate blood pressure and blood flow is imperative to deliver oxygen and nutrients to body cells and tissues, both healthy and injured. Water also plays a role in maintaining good skin turgor, which can help to diminish skin breakdown. Adequate hydration is necessary to sustain normal body temperature and to prevent excessive dehydration during fever and/or exposure to high environmental temperatures. Additionally, water is integral to maintaining normal acid-base balance, partly through the urinary excretion of electrolytes and metabolic byproducts.

The advent of air-fluidized beds inadvertently created a challenge to maintaining adequate hydration in some individuals with wounds (68). Patients with burns, decubitus ulcers, various traumas, and generalized debility placed in these beds were found to have higher insensible water losses than occurred with regular hospital beds. A continuous stream of warm air flowing across the patient was found to increase insensible evaporative water loss, primarily due to the wide range of operating temperatures, ranging from 82° to 102°F (68). However, quantification of evaporative water loss at various temperatures is a challenge. A nomogram created by McNabb and Hyatt to assist in estimating insensible water loss in patients in air-fluidized beds may be a helpful measure to the clinician managing hydration status (68).

Water loss can occur through a variety of media and all sources of loss should be considered in adequately assessing and managing hydration status. Additional sources of loss the clinician is cautioned to consider include, but are not limited to: elevated body temperature secondary to infection; elevated environmental temperature and/or humidity; abnormal sweating; respiratory difficulties; open and/or draining wounds; vomiting; diarrhea; excessive urination, regardless of cause; and intense physical activity. Water replacement to achieve the desired hydration status is necessary to avoid the general and metabolic consequences of dehydration.

General fluid recommendations for the adult range from 1.0 to 1.5 mL/ kilocalorie expended or approximately 25–40 mL/kg, dependent on age (10,67). However, these are broad guidelines only, and concomitant atypical sources of fluid loss must be recognized and counted in estimating total fluid needs.

MICRONUTRIENTS AND WOUND CARE

Numerous vitamins and minerals have been postulated to have crucial roles in wound healing, often in amounts exceeding prevailing recommended amounts for general good health. Although the physiologic function(s) of the various vitamins and minerals are known, the precise amounts needed to positively contribute to wound healing are largely unknown. The specific micronutrients given the most attention in wound healing are vitamins A, E, and C, and the mineral zinc.

Vitamin A

Vitamin A is a fat-soluble vitamin that has numerous roles in wound healing (69). Vitamin A functions to maintain integrity of epithelial and mucosal surfaces and to enhance fibroplasia that increases collagen synthesis and epithelialization (10). It also acts as an immunostimulant in humans and may enhance wound healing by increasing the number of monocytes and macrophages in the wound or by stabilizing the intracellular lysosomes of leukocytes (67). Additionally, vitamin A is known for its antagonistic effect on the anti-inflammatory consequences of glucocorticoids, which are often given in the first few days after wounding and can impair the initial phase of wound healing (10,69). However, the exact mechanism(s) by which vitamin A affects the healing process is unknown (10,67).

Supplementation of vitamin A to promote wound healing may not be warranted. If no deficiency is identified and wound healing appears to be occurring, supplementation is most likely unnecessary. If, however, wound healing has been slow or incomplete, particularly in the presence of glucocorticoid use, *short-term* supplementation may be justified. Glucocorticoids impair most aspects of wound healing: inflammatory response, fibroblast proliferation, collagen deposition, wound contraction, and epithelial migration (10). Although it remains controversial, some clinicians concurrently provide supplemental vitamin A in conjunction with glucocorticoid administration. Suggested supplemental dosages range from 10,000–15,000 IU orally for up to 7 days or approximately 5000–7500 IU parenterally for the same time period (10,67). In individuals with fat malabsorption, a water-soluble form of vitamin A should be considered. Caution must be exercised with supplementation, though, because large amounts of vitamin A are potentially toxic, particularly in renal and hepatic dysfunction, and may reactivate the inflammatory process for which the glucocorticoid was originally given, essentially creating a chasing-the-tail scenario (10,67). Monitoring vitamin A status during supplementation is suggested. Although serum vitamin A levels are not the most accurate method by which to determine existing vitamin A status, they are the most common and readily available (67).

For individuals not receiving glucocorticoids who appear to have slow or delayed wound healing, assessment of vitamin A intake/delivery relative to the dietary reference intake (DRI)/recommended dietary allowance (RDA) should be undertaken. The DRI/RDA for adults 19 years old and older is 700–900 µg (RAE)/day retinol activity equivalents, which is approximately 2330–3000 IU/day (70). If vitamin A intake/delivery is determined to be inadequate, supplementation to RDA levels may be beneficial.

Vitamin E

Vitamin E (tocopherol) is a fat-soluble vitamin that maintains and stabilizes cellular membrane integrity, mainly by protection against destruction by oxidation (38). It has anti-inflammatory properties similar to those of glucocorticoids in that it inhibits collagen synthesis and decreases tensile strength of wounds (38,67). The anti-inflammatory effects of high doses of vitamin E can be attenuated with concurrent vitamin A administration, but it may be wise to defer vitamin E supplementation unless a confirmed deficiency exists. At this time, there appears to be no definitive justification for vitamin E supplementation in wound healing. If a deficiency in this nutrient is suspected, and nutrient intake assessment is supportive, provision of supplemental vitamin E in an amount not to exceed the DRI/RDA for adults 19 to greater than 70 years old, 15 mg/day of α-tocopherol may be of benefit (71).

Vitamin C

Unlike vitamins A and E, the role of vitamin C, or ascorbic acid, in wound healing has been more clearly identified. Vitamin C is a cofactor in the hydroxylation of proline and lysine to hydroxyproline and hydroxylysine in collagen formation. Without adequate cross-linking of collagen fibers, which can occur in a vitamin C deficient state, the resulting collagenous structure is weakened, and inadequate wound closure can occur. This state can predispose the wound to infectious insults and increase susceptibility to infection. Adequate and appropriate collagen production helps to prevent infection by acting as a physical barrier to pathogens (38,67). Vitamin C also enhances neutrophil function, which aids in decreasing susceptibility to infection and participates in the synthesis of the microvascular structure (angiogenesis) that is needed to supply the new tissues with nutrients and oxygen (38,67).

Supplementation of vitamin C to promote wound healing has been shown to be beneficial in ascorbic acid-deficient individuals, but the effect in nondeficient individuals is controversial (72,73). It is unlikely, however, that vitamin C supplementation in this population will accelerate wound healing (10). Assessment of vitamin C status to determine the presence or absence of a deficiency can be challenging, given that vitamin C assays are expensive and interpretation of the findings can be difficult. Serum vitamin C levels may be determined to be substandard, but that finding cannot be extrapolated to leukocyte and platelet concentrations.

Recommendations for supplemental vitamin C in wound healing have great variability, ranging from 100 to 4000 mg/day (67). The current DRI for vitamin C ranges from 75–90 mg/day in adults, dependent upon gender and age (71). The tolerable upper intake level for adults is 2000 mg/day; dosages above that amount may elicit undesirable gastrointestinal effects (nausea, abdominal cramping, and diarrhea) (10,71). Although higher intakes of vitamin C may not be detrimental in some individuals, the potential for adverse outcomes is magnified. Of particular concern is the possible release of free iron from ferritin, augmenting an increased risk for iron-associated infection (14). In individuals with renal failure and undergoing hemodialysis or peritoneal dialysis, vitamin C supplementation of 500 mg to 1000 mg/day can precipitate renal oxalate stone formation (74,75). Some clinicians suggest, if vitamin C supplementation is necessary in this population, that no more than a total of 100–500 mg per day be given and that the total dosage be administered in divided amounts (10,69).

Vitamin K

Vitamin K, also known as the antihemmorrhage vitamin, is one of the four fat-soluble vitamins. It occurs primarily in two forms: phylloquinone (vitamin K_1), a compound found in green plants, and menaquinone (vitamin K_2), a compound synthesized by gut microflora (76). Of the two forms, vitamin K_1 is slightly more biologically active than vitamin K_2. In humans, vitamin K is essential for the post-translational carboxylation of glutamic acid residues in proteins to form γ-carboxyglutamate (GLA) residues (76,77). The GLA protein residues function in both the blood coagulation processes and bone metabolism. Four GLA proteins have been identified as necessary in blood coagulation: clotting factors II, VII, IX, and X (38,76). In bone metabolism, osteocalcin and matrix are structurally related vitamin K-dependent GLA proteins (76).

Although vitamin K does not play a direct role in wound healing, it does participate through its effects on blood coagulation. Its absence or deficiency leads to decreased coagulation, which has detrimental effects on the initial hemostatic, inflammatory phase of healing when hemostasis and clot formation postwounding are imperative to begin the healing process (38). However, caution must be exercised if supplemental vitamin K is provided, because both vitamins A and E antagonize the hemostatic properties of vitamin K (38). Formation of hematomas within the wound can impair healing and predispose the wound to infection

(78,79). Caution is also warranted in individuals receiving concomitant anticoagulation therapy. All sources of vitamin K, to include diet; herbal and botanical supplements; enteral tube feeding formulas; and PN solutions containing lipid and/or the newly formulated multivitamin infusions containing vitamin K, should be closely evaluated for their respective contributions to the total vitamin K amount being delivered to the body *before* supplements or alterations in anticoagulation therapy are initiated. The current DRI for vitamin K ranges from 90–120 μg/day in adults, dependent on age and gender (70).

Zinc

Zinc, the second most widely occurring trace element in the human body, functions as a cofactor in more than 100 different enzyme systems that play a role in protein and nucleic acid synthesis, cellular proliferation, collagen formation, and both cellular and humoral immunity, amongst many other physiologic functions (80). Evidence that zinc was essential to wound healing in humans was first described by Vallee in 1956 (81). Given zinc's role as a cofactor for RNA and DNA polymerase and DNA synthesis, a deficiency of this micronutrient will negatively impact various physiologic processes in wound healing. However, zinc supplementation in nondeficient individuals has not been proven to promote faster or more complete wound healing (82–84). Zinc levels in plasma initially rise after tissue injury, relative to the extent of the injury, but then decline secondary to redistribution of zinc to the liver (52,85,86). However, determination of a true zinc deficiency may be difficult to achieve in this environment, because plasma levels do not always positively correlate with tissues stores (69). Assessment of other zinc compartments, such as erythrocytes, leukocytes, and hair may be accomplished, but their validity in determining zinc deficiency or adequacy has not been demonstrated (69).

At present, recommendations for zinc supplementation in wound healing are limited only to those individuals who concurrently have wounds and are zinc deficient. The DRI for zinc ranges from 8–11 mg/day in adults, dependent on age and gender (70). The tolerable upper intake level is 40 mg/day, for both males and females. If zinc supplementation is undertaken, caution must be exercised because zinc is a toxic metal and oversupplementation may result in toxicity, immobilization of macrophages and inhibition of phagocytosis, and copper deficiency (87,88). To avoid possible deleterious outcomes with zinc supplementation, zinc should not be administered at doses >220 mg zinc sulfate (50 mg elemental zinc) for longer than 2 to 3 weeks, unless ongoing losses are confirmed and no subclinical signs of toxicity are present (10,69). It is also imperative to be aware of the differences in zinc bioavailability between oral and parenteral dosage forms. Approximately 20% of zinc sulfate ingested orally is bioavailable, whereas intravenously administered zinc is 100% bioavailable (10,67). For individuals receiving PN, the recommended dose for zinc is 2.5 to 4.0 mg/day for stable conditions and 4.5 to 6.0 mg/day in severely catabolic states (67,69). Some clinicians also provide additional zinc in the presence of small intestine fluid loss (12.2 mg zinc/liter fluid loss) and 17.1 mg/zinc per kilogram of stool or ileostomy output (67,69).

ADDITIONAL MICRONUTRIENTS

The preceding discussion by no means implies that only the micronutrients mentioned are involved in the various aspects of wound healing. The role(s) of other micronutrients continue to be researched for function, activity, and required amounts in the wounded condition. Copper, as part of the metalloenzyme lysyl oxidase, may influence wound healing by catalyzing the oxidation of lysyl residues on collagen. It may also be influential through its function in the superoxide dismutase enzyme system (52).

Iron is required for the hydroxylation of proline and lysine, and a deficiency, dependent on degree, may impair collagen production. Given iron's role in oxygen transportation, a deficiency can potentially negatively affect wound healing through insufficient oxygen delivery to the site (38). However, supplementation of iron in a presumed or confirmed deficiency, particularly in critical illness, should be undertaken only with extreme care. Iron is initially redistributed in severe injury, stress, and sepsis and can be sequestered in the liver as a component of ferritin, where it becomes a readily available food source for bacteria (89,90). Also to be considered is the possible release of free iron from ferritin in vitamin C supplementation in dosages greater than the DRI, again providing a possible breeding ground for microorganisms and infection (14,91).

Magnesium, through its role in protein synthesis, also participates in wound healing. It is a cofactor for numerous enzymes involved in protein synthesis and provides structural stability to ATP, which drives many of the processes involved in collagen synthesis (45). At this time, there are no recommendations for supplementation in wound healing.

The B vitamins thiamin, riboflavin, pyridoxine, pantothenic acid, and folate are also involved in wound healing through their various roles in energy release and carbohydrate, fat, and protein metabolism. A deficiency or insufficiency of any one or more of these necessary micronutrients may delay or interfere with adequate wound healing. A study by Neiva et al. on the effects of vitamin B-complex supplementation (thiamine, riboflavin, niacin, pantothenate, pyridoxine, biotin, cyanocobalamin, and folate) on periodontal wound healing in individuals with moderate to severe chronic peridontitis concluded that a vitamin-B–complex supplement, in combination with access flap surgery, resulted in a statistically significant wound healing response as compared to the placebo group (92). However, this vitamin-B complex, in both constituents and amounts, as well as response, remains to be studied in other wounded populations. Provision of a daily multivitamin containing these water-soluble vitamins in amounts approximately 100% of the DRI will not assure wound healing, but it may be a reasonable adjunct therapy, particularly in individuals with poor or marginal oral intake, such as can occur in drug and alcohol abuse and in the elderly (52).

GENERAL ENERGY AND NUTRIENT RECOMMENDATIONS

Despite the many advances in correlating nutrition's role to health and disease, nutrition remains an inexact science, outfitted with fine art—that is, there remains a great deal to discover about the interaction of nutrition in health and disease, at many different physiologic, emotional, and mental levels. The many tasks of nutrition in wound healing and wound care have yet to be identified, let alone quantified, and, most likely, qualified. With regards to macro- and micronutrient needs in wound healing, they are many; yet they are so difficult to identify, classify, and quantify. However, general recommendations can be made for intervention and maintenance. Still, as with many facets of science and medicine, generalities do not apply to everyone, nor are they intended to encompass every individual. Deviations from recommendations may be necessary, given the individual's preexisting and/or existing medical/surgical/metabolic condition(s). The clinician must utilize his or her best clinical judgment in the use and monitoring of the nutritional aspects and interventions of wound-care management. While the optimal end point is a completely healed wound, that goal may not always be realized. However, as more research is performed, preferably utilizing standardized surrogate markers, interventions, and homogenous populations, the knowledge base in this area will expand and treatment methods will become more focused and, hopefully, more successful.

The suggested guidelines for daily energy and nutrient provision in adult wound-care management are outlined in Table 14–6. As a summary, though, it appears that nutrition regimens balanced in energy, macronutrients, and micronutrients in amounts to meet, but not exceed, estimated or calculated needs is the most reasonable course of action to employ until scientific research clearly defines otherwise.

ROUTE AND TIMING OF NUTRITION SUPPORT

There has been debate as to whether the route of nutrition support (enteral oral, enteral tube, parenteral) and/or the timing of nutrition intervention play significant roles in the response to an imposed or acquired physiologic stress. Individuals determined to be malnourished before wounding occurred have been observed to have increased rates of pressure ulcer development (93,94). Conversely, individuals deemed to have adequate oral intake prior to surgical wounding were noted to have improved wound healing parameters postoperatively (95). A meta-analysis of studies performed on elective gastrointestinal surgery patients receiving early postoperative enteral tube feeding as compared to those for whom the traditional postoperative nutrition measures were ordered (NPO, IV hydration, oral diet progression as tolerated) determined that early nutrition intervention significantly reduced the risk of infection and hospital mean length of stay (96). Unfortunately,

Table 14–6 Suggested Guidelines for Daily Energy and Nutrient Provision in Adult Wound Care

Component	Suggested Guideline
Energy	30–35 kcal/kg realistic body weight
	Undernourished/underfed: 35–40 kcal/kg realistic body weight → use cautiously
Fluid	25–40 mL/kg
	1.0–1.5 mL per calorie expended
Protein	1.0–2.0 grams/kg reasonable body weight
	Determine adequacy of renal and hepatic function before providing >~1.5 grams/kg
Vitamin A	No supplementation if deficiency unconfirmed and/or wound healing is occurring
	If high dose steroid therapy is used, may consider *short term* supplementation:
	10,000–25,000 IU enterally for 7–10 days
	(<50% enteral amount if delivered parenterally
	Use cautiously if renal compromise exists
Vitamin C	No supplementation if deficiency is unconfirmed
	Deficiency known or strongly suspected: 100–500 mg BID enterally for 7–10 days; follow with DRI for age and gender thereafter
	Parenterally, 500 mg for 7–10 days; follow with DRI for age and gender thereafter
	Use caution if renal compromise exists
Vitamin E	Supplementation no longer justified
Vitamin K	Supplement only if deficiency confirmed; determine contribution of all sources of vitamin K *before* initiating supplementation and/or alterations in anticoagulation therapy
	DRI: 90 µg per day for adult females
	120 µg per day for adult males
	Parenterally, determine contribution of vitamin K from lipid infusion (if used); determine if vitamin K-containing MVI is being used in the parenteral nutrition solution
Zinc	No supplementation if deficiency is unconfirmed
	Range: RDA: 8 mg/day for women
	11 mg/day for men
	Can consider 50 mg/day elemental zinc for 7–10 days
	Parenterally, 10 mg/day for ~10 days
Arginine	Supplemental maximum safe dose: not established
	Supplementation not recommended at this time
Glutamine	No recommendation
	However, if used, maximum safe dosage is 0.57 grams/kg/day
β-hydroxy β-methyl-butyrate (HMB)	No recommendation at this time

(continues)

Table 14–6 Continued

Component	Suggested Guideline
Note:	A general multivitamin-mineral supplement containing micronutrients in amounts ≤100% of the DRI for each micronutrient may be provided in lieu of individual nutrient supplementation and/or confirmed deficiency
	Caution: If nutrient supplementation is occurring both singly and in a combination multivitamin-mineral form, total micronutrient dosage must be calculated and evaluated to avoid exceeding maximum recommended safe dosage

DRI = dietary reference intake; RDA = recommended dietary allowance

though, studies done to define the relationship(s), if any, among nutritional status at the time of wounding, nutrition intake/delivery immediately prior to and post-wounding, and wound healing have been so diverse in populations, surrogate markers, and interventions that clear and concise conclusions cannot be derived from their findings (10). However, given those limitations, some authors propose that pre-operative nutrition support in malnourished individuals may have positive effects on wound healing by reducing the occurrence of wound infections and promoting more timely wound healing (10,38). This would seem instinctively sensible and a reasonable approach to overall good medical care in the malnourished population.

CONCLUSION

The relationship between nutrition and wound healing is a complex one. Although various aspects of this relationship have been studied for centuries and have become more refined in methodology with advancements in technology and knowledge, the relationship remains an unsettled one. It seems intuitive that malnutrition would negatively impact wound healing processes and, perhaps, be a precursor for wound initiation, such as in pressure ulcer formation. Conversely, it would appear that a well-nourished state would positively influence wound healing and, as with pressure ulcer formation, possibly prevent occurrence. However, neither the malnourished nor well-nourished states have been conclusively proven to initiate or prevent wounds; to significantly retard or promote wound healing; or to invite or to deflect infectious complications. The intricacies of human physiology and metabolism in wounds, immunity, and healing processes are immense and extensively intertwined within and among each other. High-quality research, with consistent and congruent populations, well-defined end points, and standardized nutrition therapies are needed to more clearly identify feasible interventions that will promote wound health, if possible, and clarify those interventions that are potentially harmful. Until that time, clinicians who are involved in the nutrition and wound care of patients/ clients must continually update their knowledge base in this arena. They frequently may find themselves in situations where the use of best clinical judgment in wound-care management interventions and subsequent evaluation for effectiveness is the most appropriate course of action.

REFERENCES

1. Anderson DM, Keith J, Novak PD, Elliot MA. *Mosby's Medical, Nursing, & Allied Health Dictionary*. 6th ed. St. Louis, Mo.: Mosby, Inc.; 2002.

2. Thibodeau GA, Patton KT. Skin and its appendages. In: Thibodeau GA, Patton KT. *Anatomy & Physiology*. 5th ed. St. Louis, Mo.: Mosby; 2003:160–188.

3. Stillman RM. Wound care. Available at: www.emedicine.com/med/topic2754.htm. Accessed December 29, 2004.

4. National Pressure Ulcer Advisory Panel. Pressure ulcer definition and etiology. Available at: www.npuap.org/pressureulcerdef.html. Accessed January 5, 2005.

5. National Pressure Ulcer Advisory Panel. About the NPUAP. Available at: www.npuap.org/about.html. Accessed October 2, 2005.

6. National Pressure Ulcer Advisory Panel. NPUAP staging report. Available at: www.npuap.org/positn6.html. Accessed October 2, 2005.

7. Mayes T, Gottschlich MM. Burns and wound healing. In: Matarese LE, Gottschlich MM, eds. *Contemporary Nutrition Support Practice*. 2nd ed. St. Louis, Mo.: Saunders; 2003:595–615.

8. Mathus-Vliegen EMH. Nutritional status, nutrition, and pressure ulcers. *Nutr Clin Prac*. 2001;16:286–291.

9. Armstrong M. Obesity as an intrinsic factor affecting wound healing. *J Wound Care*. 1998;7:220–221.

10. Thompson C, Fuhrman MP. Nutrients and wound healing: Still searching for the magic bullet. *Nutr Clin Prac*. 2005;20:331–347.

11. Wooley JA, Sax HC. Indirect calorimetry: Applications to practice. *Nutr Clin Prac*. 2003;18:434–439.

12. Flancbaum L, Choban PS, Sambucco S, Verducci J, Burge JC. Comparison of indirect calorimetry, the Fick method, and prediction equations in estimating the energy requirements of critically ill patients. *Am J Clin Nutr*. 1999;69:461–466.

13. Malone AM. Methods of assessing energy expenditure in the intensive care unit. *Nutr Clin Prac*. 2002;17:21–28.

14. Fuhrman MP. Wound healing and nutrition. *Top Clin Nutr*. 2003;18:100–110.

15. Dharmarajan TS, Ahmed S. The growing problem of pressure ulcers: Evaluation and management for an aging population. *Postgrad Med*. 2003;113:77–90.

16. Beyer PL. Complications of enteral nutrition. In: Matarese LE, Gottschlich MM, eds. *Contemporary Nutrition Support Practice: A Clinical Guide*. 2nd ed. St. Louis, Mo.: Saunders; 2003:215–226.

17. Fuhrman, MP. Complication management in parenteral nutrition. In: Matarese LE, Gottschlich MM, eds. *Contemporary Nutrition Support Practice: A Clinical Guide*. 2nd ed. St. Louis, Mo.: Saunders; 2003:242–262.

18. Kraft MD, Btaiche IF, Sacks GS. Review of the refeeding syndrome. *Nutr Clin Prac*. 2005;20:625–633.

19. McMahon MM. Management of parenteral nutrition in acutely ill patients with hyperglycemia. *Nutr Clin Prac*. 2004;19:120–128.

20. McCowen KC, Bistrian BR. Hyperglycemia and nutrition support: Theory and practice. *Nutr Clin Prac*. 2004;19:235–244.

21. American Diabetes Association. *American Diabetes Association Complete Guide to Diabetes*. 3rd ed. Alexandra, Va.: American Diabetes Association, Inc.; 2002.

22. Wolk R. Nutrition in renal failure. In: Gottschlich MM, ed. *The Science and Practice of Nutrition Support: A Case-based Core Curriculum*. Dubuque, Iowa: Kendall/Hunt; 2001:575–599.

23. National Pressure Ulcer Advisory Panel. Nutritional support for patients. Available at: www.npuap.org/npuap_faq.html. Accessed January 5, 2005.

24. Daly JM, Heymsfield SB, Head CA, et al. Human energy requirements: Overestimation by widely used prediction equation. *Am J Clin Nutr*. 1985;42:1170–1174.

25. Frankenfield DC, Muth ER, Rowe WA. The Harris-Benedict studies of human basal metabolism: History and limitations. *J Am Diet Assoc*. 1998;98:439–445.

26. Mifflin MD, St Jeor ST, Hill LA, Scott BJ, Daugherty SA, Koh YO. A new predictive equation for resting energy expenditure in healthy individuals. *Am J Clin Nutr*. 1990;51:241–247.

27. Frankenfield DC, Rowe WA, Smith JS, Cooney RN. Validation of several established equations for resting metabolic rate in obese and nonobese people. *J Am Diet Assoc*. 2003;103:1152–1159.

28. Haydock DA, Hill GL. Impaired wound healing in surgical patients with varying degrees of malnutrition. *JPEN*. 1986;10:550–554.

29. Jorgensen LN, Sorensen LT, Kallehave F, Schulze S, Gottrup F. Increased wound collagen deposition in an uncomplicated surgical wound compared to a minimal subcutaneous test wound. *Wound Repair Regen*. 2001;9:194–199.

30. Gore DC, Chinkes DL, Wolf SE, Sanford AP, Herndon DN, Wolfe RR. Quantification of protein metabolism *in vivo* for skin, wound, and muscle in severe burn patients. *JPEN*. 2006;30:331–338.

31. Biolo G, Fleming RY, Maggi SP, Nguyen TT, Herndon DN, Wolfe RR. Inverse regulation of protein turnover and amino acid transport in skeletal muscle of hypercatabolic patients. *J Clin Endocrinol Metab*. 2002;87:3378–3384.

32. Russell MK. Laboratory monitoring. In: Matarese LE, Gottschlich MM, eds. *Contemporary Nutrition Support Practice: A Clinical Guide*. 2nd ed. St. Louis, Mo.: Saunders; 2003:45–62.

33. Blackburn GL, Bistrian BR, Maini BS, et al. Nutritional and metabolic assessment of the hospitalized patient. *JPEN*. 1977;1:11–22.

34. Gottschlich M. Burns. In: Gottschlich M, Matarese L, Shronts E, eds. *Nutrition Support Dietetics Core Curriculum*. 2nd ed. Silver Spring, Md.: American Society for Parenteral and Enteral Nutrition; 1993:341–349.

35. Bergstrom N, Bennett MA, Carlson CE, et al. Treatment of pressure ulcers. Assessment: Nutritional assessment and management. In: *AHCPR Supported Clinical Practice Guidelines, Treatment of Pressure Ulcers: Clinical Guideline No. 15*. Rockville, Md.: U.S. Department of Health and Human Services, Agency for Health Care Policy and Research; 1994. AHCPR Publication Number 95-0652. Available at: www.ncbi.nlm.nih.gov/books/bv.fcgi?rid=hstat2.section.5393. Accessed July 10, 2006.

36. ASPEN Board of Directors and the Clinical Guidelines Task Force. Guidelines for the use of parenteral and enteral nutrition in adult and pediatric patients. *JPEN*. 2002;26(suppl):1SA–138SA.

37. Luiking YC, Poeze M, Dejong CH, Ramsay G, Deutz NE. Sepsis: An arginine deficiency state? *Crit Care Med*. 2004;32:2135–2145.

38. Williams JZ, Barbul A. Nutrition and wound healing. *Surg Clin N Am*. 2003;83:571–596.

39. Stechmiller JK, Childress B. Arginine supplementation and wound healing. *Nutr Clin Prac*. 2005;20:52–61.

40. Seifter E, Rettura G, Barbul A, et al. Arginine: An essential amino acid for injured rats. *Surgery.* 1978;84:224–230.

41. Barbul A, Lazarou SA, Efron DT, Wasserkrug HL, Efron G. Arginine enhances wound healing and lymphocyte immune responses in humans. *Surgery.* 1990;108:331–337.

42. Zaloga GP, Siddiqui R, Terry C, Marik PE. Arginine: Mediator or modulator of sepsis? *Nutr Clin Prac.* 2004;19:201–215.

43. Nijveldt RJ, Teerlink T, Van Der Hoven B, et al. Asymmetrical dimethylarginine (ADMA) in critically ill patients: High plasma ADMA concentration is an independent risk factor of ICU mortality. *Clin Nutr.* 2003;22:23–30.

44. Annane D, Sanquer S, Sebille V, et al. Compartmentalised inducible nitric-oxide synthase activity in septic shock. *Lancet.* 2000;355:1143–1148.

45. Williams JZ, Abumrad N, Barbul A. Effect of a specialized amino acid mixture on human collagen deposition. *Ann Surg.* 2002;236:369–374.

46. Young LS, Stoll S. Proteins and amino acids. In: Matarese LE, Gottschlich MM, eds. *Contemporary Nutrition Support Practice.* 2nd ed. St. Louis, Mo.: Saunders; 2003:94–104.

47. Ziegler TR, Benfell K, Smith RJ, et al. Safety and metabolic effects of L-glutamine administration in humans. *JPEN.* 1990;14(suppl 4);137S–146S.

48. McCauley R, Platell C, Hall J, et al. Effects of glutamine on colonic strength anastomosis in the rat. *JPEN.* 1991;15:437–439.

49. Clark RH, Feleke G, Din M, et al. Nutritional treatment for acquired immunodeficiency virus-associated wasting using beta-hydroxy beta-methylbutyrate, glutamine, and arginine: A randomized, double-blind, placebo-controlled study. *JPEN.* 2000;24:133–139.

50. May PE, Barber A, D'Olimpio JT, Hourihane A, Abumrad NN. Reversal of cancer-related wasting using oral supplementation with a combination of beta-hydroxy-beta-methylbutyrate, arginine, and glutamine. *Am J Surg.* 2002;183:471–479.

51. Marcora S, Lemmey A, Maddison P. Dietary treatment of rheumatoid cachexia with beta-hydroxy-beta-methlybutyrate, glutamine and arginine: A randomised controlled trial. *Clin Nutr.* 2005;24:442–454.

52. Lewis B. Nutrition and wound healing. In: Kloth LC, McCulloch JM, eds. *Wound Healing: Alternatives in Management.* 3rd ed. Philadelphia, Pa.: F.A. Davis Company; 2002:35–67.

53. Barbul A, Purtill WA. Nutrition in wound healing. *Clinics in Dermatology.* 1994;12:133–140.

54. Ettinger S. Macronutrients: Carbohydrates, proteins, and lipids. In: Mahan LK, Escott-Stump S, eds. *Krause's Food, Nutrition, & Diet Therapy.* 11th ed. Philadelphia, Pa.: Saunders; 2004:37–74.

55. Caffrey BB, Jonnson JT Jr. Role of essential fatty acids in wound healing in rats. *Prog Lipid Res.* 1981;20:641–647.

56. Hulsey TK, O'Neill JA, Neblett WR, Meng HC. Experimental wound healing in essential fatty acid deficiency. *J Pediatr Surg.* 1980;15:505–508.

57. Caldwell MD, Jonsson HT, Othersen HB Jr. Essential fatty acid deficiency in an infant receiving prolonged parenteral alimentation. *J Pediatr.* 1972;81:894–898.

58. Wene JD, Connor WE, DenBesten L. The development of essential fatty acid deficiency in men fed fat free diets intravenously and orally. *J Clin Invest.* 1975;56:127–134.

59. Albina JE, Gladden P, Walsh WR. Detrimental effects of an omega-3 fatty acid-enriched diet on wound healing. *JPEN.* 1993;17:519–521.

60. Sperling RI, Robin JL, Kylander KA, Lee TH, Lewis RA, Austen KF. The effects of N-3 polyunsaturated fatty acids on the generation of platelet-activating factor by human monocytes. *J Immunol.* 1987;139:4186–4191.

61. Endres S, Ghorbani R, Kelly VE, et al. The effect of dietary supplementation with N-3 polyunsaturated fatty acids on the synthesis of interleukin-1 and tumor necrosis factor by mononuclear cells. *N Engl J Med.* 1989;320:265–271.

62. Goodson III WH, Hunt TK. Wound collagen accumulation in obese hyperglycemic mice. *Diabetes*. 1986;35:491–495.

63. Langouche L, Vanhorebeek I, Vlasselaers D, et al. Intensive insulin therapy protects the endothelium of critically ill patients. *J Clin Invest*. 2005;115:2277–2286.

64. Furnary AP, Zerr KJ, Grunkemeier GL, Starr A. Continuous intravenous insulin infusion reduces the incidence of deep sternal wound infection in diabetic patients after cardiac surgical procedures. *Ann Thorac Surg*. 1999;67:352–362.

65. Van den Berghe, Wouters P, Weekers F, et al. Intensive insulin therapy in critically ill patients. *N Engl J Med*. 2001;345:1359–1367.

66. Van den Berghe G, Wouters PJ, Bouillon R, et al. Outcome benefit of intensive insulin therapy in the critically ill: Insulin dose versus glycemic control. *Crit Care Med*. 2003;31:359–366.

67. Scholl D, Langkamp-Henken B. Nutrient recommendations for wound healing. *J Intraven Nurs*. 2001;24:124–132.

68. McNabb LJ, Hyatt J. Effect of an air-fluidized bed on insensible water loss. *Crit Care Med*. 1987;15:161–162.

69. Ross V. Micronutrient recommendations for wound healing. *Support Line*. 2002;24:3–9.

70. Institute of Medicine, Food and Nutrition Board. *Dietary Reference Intakes: Vitamin A, Vitamin K, Arsenic, Boron, Chromium, Copper, Iodine, Iron, Manganese, Molybdenum, Nickel, Silicon, Vanadium, and Zinc*. Washington, D.C.: National Academy Press; 2001.

71. Institute of Medicine, Food and Nutrition Board. *Dietary Reference Intakes for Vitamin C, Vitamin E, Selenium, and Carotenoids*. Washington, D.C.: National Academy Press; 2000.

72. Hodges RE, Baker EM, Hood J, Sauberlich HE, March SC. Experimental scurvy in man. *Amer J Clin Nutr*. 1969;22:535–548.

73. ter Riet G, Kessels GH, Knipschild PG. Randomized clinical trial of ascorbic acid in the treatment of pressure ulcers. *J Clin Epidemiol*. 1995;48:1453–1460.

74. Tomson CR, Channon SM, Parkinson IS, et al. Correction of subclinical ascorbate deficiency in patients receiving dialysis: Effects on plasma oxalate, serum cholesterol, and capillary fragility. *Clin Chim Acta*.1989;180:225–264.

75. Rolton HA, McConnell KM, Modi KS, Macdougall AI. The effect of vitamin C intake on plasma oxalate in patients on regular haemodialysis. *Nephrol Dial Transplant*. 1991;6:440–443.

76. Boosalis MG. Vitamins. In: Matarese LE, Gottschlich MM, eds. *Contemporary Nutrition Support Practice*. 2nd ed. St. Louis, Mo.: Saunders; 2003:145–163.

77. Gallagher ML. Vitamins. In: Mahan LK, Escott-Stump S, eds. *Krause's Food, Nutrition, & Diet Therapy*. 11th ed. Philadelphia, Pa.: Saunders; 2004:75–119.

78. Hadley SA, Fitzsimmons L. Nutrition and wound healing. *Top Clin Nutr*. 1990;5:72–81.

79. Ruberg RL. Role of nutrition in wound healing. *Surg Clin North Am*. 1984;64:705–714.

80. Mayes T, Gottschlich MM. Burns and wound healing. In: Matarese LE, Gottschlich MM, eds. *Contemporary Nutrition Support Practice*. 2nd ed. St. Louis, Mo.: Saunders; 2003:595–615.

81. Vallee BL. Metabolic role of zinc. *JAMA*. 1956;162:1053–1057.

82. Hallbook T, Lanner E. Serum zinc and healing of leg ulcers. *Lancet*. 1972;2:780–782.

83. Floersheim GL, Lais E. Lack of effect of oral zinc sulfate on wound healing in leg ulcer. *Schweiz Med Wochenschr*. 1980;110:1138–1145.

84. Wilkinson EA, Hawke CI. Oral zinc for arterial and venous leg ulcers. *Cochrane Database Syst Rev*. 2000;2:CD001273.

85. Agay D, Anderson RA, Sandre C, et al. Alterations of antioxidant trace elements (Zn, Se, Cu) and related metallo-enzymes in plasma and tissues following burn injury in rats. *Burns*. 2005;31: 366–371.

86. Kozar RA, McQuiggan MM, Moore FA. Trauma. In: Merritt R, ed. *The ASPEN Nutrition Support Practice Manual.* 2nd ed. Silver Spring, Md.: American Society for Parenteral and Enteral Nutrition; 2005:271–276.

87. Fosmire GJ. Zinc toxicity. *Amer J Clin Nutr.* 1990;51:225–227.

88. Chandra RK. Excessive intake of zinc impairs immune responses. *JAMA.* 1984;21:1443–1446.

89. Robien MA. Iron and microbial infection. *Support Line.* 2000;22:23–27.

90. Bullen J, Griffiths E, Rogers H, Ward G. Sepsis: The critical role of iron. *Microbes Infect.* 2000; 2:409–415.

91. Tarng DC, Wei YH, Huang TP, Kuo BIT, Yang WC. Intravenous ascorbic acid as an adjuvant therapy for recombinant erythropoietin in hemodialysis patients with hyperferritinemia. *Kidney Int.* 1999;55:2477–2486.

92. Neiva RF, Al-Shammari K, Nociti FH Jr, Soehren S, Wang HL. Effects of vitamin-B complex supplementation on periodontal wound healing. *J Periodontol.* 2005;76:1084–1091.

93. Perier C, Granouillet R, Chamson A, Gonthier R, Frey J. Nutritional markers, acute phase reactants and tissue inhibitor of matrix metalloproteinase 1 in elderly patients with pressure sores. *Gerontology.* 2002;48:298–301.

94. Pinchcofsky-Devin GD, Kaminski Jr MV. Correlation of pressure sores and nutritional status. *J Am Geriatr Soc.* 1986;34:435–440.

95. Windsor JA, Knight GS, Hill GL. Wound healing response in surgical patients: Recent food intake is more important than nutrition status. *Br J Surg.* 1988;75:135–137.

96. Lewis SJ, Egger M, Sylvester PA, Thomas S. Early enteral feeding versus "nil by mouth" after gastrointestinal surgery: Systematic review and meta-analysis of controlled trials. *BMJ.* 2001; 323:773–776.

97. DRI Macronutrient Symposium. Carbohydrates. Food and Nutrition Board. December 16, 2002. Available at: www.iom.edu/Object.File/Master/7/317/0.pdf. Accessed October 10, 2005.

Index

341